Complete Revision
for the Intercollegiate MRCS

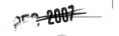
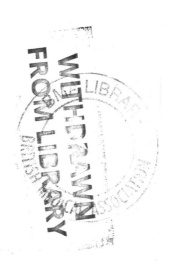

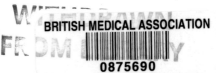

Commissioning Editor: Laurence Hunter
Development Editor: Hannah Kenner
Project Manager: Nancy Arnott
Design Direction: Erik Bigland
Illustration Buyer: Gillian Murray
Illustrator: Oxford Illustrators

Complete Revision for the Intercollegiate MRCS

K Conway MB BCh MD MRCSEd MRCSI
Specialist Registrar on the All-Wales Higher Surgical Training Programme
Regional Vascular Unit
University Hospital of Wales
Cardiff, UK

S Enoch MB BCh MRCSEd MRCS (Eng)
Surgical Research Fellow of Royal Colleges of Surgeons of England,
Edinburgh and Ireland
Wound Healing Research Unit
University Hospital of Wales
Cardiff, UK

S Kumar MBBS MS FRCS(Ed)
Specialist Registrar in Surgery
Department of Surgery
University College London Hospital
London, UK

D Leaper MD ChM FRCS FACS
Emeritus Professor of Surgery
University of Newcastle upon Tyne
Visiting Professor
University of Cardiff
Cardiff, UK

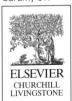

ELSEVIER
CHURCHILL
LIVINGSTONE

Edinburgh London New York Oxford Philadelphia St Louis Sydney Toronto 2007

ELSEVIER
CHURCHILL LIVINGSTONE

An imprint of Elsevier Limited

© 2007, Elsevier Limited. All rights reserved.

The rights of K Conway, S Enoch, S Kumar and D Leaper to be identified as authors of this work have been asserted by them in accordance with the Copyright, Designs and Patents Act 1988

First published 2007

ISBN-13: 978-0-443-10187-8
ISBN-10: 0-443-10187-6

British Library Cataloguing in Publication Data
A catalogue record for this book is available from the British Library

Library of Congress Cataloging in Publication Data
A catalog record for this book is available from the Library of Congress

Notice
Knowledge and best practice in this field are constantly changing. As new research and experience broaden our knowledge, changes in practice, treatment and drug therapy may become necessary or appropriate. Readers are advised to check the most current information provided (i) on procedures featured or (ii) by the manufacturer of each product to be administered, to verify the recommended dose or formula, the method and duration of administration, and contraindications. It is the responsibility of the practitioner, relying on their own experience and knowledge of the patient, to make diagnoses, to determine dosages and the best treatment for each individual patient, and to take all appropriate safety precautions. To the fullest extent of the law, neither the Publisher nor the Authors assume any liability for any injury and/or damage to persons or property arising out or related to any use of the material contained in this book.

The Publisher

Printed in China

Preface

Success in an examination, among other things, depends on a focussed systematic preparation, developing the skills of logical analysis and structured ordering of gathered information during the preparation process, and a well-rehearsed routine of presentation of the knowledge given a situation under test conditions. So the better you are prepared in these key domains, the greater are your chances of success in the MRCS. This book is written and presented in a way that incorporates the above values and supports consolidation of acquired factual knowledge.

Knowledge of the exam conditions is important to have a tailored approach which is time saving and efficient. This book has been written by a team of junior surgeons who have recently passed the MRCS and by an experienced MRCS and Intercollegiate Fellowship examiner. The MRCS is comprised of three parts: Part 1 MCQs (Principles of Surgery-in-General); Part 2 EMQs (Surgical Specialties); and Part 3 Oral (Basic Sciences) and Clinical. This book covers all of these sections in the style in which they will be examined. In addition the book has been reviewed by a panel of experts to ensure accuracy and relevance.

This book differs from other MRCS texts in that it covers all headings in the Intercollegiate MRCS syllabus in the style in which you will be examined. Therefore it may be used as a textbook which you can work through in a logical manner as you prepare for the MRCS; or as a revision aid to prepare you for the style in which questions are asked and the level of response which the examiners will expect in return.

We advise you to start using this book early on in your post-graduate surgical training so that you can become familiar with the text. The book may then also be used as a revision and preparation tool for the exam.

The comprehensive coverage of the topics should give you the confidence as the exams approach. As all headings from the Intercollegiate MRCS syllabus have been covered, you can therefore be sure that you will have covered all subjects which you are likely to be questioned on in the exam. The layout of the book enables you to cover subjects which are most likely to come up in a given part of the exam therefore avoiding subjects which are less likely to come up.

The questions are asked in similar style to the examination, therefore enabling you to feel better prepared as the questioning style will be more familiar. Each question is answered by an explanation to the expected level and depth expected by the MRCS examiners.

We wish you every success.

KC
SE
SK
DL

Acknowledgement

The authors wish to especially thank Aisling Butler and Mark Haynes for their help in compiling this book. Thanks are also extended to those who reviewed individual sections.

Reviewers

A J Collins MB BCh BAO FRCSI FRCR
Consultant Radiologist
Radiology Department
Royal Victoria Hospital
Belfast

K G Harding MB MRCGP FRCS
Professor of Rehabilitation Medicine
Director Wound Healing Research Unit
Wound Healing Research Unit
Cardiff University
Cardiff

S Hill MA MS MB BS FRCS
Consultant Vascular Surgeon
Cardiff Regional Vascular Unit
University Hospital of Wales
Cardiff

K A R Hutton MB ChB FRCS(Paed) ChM
Consultant Paediatric Surgeon and Urologist
Department of Paediatric Surgery
University Hospital of Wales
Heath Park
Cardiff

H Jain MBBS MS FRCS (Neurosurgery)
Consultant Neurosurgeon
Apollo Gleneagles Hospital
Calcutta
India

P Kumar MS DNBE FRCS(Ed)
Consultant Surgeon
University Hospital of North Tees
Stockton-on-Tees

J A McAteer MB BCh FRCA
Consultant Anaesthetist
Department of Anaesthetics and Intensive Care
Ulster Hospital
Belfast

P E Price BA(Hons) PhD AFBPsS CHPsychol
Research Director
Wound Healing Research Unit
Cardiff University
Cardiff

D Scott-Coombes MS FRCS
Consultant Endocrine Surgeon
Department of Endocrine Surgery
University Hospital of Wales
Cardiff

S Tolan MB BCh MRCP
Specialist Registrar
Department of Clinical Oncology
The Christie Hospital
Manchester

J Torkington MS MB BS FRCS
Consultant Colorectal Surgeon
Department of Colorectal Surgery
University Hospital of Wales
Cardiff

Contents

CHAPTER 1: APPLIED BASIC SCIENCES
MRCS Part 1 – MCQs: Principles of Surgery-in-General

CONTENTS

CHAPTER 2: CLINICAL PROBLEM SOLVING
MRCS Part 2 – EMQs: Surgical Specialties

CHAPTER 3: THE VIVA
MRCS Part 3 – Oral: Basic Sciences

CHAPTER 4: CLINICAL CASE SCENARIOS
MRCS Part 3 – Clinical

MCQs

Applied Basic Sciences

QUESTIONS

Perioperative care

Q1.1 Perioperative risk scoring systems
Preoperative prognostic scoring systems include:
- **A** APACHE II
- **B** ASA
- **C** GCS
- **D** Imrie
- **E** POSSUM

Q1.2 Assessment of fitness for surgery (spirometry)
Spirometry directly measures:
- **A** forced expiratory volume in 1 second (FEV_1)
- **B** forced vital capacity (FVC)
- **C** physiological dead space
- **D** residual volume (RV)
- **E** diffusing capacity of the lung (D_L)

Q1.3 Management of the diabetic patient
Diabetic patients on an ambulatory care unit list should:
- **A** take their diabetic medication as usual on the morning of surgery
- **B** be prescribed an insulin/dextrose sliding scale
- **C** be placed first on the list
- **D** omit diabetic medication the evening following surgery
- **E** remain in hospital overnight for observation

Q1.4 Perioperative cardiac events
Which of the following are risk factors with a high likelihood for a perioperative cardiac event in a patient with known ischaemic heart disease?:
- **A** abdominal surgery
- **B** age >50 years
- **C** aortic incompetence
- **D** emergency procedure
- **E** myocardial infarction 2 years previously

Q1.5 Issues related to medications
The following medications should be stopped prior to surgery:
- **A** corticosteroids
- **B** aspirin
- **C** antihypertensives
- **D** combined oral contraceptive pill
- **E** potassium-sparing diuretics

Answer found on pp. 17-19.

Q1.6 Informed consent
Informed consent requires:
- **A** assessment of patient's mental competence
- **B** description of the procedure
- **C** likely outcome and prognosis
- **D** national rate of complications
- **E** other alternative treatments

Q1.7 Pre-medication
Pre-medication may cause:
- **A** drying of secretions
- **B** reduced anxiety
- **C** impaired respiratory function
- **D** amnesia
- **E** reduced postoperative pain

Q1.8 General anaesthesia
The following drugs are used during the induction of general anaesthesia:
- **A** etomidate
- **B** isoflurane
- **C** neostigmine
- **D** propofol
- **E** suxamethonium

Q1.9 Local anaesthesia
Toxic effects of local anaesthetics include:
- **A** circumoral paraesthesia
- **B** light headedness
- **C** tachycardia
- **D** urticarial rash
- **E** vomiting

Q1.10 Regional anaesthesia
Complications of regional anaesthesia include:
- **A** aspiration of gastric contents
- **B** hypotension
- **C** increased intracranial pressure
- **D** respiratory depression
- **E** spread of sepsis

Q1.11 Positioning of the patient in surgery
Poor positioning on the operating table may result in injury to the:
- **A** brachial plexus
- **B** femoral nerve
- **C** hypoglossal nerve
- **D** lateral popliteal nerve
- **E** ulnar nerve

Answer found on pp. 20-22. 3

Q1.12 Haemolytic disorders

Causes of haemolytic anaemia include:

A glucose-6-phosphate dehydrogenase deficiency
B long-distance running
C myeloma
D pregnancy
E prosthetic heart valves

Q1.13 Disorders of coagulation

Congenital risk factors for thrombosis include:

A antithrombin deficiency
B homocystinuria
C protein C deficiency
D protein S deficiency
E resistance to activated protein C

Q1.14 Preparation and components of blood products

Fresh frozen plasma:

A contains all coagulation factors
B contains white blood cells
C is indicated in bleeding from Haemophilia A
D is associated with bronchospasm
E is obtained from a pool of blood donors

Q1.15 Blood transfusion

The following may occur as a result of blood transfusion:

A acute haemolytic reaction
B air embolism
C endotoxic shock
D hypercalcaemia
E hypokalaemia

Postoperative management and critical care

Q1.16 Postoperative monitoring

With regard to patient monitoring in the postoperative period:

A the pulse oximeter gives a useful measure of the adequacy of ventilation
B a rising pulse rate is rarely a sign of poorly managed pain
C hourly urine output provides an indication of fluid balance
D manual central venous pressure measurements on the general ward provide accurate assessment of postoperative fluid requirements
E drain output should be monitored as a sign of bleeding in the post-operative period

 Answer found on pp. 23-25.

Q1.17 Pain control

Pain in the postoperative period:

A increases the risks of postoperative cardiac ischaemia

B is associated with an increased risk of deep vein thrombosis

C is best managed with "as required analgesia"

D may improve respiratory function

E is almost similar in patients who have undergone the same procedure

Q1.18 Fluid and electrolyte management

In a healthy 70 kg male patient, who is stable after major elective surgery, the fluid and electrolyte requirements in the first 24–48 hours will be met by the following fluid regimens:

A 2.5 litres of 4% dextrose/0.18% saline per 24 hours

B 0.5 litres of normal saline and 2 litres of 5% dextrose per 24 hours

C 1.5 litres of normal saline and 1 litre of 5% dextrose per 24 hours

D 2.5 litres of normal saline per 24 hours

E 2.5 litres of Hartmann's solution per 24 hours

Q1.19 Nutrition in the surgical patient

Postoperative nutritional support:

A is indicated in all patients undergoing major abdominal surgery

B may be complicated by problems with venous access when administered enterally

C results in metabolic complications in approximately 5% of patients who are parenterally fed

D when administered enterally may be complicated by problems of absorption

E in the immediate postoperative period should be preferably administered parenterally for a short period

Q1.20 Thromboembolic disease

The following patients have an increased risk of developing thromboembolic disease:

A 68-year-old male undergoing a radical prostatectomy

B 61-year-old male undergoing a day-case inguinal hernia repair

C 23-year-old obese female on the oral contraceptive pill, admitted with gallstone pancreatitis

D 22-year-old male who sustained a fractured femoral shaft in a motorbike accident

E 46-year-old female with advanced breast cancer

Answer found on pp. 25-28.

Q1.21 Diagnosis of postoperative renal failure

The following statements regarding renal function are true:

A optimal postoperative urine output in an adult should be >0.5 ml/kg per hour

B oliguria is defined as a urine output of less than 30 ml/hour for 2 consecutive hours

C initial management of renal dysfunction in the postoperative patient should comprise intravenous furosemide

D a rise in serum creatinine is an early sign of impending renal failure

E pre-existing renal disease makes postoperative renal dysfunction more likely

Q1.22 Systemic inflammatory response syndrome (SIRS)

Systemic inflammatory response syndrome (SIRS):

A can only be identified in a patient with a documented infection

B in the presence of documented infection and haemodynamic compromise is called severe sepsis

C is suspected in a patient with a pulse of 95 bpm and a white cell count of 3×10^9/L

D progresses to multi-organ failure if left untreated

E results in end-organ tissue damage through hypoxia

Q1.23 Multiple organ dysfunction syndrome (MODS)

With regard to the multiple organ dysfunction syndrome (MODS) and multiple organ failure (MOF):

A pulmonary failure, presenting as acute respiratory distress syndrome (ARDS) typically occurs first in the development of MOF

B the body organs are not capable of maintaining homeostasis

C the progression of MODS to MOF is unaffected by periods of hypotension

D there is a generalised catabolic state

E where four organs are affected by MOF the mortality rate is approximately 50%

Q1.24 Pathophysiology of wound healing

A cutaneous wound heals by:

A delayed primary healing if the patient has a history of poor wound healing

B first intention if closed within 24 hours of its creation

C secondary intention if the wound is closed following a period of packing

D the action of myofibroblasts in primary healing

E secondary intention in the split-thickness skin graft donor sites

Q1.25 Hidradenitis suppurativa

Hidradenitis suppurativa:

A is caused by inflammation of the exocrine glands
B is associated with sinus formation
C requires biopsy to confirm the diagnosis in the acute stages
D can be successfully treated with prolonged courses of oral antibiotics
E can lead to dermal fibrosis and contractures

Q1.26 Hypertrophic scars

Hypertrophic scars:

A are confined to the margins of the original scar
B are usually seen over the flexor surfaces
C have a strong genetic predisposition
D may result from excessive wound tension
E respond to conservative treatment and subside with time

Q1.27 Lasers

Lasers:

A absorption depth is dependent upon the wavelength of the laser
B beams are mostly red
C contain light over a wide range of wavelengths
D may cause retinal burns and cataracts
E used most commonly in surgical practice is the diode laser

Q1.28 Diathermy

Regarding diathermy:

A alternating currents applied at a frequency of 50 Hz result in muscle contraction
B at low frequencies, currents of 100 mA may cause serious heart arrhythmias
C high frequency alternating current applied with a low current density produces high local temperatures
D the patient plate should be applied well away from the site of operation
E monopolar diathermy should always be used when operating on appendages

Q1.29 Suture and ligature materials

The following are examples of synthetic absorbable sutures:

A Monocryl (poliglecaprone)
B PDS (polydioxanone)
C Prolene (polypropylene)
D Silk
E Vicryl (polyglactin)

Answer found on pp. 30–33.   7

Q1.30 Basic surgical instruments

A mini operation set contains:

A 2 Babcock tissue forceps
B 1 fine-toothed forceps
C 2 Langenbeck retractors
D 1 McIndoe scissors
E 1 Morris retractor

Q1.31 Minor surgical procedures

When suturing any wound it is important to:

A achieve haemostasis
B close deeper tissues
C invert the skin edge
D tie sutures tightly
E wipe the wound before closing to remove blood

Q1.32 Tourniquets

A tourniquet during surgery is indicated:

A to create a bloodless surgical field
B to occlude inflow when creating a vascular anastomosis
C to prevent haematoma when reducing distal limb fractures
D to secure haemostasis in uncontrolled bleeding
E to isolate the distal limb for infusion of local anaesthetic

Management and legal issues in surgery

Q1.33 Decision making in surgery based on evidence

Regarding levels of evidence-based medicine:

A Ia – evidence from at least one randomised controlled trial
B Ib – evidence from a trial which is not randomised
C IIa – case control study results
D IIb – evidence from an expert committee
E III – evidence from a meta-analysis of randomised controlled trials

Q1.34 Statistics

The following statistical tests are for parametric data:

A Kruskal–Wallis
B Mann–Whitney U
C Pearson's correlation coefficient
D *t*-tests
E Wilcoxon signed rank test

Answer found on pp. 33-35.

Q1.35 Principles of clinical trials

A clinical trial requires:

A a placebo control
B a protocol
C ethics committee approval
D patient matching within the trial
E randomisation

Q1.36 Audit

The following are examples of audit projects:

A a study comparing the outcomes of a new laser surgery technique to the prostate with the gold standard of monopolar transurethral resection
B a study of the application of a new hospital guideline on the use of an intravenous cannula
C a study of the treatment pathway for a patient referred with rectal bleeding, from referral to definitive treatment
D a review of the management of patients with acute pancreatitis compared with the gold standard of the British Society of Gastroenterology guidelines
E a randomised study comparing patient's discomfort on insertion of an intravenous cannula with or without topical local anaesthetic

Q1.37 Clinical governance

Clinical governance requires:

A clinical risk reduction programme to be in place
B consultants to be responsible for the clinical actions of their juniors
C evidence based practice should be employed in day-to-day practice
D poor clinical performance to be monitored and reviewed regularly
E participation in regular mortality and morbidity meetings

Q1.38 Medical litigation: avoidance of errors

The following methods are employed in theatre to avoid errors:

A on the operating list left and right are signified by 'L' and 'R' respectively
B patients are sent for by name
C the anaesthetist is responsible for checking the patient's identity
D the side to be operated is marked by the operating surgeon
E the surgeon sees the patient and reviews the notes following induction of anaesthesia

Answer found on pp. 36-38.

Clinical microbiology

Q1.39 Sources of surgical infection

The following patients should receive antibiotic prophylaxis prior to inserting a urethral catheter:

A a 72-year-old male who underwent a total hip replacement 2 months previously

B a 62-year-old female with rheumatic heart disease

C a 48-year-old male with a mechanical aortic valve

D a 56-year-old male who is being treated with steroids and azathioprine for retroperitoneal fibrosis

E a 33-year-old female receiving a bone marrow transplant

Q1.40 Surgically important microorganisms

The following bacteria are likely to be the causative organisms in the corresponding disease:

A *Escherichia coli* and urinary tract infection

B *Neisseria meningitidis* and post splenectomy sepsis

C *Pseudomonas aeruginosa* and a wound infection of an inguinal hernia repair

D *Staphylococcus aureus* and cholangitis

E *Streptococcus faecalis* and lower lobe pneumonia

Q1.41 Surgical infection and its prevention

The following are proven to reduce the risk of surgical infection:

A admission to hospital on the day of surgery

B early mobilisation and physiotherapy

C removal of all indwelling lines and catheters at the earliest opportunity

D shaving of the operation site by the patient prior to admission to hospital

E use of appropriate antibiotic prophylaxis

Q1.42 Pathophysiology of sepsis

The response to infection and the development of the systemic inflammatory response syndrome (SIRS):

A during phase 1, there is commonly a tachycardia and pyrexia >38°C

B in phase 3 the release of inflammatory mediators becomes destructive resulting in dysfunction of various end organs

C normal resolution occurs without progression beyond phase 2

D the earliest response involves the local production of cytokines and recruitment of monocytes and macrophages to the site of injury

E this acute phase response is kept in check by the simultaneous release of pro-inflammatory mediators and endogenous antagonists

Q1.43 Principles of asepsis and antisepsis

When preparing a patient's skin for surgery:

A a preoperative shower with chlorhexidine reduces wound infections

B pre-existing skin infections should be pre-treated

C preoperative shaving should be performed the night before surgery

D the patient's skin should be prepared using an antiseptic solution which is rubbed onto the skin and then immediately wiped dry with a clean swab

E the use of incisional plastic drapes over the operative site results in significantly reduced wound infection rates

Q1.44 Sterilisation in surgical practice

Surgical practice sterilisation:

A is achieved using dry heat at 160°C for 1 hour

B of flexible endoscopes is achieved with glutaraldehyde (2%)

C of reusable instruments is achieved with gamma radiation

D of the skin is commonly achieved using an alcoholic solution of chlorhexidine

E using autoclaves is achieved by the utilisation of steam at pressure

Q1.45 Antibiotic prophylaxis

Antibiotic prophylaxis:

A should be used in all elective and emergency surgical procedures

B administered topically at wound closure reduces the rate of deep surgical site infection (SSI)

C should be administered parenterally immediately prior to surgery (at induction of anaesthesia)

D should be appropriate to the procedure being undertaken

E is more effective if prescribed for 5 days

Q1.46 Antibiotic resistance

Antibiotic resistance by bacteria may be developed by the following mechanisms:

A β-lactamase producing organisms are resistant to quinolones as the enzyme inactivates the antibiotic

B partial treatment of an infection may select out a resistant subpopulation which then proliferates

C plasmids encoding genes conferring resistance may be transferred from one organism to another by conjugation

D tetracycline resistance occurs by changes in the cell membrane becoming impermeable to the drug

E trimethoprim resistance is acquired through the production of an alternative form of dihydrofolate reductase which has no affinity for the drug

Answer found on pp. 40-43.

Q1.47 Surgery in the high-risk patient

When operating on a high-risk surgical patient:

A an additional assistant is required to improve exposure

B disposable protective clothing (impervious gowns, eye protectors etc.) should be worn

C gloves offer some protection from needle stick injury

D scalpels should be passed hand to hand to avoid risk of injury to the surgeon

E solid needles have a higher rate of blood transfer than hollow needles

Q1.48 Universal precautions

The following statements regarding universal precautions are true:

A intraoperatively-fixed retraction devices reduce the risk of sharps injuries

B masks and water repellent clothing should be worn during all surgical procedures

C needles should be re-sheathed before handing back to the scrub nurse

D scalpels should be passed in a kidney bowl

E wearing rubber gloves protects against sharps injury

Q1.49 Management of sharps injuries

After sustaining a sharps injury during a surgical procedure:

A an incident report should be completed and filed

B blood tests for HIV and Hepatitis should be obtained from the patient while still in theatre

C post-exposure prophylaxis for HIV should be administered ideally within 1 hour of the injury if the patient is in a high risk group

D the healthcare worker who has failed to respond to a Hepatitis B vaccination should receive a booster vaccination soon after

E the wound should be washed liberally with soap and water once the case is finished

Emergency medicine and management of trauma

Q1.50 Hypovolaemic shock

Class II hypovolaemic shock in a fit young man results in:

A a pulse rate >140 bpm

B a raised diastolic pressure but normal systolic blood pressure

C a urine output of 10 ml/hour

D confusion

E widened pulse pressure

 Answer found on pp. 43-45.

Q1.51 Definitive airways

The following are definitive airways:

A nasopharyngeal
B nasotracheal
C oropharyngeal
D orotracheal
E tracheostomy

Q1.52 Chest trauma

Myocardial contusions from blunt trauma:

A are associated with valvular disruption
B are diagnosed on echocardiogram
C result in cardiogenic shock
D require early surgical intervention
E require monitoring by serial cardiac enzymes

Q1.53 Cervical spine fractures

Regarding cervical spine fractures:

A a Jefferson fracture affects the axis
B atlantoaxial fracture dislocation is associated with sudden death
C the odontoid process is affected in 60% of axis fractures
D type I odontoid fractures occur through the base of the dens
E type II odontoid fractures require surgical fixation

Q1.54 Cerebral blood flow and brain injury

Cerebral blood flow is:

A approximately 250 ml/100 g of brain tissue/min in an adult
B higher in adults compared with children
C autoregulated in response to mean systolic blood pressure
D autoregulated in response to changes in PaO_2
E reduced by <10% if a brain injury is severe enough to cause unconsciousness

Q1.55 Management of burns

Early management of partial thickness burns affecting 5% of the total body surface require:

A clothing to be left intact until the patient is transferred to the operating theatre
B aggressive intravenous fluid management
C application of icy cold water to burnt areas
D intravenous antibiotics
E transfer to the specialised burns unit

Answer found on pp. 45-48.   **13**

Principles of surgical oncology

Q1.56 Normal cell replication
The phases of the normal cell cycle include:
A G_2
B M
C R
D S
E T

Q1.57 Disordered cell replication
Disordered cell replication results from the presence of:
A CDKs
B E2F
C p53
D RB1
E R points

Q1.58 Behaviour of cancer cells
In a neoplasm the:
A cell cycle time is increased
B cell differentiation is increased
C cell loss coefficient is reduced
D growth fraction is reduced
E total cell number is increased

Q1.59 Cancer genes
Which of the following associations between a cancer and gene are true:
A breast – BRCA1
B familial adenomatosis polyposis – FAA
C gastric cancer – TP53
D multiple endocrine neoplasia 2 (MEN II) – RET
E papillary renal cell cancer – MET

Q1.60 Mechanisms and pathways of tumour genesis
DNA mutations are:
A heritable
B permanent
C repairable
D silent
E spontaneous

Answer found on pp. 49-51.

Q1.61 Tumour markers

The association between the following tumour markers and tumours are recognised:

A α-fetoprotein (AFP) – hepatoma
B CA125 – gastric carcinoma
C CA19-9 – pancreatic carcinoma
D CA15-3 – breast carcinoma
E CA27.29 – bronchial carcinoma

Q1.62 Cellular mechanisms of invasion and metastasis

Prerequisites for a tumour to metastasise include:

A angiogenesis
B cell adhesion
C dismantle cell–cell adhesions
D extra-cellular matrix degradation
E motogenesis

Q1.63 Cancer Registries

The main functions of Cancer Registries are:

A distributing information on palliative care
B evaluation of the impact of treatment
C investigations of links between environmental factors and cancer formation
D monitoring trends in cancer
E organisation and funding screening programmes

Q1.64 Common cancers survival rates

The 5-year survival rates of:

A breast cancer is 86%
B Duke's B colonic cancer is 67%
C Stage I gastric cancer is 22%
D oesophageal cancer is 45%
E prostatic cancer is 41%

Q1.65 Screening programmes

NHS screening programmes exist for:

A breast
B cervix
C colon
D oesophagus
E prostate

Answer found on pp. 51-54.   **15**

Q1.66 Chemotherapy

The following statements regarding chemotherapeutic agents are true:

A Cisplatin is used in bladder and lung cancers and the dosage used is dependent upon renal function

B Cyclophosphamide, used to treat haematological malignancies, may cause significant haematuria

C Docetaxel is used in breast cancer and works by linking the alkyl group to chemical groups in proteins and nucleic acids

D Doxorubicin inhibits topoisomerase II and is used in breast cancer chemotherapy

E 5-Fluorouracil blocks DNA synthesis/replication and is used in colorectal cancer

Q1.67 Hormone therapy

With regard to hormone therapy in prostate cancer:

A adverse effects of hormone treatment are minimal

B chemical castration, in the form of LHRH analogues, causes an initial rise in serum testosterone levels

C oestrogen therapy (oestradiol) is effective at controlling prostate cancer

D prostate cancers do not grow in the absence of testosterone and hormone treatment offers patients a long-term cure

E surgical and chemical castration have similar long-term outcomes in terms of disease control

Answer found on pp. 54-55.

ANSWERS

Perioperative care

A1.1 Preoperative prognostic scoring systems include:
A APACHE II
B ASA
C GCS
D Imrie
E POSSUM

A1.1 **A** = T **B** = T **C** = F **D** = F **E** = T

Preoperative prognostic scoring systems have been developed to quantify a patient's illness severity and to evaluate their ability to tolerate surgery. Other uses of scoring systems include stratification of patients (so that fair comparisons can be made between comparable risk groups in outcomes assessment or in audit) and in objective documentation of the clinical condition of a patient being sequentially observed for disease progression or effect of an intervention, usually in an intensive care setting. A number of systems have been developed, with no system having universal application. Acute Physiology Assessment and Chronic Health Evaluation (APACHE II) is the most widely used system in the UK, in which a sum of scores of 12 physiological parameters (called the acute physiology score) is added to the Glasgow Coma Score, points for age, points for co-morbidity and points for the type of management (emergency surgery or conservative management) to give the total APACHE score. The American Society of Anesthesiologist scoring system is a more simplified system categorising the patients 1–5 (1, healthy; 2, mild systemic disease; 3, severe systemic disease; 4, life-threatening disease; 5, unlikely to survive with or without surgery). The Glasgow Coma Score is an assessment of the level of consciousness. The Glasgow–Imrie scoring system is used to stratify acute pancreatitis into mild and severe. The Physiological and Operative Severity Score for enUmeration of Mortality and Morbidity (POSSUM) is a scoring system based on 12 clinical and laboratory parameters and an operative score assessing six surgery related parameters to produce an estimated risk of morbidity and mortality. Following surgery, the estimated risk is compared with the observed outcome.

A1.2 Spirometry directly measures:
A forced expiratory volume in 1 second (FEV_1)
B forced vital capacity (FVC)
C physiological dead space
D residual volume (RV)
E diffusing capacity of the lung (D_L)

A1.2 **A** = T **B** = T **C** = F **D** = F **E** = F

The respiratory system is assessed by pulmonary function tests. Pulmonary function tests usually include spirometry, measurement of airflow rates and the calculation of lung volumes. A spirometer directly measures only the air volumes. Airflow rates are derived parameters calculated electronically based on volume changes and time. Lung capacities are calculated by a helium or nitrogen washout technique. Forced vital capacity (FVC) is the amount of air that can be expelled when the lungs are maximally inflated. FEV_1 is the volume of air exhaled in the first second of FVC. An FVC/FEV_1 ratio of less than 80% is consistent with chronic obstructive pulmonary disease and is a good measure of its severity. The physiological dead space is the air in the upper airways which is not available for alveolar gas exchange. The residual volume (RV) is the volume of air remaining in the lungs following maximal expiration. The volume of gas exchanged across the alveolar-capillary membrane per minute (D_L) is calculated to provide a measure of abnormal gas exchange, e.g. congestive heart failure.

A1.3 Diabetic patients on an ambulatory care unit list should:
A take their diabetic medication as usual on the morning of surgery
B be prescribed an insulin/dextrose sliding scale
C be placed first on the list
D omit diabetic medication the evening following surgery
E remain in hospital overnight for observation

A1.3 **A** = F **B** = F **C** = T **D** = F **E** = F

Diabetes mellitus is not a contraindication for ambulatory (day-case) surgery. Patients with type I diabetes are more difficult to manage than those with type II. A prerequisite for diabetic patients to undergo day-case surgery is good glycaemic control in the months prior to surgery. Diabetic patients are suitable for most surgery performed in the ambulatory care unit. However, more major surgery requires admission to the general ward and the surgery performed in the main theatre suite. Regional anaesthetics should be employed where possible to avoid the longer periods of starvation required with a general anaesthetic. The patient should omit their diabetic medication on the morning of surgery and be placed at the start of the operating list. Following surgery, the patient should eat early, if not nauseated, and recommence their diabetic medication as normal. Diabetic patients do not require overnight in-hospital observation in the absence of any perioperative problem.

A1.4 **Which of the following are risk factors with a high likelihood for a perioperative cardiac event in a patient with known ischaemic heart disease?:**
A abdominal surgery
B age >50 years
C aortic incompetence
D emergency procedure
E myocardial infarction 2 years previously

A1.4 **A** = T **B** = F **C** = F **D** = T **E** = F

Patients with a history of ischaemic heart disease are at an increased risk of developing perioperative cardiac problems including myocardial infarction and cardiac failure. The Goldman's Cardiac Risk Index is a prognostic indicator for predicting the likelihood of developing a perioperative life-threatening cardiac event in a patient with ischaemic heart disease. Risk factors with a high likelihood of resulting in cardiac event include: age >70 years, raised jugular venous pressure, third heart sound, myocardial event in the preceding 6 months, surgery on the abdomen or thorax, symptomatic aortic stenosis, poor general condition and emergency surgery. Cardiopulmonary exercise test (which measures metabolic parameters while the patient exercises on a bicycle ergometer) is an objective method of assessing cardiac risk and provides more information than a treadmill test. Serum Brain Natriuretic Peptide (BNP) is being evaluated as a laboratory test for prediction of cardiac events.

A1.5 **The following medications should be stopped prior to surgery:**
A corticosteroids
B aspirin
C antihypertensives
D combined oral contraceptive pill
E potassium-sparing diuretics

A1.5 **A** = F **B** = F **C** = F **D** = T **E** = T

The risk of stopping a long-term medication preoperatively is usually greater than continuing it intraoperatively. Concomitant medications may alter the action of drugs administered during surgery and it is therefore vital that the anaesthetist is made aware of all the patient's medications. Patients on long-term corticosteroid therapy develop adrenal atrophy and will require an increased dose of steroids in the perioperative period. Withdrawal of the steroids could result in an Addisonian crisis (tachycardia, hypotension, oliguria and confusion). Antiplatelet therapy results in an increased anaesthetic and surgical risk; however, stopping this therapy usually increases the overall risk to the patient. Antihypertensives should be continued as normal and be recommenced soon after surgery if the patient is normotensive. Oestrogen-containing contraceptives should be discontinued 4 weeks prior to surgery due to the risk of thromboembolic disease; they should be recommenced 2 weeks following surgery. Potassium-sparing diuretics are withheld on the morning of surgery due to the risk of perioperative hyperkalaemia.

A1.6 Informed consent requires:

A assessment of patient's mental competence
B description of the procedure
C likely outcome and prognosis
D national rate of complications
E other alternative treatments

A1.6 **A** = T **B** = T **C** = T **D** = F **E** = T

Informed consent is only obtained when the patient is able to make a considered choice for what is in his/her best interest. Informed consent therefore requires an assessment of the patient's mental competence and accurate information delivered in a way that is best understood by the patient. The patient requires information on the specific aspects and the general aspects of the procedure, e.g. type of anaesthetic. The patient should also be given an accurate assessment of the possible outcomes and prognosis following the procedure. The patient should be informed of the surgeon's own complication rate for the procedure. The patient should also be provided information about alternative medical treatments and their likely outcomes.

A1.7 Pre-medication may cause:

A drying of secretions
B reduced anxiety
C impaired respiratory function
D amnesia
E reduced postoperative pain

A1.7 **A** = T **B** = T **C** = T **D** = T **E** = T

Pre-medication is given in order to reduce anxiety, to dry secretions and to reduce peri- and postoperative pain. This allows lighter anaesthesia resulting in reduced recovery times. Drying of secretions by hyoscine is particularly useful in dental, pulmonary and paediatric surgery and for bronchoscopy. Anxiolysis is often achieved by using a benzodiazepine such as temazepam. Some of the drugs used for pre-medication, particularly the opiates, may cause respiratory depression; impair consciousness and induce some amnesia. Unless they have a short duration of action this could be a disadvantage for short general anaesthetics. The patient should be consented for surgery prior to receiving their pre-medication. Consent taken under the influence of any drugs may be considered invalid in any subsequent medico-legal action. Analgesia administered intraoperatively in the form of opioids or NSAIDs reduces the postoperative analgesic requirements.

A1.8 **The following drugs are used during the induction of general anaesthesia:**
A etomidate
B isoflurane
C neostigmine
D propofol
E suxamethonium

A1.8 **A** = T **B** = F **C** = F **D** = T **E** = T

General anaesthesia produces a loss of sensation and consciousness. It is divided into three phases: induction, maintenance and reversal. Induction is achieved by the action of a single or combination of drugs. Propofol and etomidate are both short-acting intravenous induction agents. At induction, muscle relaxation is required to enable endotracheal intubation. An alternative to endotracheal intubation is the placement of a laryngeal mask, which does not require muscle relaxation. Suxamethonium is used to produce muscle relaxation at induction of anaesthetic as it has a short duration of action of approximately 5 minutes. Anaesthesia is maintained using inhaled volatile agent, i.e. isoflurane. Longer acting muscle relaxants are used intraoperatively to allow mechanical ventilation or access to the abdominal cavity. Reversal of muscle relaxation is achieved with neostigmine.

A1.9 **Toxic effects of local anaesthetics include:**
A circumoral paraesthesia
B light headedness
C tachycardia
D urticarial rash
E vomiting

A1.9 **A** = T **B** = T **C** = T **D** = F **E** = F

Local anaesthetics create a temporary loss of sensation due to blockade of nerve transmission in the peripheral nerves. The action of local anaesthetics is by the blockade of the sodium channels in the nerve cell membrane, preventing propagation of the action potential. Local anaesthetic toxicity results from inadvertent intravenous injection or from overdose. Toxic effects relate from membrane stabilisation in the central nervous or cardiovascular systems. Initial effects include a feeling of inebriation and light headedness followed by sedation, tingling around the mouth (circumoral paraesthesia) and twitching. Cardiovascular toxicity is most frequently associated with bupivacaine overdose. Initially the patient becomes hypertensive and tachycardic, followed by a phase of cardiovascular depression in which cardiac output drops and hypotension develops. Later bradycardia, respiratory depression and convulsions occur. When infiltrating local anaesthetic it is important to draw the plunger of the syringe back before injecting to ensure the needle is not in a blood vessel. Adequate resuscitation equipment must be readily accessible.

A1.10 Complications of regional anaesthesia include:
A aspiration of gastric contents
B hypotension
C increased intracranial pressure
D respiratory depression
E spread of sepsis

A1.10 **A** = F **B** = T **C** = F **D** = T **E** = T

Regional anaesthesia avoids some of the complications associated with general anaesthesia but has its own procedure specific and drug specific complications. As regional anaesthetics only involve part of the body, the patient remains conscious and is able to protect his/her own airway, i.e. avoiding aspiration of gastric contents. Hypotension may result from epidural or spinal anaesthesia due to autonomic blockade producing vasodilation below the level of the block. Increased intracranial pressure is a complication of general anaesthesia and is not seen with regional anaesthesia. Respiratory depression results from doses of local anaesthetic in excess of the safe dose. A major concern with regional anaesthesia is inoculation of skin commensals or skin pathogens into sterile locations such as the epidural space. Despite these concerns, regional anaesthesia provides excellent postoperative analgesia and avoids the common complication of postoperative nausea and vomiting seen with general anaesthesia.

A1.11 Poor positioning on the operating table may result in injury to the:
A brachial plexus
B femoral nerve
C hypoglossal nerve
D lateral popliteal nerve
E ulnar nerve

A1.11 **A** = T **B** = F **C** = F **D** = T **E** = T

The patient is placed on soft synthetic pads which are attached to the operating table. These pads are designed to mould to the shape of the patient's body. Nerves are at risk of injury when it is necessary to extend the limbs. It is important not to over-stretch joints in an unconscious patient. In addition, nerves are also at risk over bony prominences. The ulnar nerve and the lateral popliteal are at particular risk as they course around a bony prominence (medial epicondyle and neck of fibula, respectively) and lie superficially. These bony prominences therefore require additional padding. The brachial plexus is at risk when the arm is over-extended on an arm-board or when the arm is extended and externally rotated above the patient's head. The femoral and hypoglossal nerves may be at risk of injury from skin retractors but not from poor positioning.

A1.12 Causes of haemolytic anaemia include:
A glucose-6-phosphate dehydrogenase deficiency
B long-distance running
C myeloma
D pregnancy
E prosthetic heart valves

A1.12 **A** = T **B** = T **C** = F **D** = F **E** = T

Haemolytic anaemia results when red blood cells do not survive their normal lifespan of approximately 120 days and are not replenished in sufficient numbers by the bone marrow. Destruction of red blood cells may occur due to intrinsic abnormalities of the blood cell (e.g. glucose-6-phosphate dehydrogenase deficiency, hereditary spherocytosis, sickle cell disease) or from an acquired cause (autoimmune disorders, sepsis and mechanical causes such as prosthetic heart valves and long-distance running). Clinically, the patient may appear anaemic and jaundiced (hyperbilirubinaemia due to increased haemoglobin breakdown). Pregnancy usually results in a dilutional anaemia (normocytic, normochromic) and myeloma results in anaemia from bone marrow failure. Patients from the Middle East, South-East Asia and Africa should be screened preoperatively for glucose-6-phosphate dehydrogenase deficiency, hereditary spherocytosis and sickle cell disease.

A1.13 Congenital risk factors for thrombosis include:
A antithrombin deficiency
B homocystinuria
C protein C deficiency
D protein S deficiency
E resistance to activated protein C

A1.13 **A** = T **B** = T **C** = T **D** = T **E** = T

Hypercoagulable states may result from a congenital deficiency of physiologically occurring anticoagulant factors. Antithrombin inactivates factors IX, X, XI, XII and thrombin. Heparin acts by binding to antithrombin to potentiate its action. Activated protein C binds to protein S to inactivate factors V and VIII. Resistance to activated protein C is also known as factor V Leiden defect. This genetic defect is present in approximately 7% of the population in the UK. All of these conditions are inherited autosomally. Homocystinuria is a genetic condition which results in a disorder of the metabolism of the amino acid methionine. Patients with this condition are at an increased risk of thromboembolic disease.

A1.14 Fresh frozen plasma:

A contains all coagulation factors
B contains white blood cells
C is indicated in bleeding from Haemophilia A
D is associated with bronchospasm
E is obtained from a pool of blood donors

A1.14 **A** = T **B** = F **C** = F **D** = T **E** = F

Fresh frozen plasma (FFP) is obtained from the supernatant liquid obtained from centrifuging a unit of whole blood obtained from a single donor and storing at −30°C. Centrifuging removes nearly all white and red blood cells. The FFP can be stored for up to 12 months and is prepared by thawing gently in a water bath. Group-specific compatibility is required although cross-matching is unnecessary. Allergic type reactions such as bronchospasm and acute respiratory distress syndrome may follow infusion. Indications for FFP transfusion include replacement of coagulation factors or other plasma proteins where their concentration is reduced, e.g. acquired deficiencies (such as in patients on warfarin who need rapid reversal prior to emergency surgery). Bleeding secondary to Haemophilia A should be reversed with Factor VIII fraction (dried).

A1.15 The following may occur as a result of blood transfusion:

A acute haemolytic reaction
B air embolism
C endotoxic shock
D hypercalcaemia
E hypokalaemia

A1.15 **A** = T **B** = F **C** = T **D** = F **E** = F

Hazards of blood transfusion may be divided into immune and non-immune complications. These complications can be acute or delayed. While a great deal of publicity surrounds the risks of viral transmission and possible risks of variant Creutzfeldt–Jakob disease (vCJD), HIV and Hepatitis transmission, the risk is small when compared with the risk of a 'wrong blood in wrong patient' incident, which occurs in approximately 1:30000 units transfused. Incompatibility of blood groups may cause death. Therefore, one of the most important aspects of day-to-day use of blood products is ensuring the correct identity of the patient at every stage of the process. Acute non-immune reactions which may occur following transfusion include hyperkalaemia, hypocalcaemia, air embolism, hypothermia (after large transfusions) and endotoxic shock (after bacterial or pyogen contamination from the blood collection process). Delayed non-immune reactions include infection with a variety of blood-borne viruses such as HIV, Hepatitis B and C and cytomegalovirus (CMV). Acute immune complications include febrile non-haemolytic reactions, ABO incompatibility (acute haemolytic reaction), allergic reactions and transfusion related acute lung injury. Delayed immune reactions include delayed haemolytic transfusion reaction, post transfusion purpura, immune modulation and transfusion-associated graft-versus-host disease.

Postoperative management and critical care

A1.16 With regard to patient monitoring in the postoperative period:

A the pulse oximeter gives a useful measure of the adequacy of ventilation

B a rising pulse rate is rarely a sign of poorly managed pain

C hourly urine output provides an indication of fluid balance

D manual central venous pressure measurements on the general ward provide accurate assessment of postoperative fluid requirements

E drain output should be monitored as a sign of bleeding in the postoperative period

A1.16 **A** = F **B** = F **C** = T **D** = F **E** = T

Monitoring in the postoperative period enables early recognition of postoperative complications and appropriate fluid and pain management. The pulse oximeter gives a useful guide of the adequacy of oxygenation but does not give any information about ventilation (it may be normal because of a high inspired oxygen level). A rising pulse rate usually indicates poorly managed pain but may also indicate bleeding or inadequate fluid maintenance. The hourly urine output in a patient with normal renal function is a useful measure of renal perfusion. This is dependent on circulatory volume and so can help guide fluid replacement. Central venous pressure measurement is the best guide to fluid management and replacement on the ICU using a Statham pressure transducer. However, on general wards it is usually measured manually using a spirit level and tape measure, resulting in significant variability and inaccuracy, and is open to a significant risk of infectious contamination. Drain output is useful in the recognition of postoperative haemorrhage and if amounts are large or persistent, they indicate the need for re-operation/re-exploration to stop the bleeding. The absence of significant bloody drainage does not make bleeding impossible as the drain may be blocked. In the face of a rising pulse rate and falling blood pressure it must not give a sense of false 'security'.

A1.17 Pain in the postoperative period:

A increases the risks of postoperative cardiac ischaemia

B is associated with an increased risk of deep vein thrombosis

C is best managed with "as required analgesia"

D may improve respiratory function

E is almost similar in patients who have undergone the same procedure

A1.17 **A** = T **B** = T **C** = F **D** = F **E** = F

Pain increases sympathetic output leading to increased myocardial oxygen demand and therefore an increased risk of myocardial ischaemia, particularly in patients with pre-existing cardiac disease. Poorly managed postoperative pain may result in delayed mobilisation and respiratory effort, particularly when analgesia use is excessive and causing an impaired conscious level.

In turn, there is an increased risk of hypostatic complications such as deep vein thrombosis. Poor management of postoperative pain impairs the patient's ability to cough, breathe deeply and cooperate with physiotherapy, leading to retention of secretions, atelectasis and pneumonia. Effective analgesia which reduces pain but does not impair mobilisation, can improve respiratory function.

PRN regimes rely on the patient requesting analgesia when in pain. This results in considerable time delays between request and administration. In addition, peak plasma levels obtained by intramuscular or intravenous opioid injections, and the time taken to reach these levels varies between patients. Pain relief and opioid levels swing between sub-optimal and excessive. The standard regime is therefore optimal for only a small number of patients. Patient controlled or, when appropriate, epidural analgesia give the gold standards of balance of analgesia and mobilisation.

The plasma concentrations of opioids required to provide effective analgesia may vary up to four-fold between patients undergoing similar procedures.

A1.18 In a healthy 70 kg male patient, who is stable after major elective surgery, the fluid and electrolyte requirements in the first 24–48 hours will be met by the following fluid regimens:

A 2.5 litres of 4% dextrose/0.18% Saline per 24 hours
B 0.5 litres of normal saline and 2 litres of 5% dextrose per 24 hours
C 1.5 litres of normal saline and 1 litre of 5% dextrose per 24 hours
D 2.5 litres of normal saline per 24 hours
E 2.5 litres of Hartmann's solution per 24 hours

A1.18 A = F **B** = F **C** = F **D** = F **E** = F

The requirements of a fit and healthy 70 kg man is approximately 2.5 litres of water (35 ml/kg), 100 mmol (1–2 mmol/kg) sodium and 70 mmol potassium (1 mmol/kg). Normal saline contains 154 mmol sodium per litre. Dextrose-saline contains 30 mmol sodium per litre. Hartmann's solution contains 131 mmol sodium and 5 mmol potassium per litre. None of the regimens described contain the optimal balance of sodium potassium or fluid requirements.

These requirements assume that no oral intake can be included and there is not any excessive loss of water or electrolytes from a drain or from the bowel. Equally, in the first 24–48 hours after surgery urine output may not match this input mainly due to the secretion of antidiuretic hormone (ADH) from the posterior pituitary. Potassium loss may be excessive after major surgery because of mineralocorticoid release, predominantly through the renin-angiotensin-aldosterone response, but this needs to be balanced against levels of potassium in blood raised following the tissue trauma of surgery. Sodium is retained by the early metabolic response to trauma but plasma levels may not reflect this because of ADH release.

A1.19 Postoperative nutritional support:

A is indicated in all patients undergoing major abdominal surgery

B may be complicated by problems with venous access when administered enterally

C results in metabolic complications in approximately 5% of patients who are parenterally fed

D when administered enterally may be complicated by problems of absorption

E in the immediate postoperative period should be preferably administered parenterally for a short period

A1.19 **A** = F **B** = F **C** = T **D** = T **E** = T

All patients undergoing major surgery should have their nutritional requirements assessed preoperatively. Those severely malnourished should be considered for preoperative nutritional support where surgical urgency allows. Normally nourished patients do not require supplementary postoperative nutritional support. However, if oral nutrition has not been started within 48 hours of surgery, then supplementation must be considered. An otherwise optimal postoperative recovery may be compromised by delayed nutrition. Total Parenteral Nutrition (TPN) feeding is given intravenously when feeding enterally is not possible due to a non-functioning gastrointestinal tract or if there is a high output gastrointestinal fistula. When possible, enteral feeding is always preferable to the parenteral route. There is some evidence that early enteral feeding reduces the risk of sepsis in the critically ill patient. Parenteral feeding may be complicated by line-related problems (e.g. air embolism, pneumothorax, TPN-thorax, infection) or metabolic complications, which occur in approximately 5% of patients. Enteral nutrition may cause gastrointestinal upset (cramps, bloating, diarrhoea) aspiration pneumonia and affect drug absorption. Enteral nutrition may be further complicated with problems with the feeding line, i.e. displacement.

A1.20 The following patients have an increased risk of developing thromboembolic disease:

A 68-year-old male undergoing a radical prostatectomy

B 61-year-old male undergoing a day-case inguinal hernia repair

C 23-year-old obese female on the oral contraceptive pill, admitted with gallstone pancreatitis

D 22-year-old male who sustained a fractured femoral shaft in a motorbike accident

E 46-year-old female with advanced breast cancer

A1.20 **A** = T **B** = T **C** = T **D** = T **E** = T

Risk factors for deep vein thrombosis include recent surgery, immobilisation, trauma, obesity, the oral contraceptive pill, heart failure, cancer and age >60 years, and in particular, a history of previous thromboembolism. All surgical patients having a general anaesthetic, even short day-case procedures, should be treated with some form of thromboprophylaxis, according to their relative risk of developing a deep vein thrombosis (DVT)/pulmonary embolism (PE). Graduated compression, thromboembolic deterrent (TED) stockings, calf or foot pumps (intermittent pneumatic compression), subcutaneous low molecular weight heparin and systemic anticoagulation are all used as prophylaxis depending on the risk. Incidence of thromboembolic complications is further reduced by early mobilisation and shorter operating times. Thromboembolic complications occur as DVT in approximately 10% of operations (detected by imaging techniques), while PE occurs in about 1% and results in death in approximately 0.1% of operations.

A1.21 The following statements regarding renal function are true:

A optimal postoperative urine output in an adult should be >0.5 ml/kg per hour

B oliguria is defined as a urine output of less than 30 ml/hour for 2 consecutive hours

C initial management of renal dysfunction in the postoperative patient should comprise intravenous furosemide

D a rise in serum creatinine is an early sign of impending renal failure

E pre-existing renal disease makes postoperative renal dysfunction more likely

A1.21 **A** = T   **B** = F   **C** = F   **D** = F   **E** = T

An ideal urine output in the postoperative patient is >0.5 ml/kg per hour. If it falls below this, the cause should be investigated and appropriate management should be instituted. Oliguria is defined as a postoperative urine output of less than 30 ml/hour for 4 consecutive hours. The most common cause of renal dysfunction in the postoperative patient is hypovolaemia and fluids should always be given first. The treatment of this usually needs admission to a high dependency unit (HDU) with fluid balance optimised by the use of central venous pressure measurement. If hypotension persists with correction of venous filling, the patient may need upstaging to intensive care, with consideration of inotropic support. Intravenous diuretics should never be given during the initial management of suspected renal dysfunction. A fall in urine output is one of the first signs of renal dysfunction; changes in serum creatinine occur later when established renal damage has not been prevented (e.g. acute tubular necrosis) and renal support such as dialysis is required. The commonest causes of postoperative renal dysfunction are hypovolaemia, hypotension, sepsis, nephrotoxic drugs and pre-existing renal disease.

A1.22 Systemic inflammatory response syndrome (SIRS):

A can only be identified in a patient with a documented infection

B in the presence of documented infection and haemodynamic compromise is called severe sepsis

C is suspected in a patient with a pulse of 95 bpm and a white cell count of 3×10^9/L

D progresses to multi-organ failure if left untreated

E results in end-organ tissue damage through hypoxia

A1.22 **A** = F **B** = T **C** = T **D** = T **E** = F

SIRS is defined as a characteristic, systemic, clinical response to inflammation (infective or non-infective) with two or more of the following: (1) temperature above 38°C or below 36°C; (2) heart rate above 90 bpm; (3) respiratory rate above 20 breaths/min or $PaCO_2$ less than 4.3 kPa; (4) white cell count above 12×10^9/L or below 4×10^9/L or 10% of immature forms. SIRS in the presence of a documented infection is called sepsis. Severe sepsis is SIRS in the presence of documented infection with haemodynamic compromise. The development of untreated SIRS, through to sepsis, leads to multiple organ dysfunction syndrome (MODS). The destructive systemic effect of SIRS is the result of cytokines and other inflammatory mediators triggering numerous humoral cascades, which result in sustained activation of the immune system, loss of integrity of the microcirculation and end-organ dysfunction.

A1.23 With regard to the multiple organ dysfunction syndrome (MODS) and multiple organ failure (MOF):
   A pulmonary failure, presenting as acute respiratory distress syndrome (ARDS) typically occurs first in the development of MOF
   B the body organs are not capable of maintaining homeostasis
   C the progression of MODS to MOF is unaffected by periods of hypotension
   D there is a generalised catabolic state
   E where four organs are affected by MOF the mortality rate is approximately 50%

A1.23 **A** = T **B** = T **C** = F **D** = T **E** = F

MODS is a state of physiological derangement in which organ function is no longer adequate to maintain homeostasis. Typically, patients progress through SIRS, sepsis and severe sepsis before developing MODS; left untreated, the patients progress to develop MOF. In MODS, the organs involved and the sequence of their dysfunction is determined by the original insult. Patients at the extremes of age are at increased risk of developing MODS. The progression of MODS to MOF is accelerated in the presence of a second insult (e.g. hypotension, infection, ischaemia). As MOF develops, the lungs are typically affected first (ARDS) followed by hepatic, intestinal, renal, haematological (coagulopathy) and finally cardiac failure. When one organ is affected, there is a 70% survival; however, the mortality rises up to 100% when four organs are affected.

A1.24 A cutaneous wound heals by:
   A delayed primary healing if the patient has a history of poor wound healing
   B first intention if closed within 24 hours of its creation
   C secondary intention if the wound is closed following a period of packing
   D the action of myofibroblasts in primary healing
   E secondary intention in the split-thickness skin graft donor sites

A1.24 **A** = F **B** = T **C** = F **D** = F **E** = F

Healing by first intention (primary healing) occurs when a wound is closed within 12–24 hours of its creation, as in a clean surgical incision. In such wounds, the wound edges are approximated using sutures, glue or a mechanical device such as staples. Delayed primary closure is recommended for contaminated or poorly delineated wound such as bites or abdominal wounds after peritoneal soiling. The wound is initially left open to prevent infection and closed after a few days when the host defences have been allowed to debride the wound. Grossly contaminated wounds, wounds with extensive soft tissue loss, or wounds after some surgical procedures, e.g. laparostomy are left to heal by secondary intention (secondary healing). The wound eventually closes by both wound contraction and matrix deposition and epithelialisation. Myofibroblasts, having structural properties of both fibroblasts and smooth muscle cells, are thought to play a key role in wounds healing by secondary intention. Healing of split-thickness donor graft sites do not occur by secondary intention but by epithelialisation from the skin edges and appendages.

A1.25 Hidradenitis suppurativa:

A is caused due to inflammation of the exocrine glands
B is associated with sinus formation
C requires biopsy to confirm the diagnosis in the acute stages
D can be successfully treated with prolonged courses of oral antibiotics
E can lead to dermal fibrosis and contractures

A1.25 **A** = F **B** = T **C** = F **D** = F **E** = T

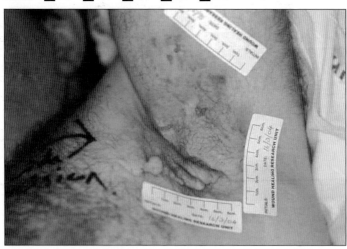

Fig. 1.25.1 Left axillary hidradenitis suppurativa

Hidradenitis suppurativa (HS) (Fig. 1.25.1) is a chronic suppurative disease of the apocrine sweat glands. It has a predilection for the inter-triginal regions such as the axilla, groin and perineum. It is manifested by recurrent abscesses, sinuses and, occasionally, fistulas. The physical nature of the apocrine glands (long narrow ducts), allows anaerobic organisms to grow and these organisms are often the cause of the flare up of the disease. The glands subsequently rupture leading to extension of infection resulting in further local inflammation, tissue destruction and skin damage. Diagnosis is largely clinical, and no investigation is indicated in the acute stages of the disease. Treatment with empirical oral antibiotics may result in resolution of the acute symptoms. However, incision and drainage of the abscess is required if the symptoms fail to subside. In addition, since local recurrences are common, wide radical resection of all apocrine glands bearing skin is strongly recommended. Radical excision also minimises the recurrence rate as opposed to limited surgical interventions. The accepted modalities to achieve coverage of the excised area include: primary closure; healing by secondary intention; skin grafting and; the use of local tissue flaps. Chronic HS leads to progressive destruction of normal skin architecture with the development of periductal and periglandular inflammation, dermal and subcutaneous fibrosis, and scarring and contractures.

A1.26 Hypertrophic scars:

A are confined to the margins of the original scar
B are usually seen over the flexor surfaces
C have a strong genetic predisposition
D may result from excessive wound tension
E respond to conservative treatment and subside with time

A1.26 **A** = T **B** = T **C** = F **D** = T **E** = T

A hypertrophic scar is a form of excessive healing resulting from over-production of many components of the healing process, including fibroblasts, collagen, elastin and proteoglycans. The incidence of hypertrophic scars is highest in: wounds crossing flexor surfaces; wounds crossing tension lines; areas of excessive skin (wound) tension and movement; deep dermal burns and; wounds left to heal by secondary intention (more than 3 weeks). Hypertrophic scars are confined to the margins of the original scar whilst keloids outgrow the wound (scar) area. Hypertrophic scars do not have a genetic predisposition; keloids are thought to have a genetic link. Hypertrophic scars respond to appropriate conservative treatment, including topical steroids and compression therapy, and subside with time. This is in contrast to keloid scarring which does not usually respond to any of the currently available conventional treatments and frequently recur, sometimes even more aggressively, after surgical excision.

A1.27 Lasers:

A absorption depth is dependent upon the wavelength of the laser
B beams are mostly red
C contain light over a wide range of wavelengths
D may cause retinal burns and cataracts
E used most commonly in surgical practice is the diode laser

A1.27 **A** = T **B** = F **C** = F **D** = T **E** = T

The laser beam emitted by a given lasing medium is of single wavelength, which is dependent upon the lasing medium used. The laser is a highly directional, coherent (monochromatic and in phase) beam of electromagnetic radiation which may or may not be visible. Lasers which do not produce light within the visible spectrum have a visible guiding beam which is usually a red helium-neon beam. Inadvertent injury may occur to anyone in the operating room, commonly with injury to the skin or eyes resulting in retinal or corneal burns and cataracts. Everyone in the room in which the laser is being used should wear eye protection specific to the laser being used. The diode laser is used most commonly in surgical practice.

A1.28 Regarding diathermy:

A alternating currents applied at a frequency of 50 Hz result in muscle contraction
B at low frequencies, currents of 100 mA may cause serious heart arrhythmias
C high frequency alternating current applied with a low current density produces high local temperatures
D the patient plate should be applied well away from the site of operation
E monopolar diathermy should always be used when operating on appendages

A1.28 **A** = T **B** = T **C** = F **D** = F **E** = F

Diathermy works via the passage of high frequency alternating current through body tissues. At the active electrode (surgical site), the current is locally concentrated (a high current density) resulting in high temperatures. At the return electrode (patient plate), the current has a low current density resulting in little heat production. The patient plate should be applied to a well vascularised area of skin (free of hair) close to the site of operation. Poor application of the patient plate is the commonest cause of inadvertent diathermy injury. Low frequency alternating current (50 Hz) results in neuro-muscular contraction, while rising currents (>80 mA) can interrupt the electrical pathways in the heart and may cause ventricular fibrillation. At higher frequencies (>50 kHz) this effect disappears. Surgical diathermy machines use frequencies of 400 kHz–10 MHz, at which frequency currents up to 500 mA may be safely used. When operating on appendages such as the penis, bipolar diathermy should be used, as monopolar diathermy produces heat at the base of the appendage, resulting in tissue damage and vessel thrombosis, due to the high current densities.

A1.29 The following are examples of synthetic absorbable sutures:

A Monocryl (poliglecaprone)
B PDS (polydioxanone)
C Prolene (polypropylene)
D Silk
E Vicryl (polyglactin)

A1.29 **A** = T **B** = T **C** = F **D** = F **E** = T

Suture materials may be: natural or synthetic; absorbable or non-absorbable and; braided or monofilament. The choice of suture material depends upon a number of factors including: the required tensile strength, ease of handling and knotting, the body's inflammatory reaction to the material, whether the material is to be absorbed and the thickness of the suture material. Synthetic polymers are tailor-made for their purpose. Non-absorbable synthetic polymers such as Prolene or Nylon (polyamide) offer long-lasting tensile strength with minimal tissue reaction, and are used for vascular anastomosis and mass closure of the abdominal wall, respectively. Braided synthetic absorbable sutures such as Vicryl offer easier handling and knotting characteristics and are often used for bowel anastomosis. Vicryl retains its strength for 28 days and is completely absorbed by hydrolysis by 90 days. Monocryl is a synthetic absorbable monofilament Vicryl, which retains its tensile strength for 20 days and is absorbed after 28 days. Silk is a non-absorbable, braided, natural suture, which offers excellent handling and knotting characteristics. However, it induces a marked inflammatory tissue reaction and is therefore only usually used for temporary fixation of a drain. PDS (Poly-Dioxanone Suture) is a synthetic, absorbable monofilament suture which is slowly absorbed by hydrolysis. It is completely absorbed in 180–210 days, has high tensile strength which remains at 70% at 2 weeks and 50% at 4 weeks.

A1.30 A mini operation set contains:

A 2 Babcock tissue forceps
B 1 fine-toothed forceps
C 2 Langenbeck retractors
D 1 McIndoe scissors
E 1 Morris retractor

A1.30 **A** = F **B** = T **C** = T **D** = T **E** = F

Surgical instruments come packed in a 'set' or are supplied separately. Instruments are packed as sets as they contain most of the instruments necessary for a given procedure and can be sterilised as a set (tray). It is more economical to pack instruments which are used less often, as 'supplements'. Instruments which come as part of a set are also packed as supplements to replace instruments which may become contaminated during a procedure. Where possible within a set, instruments are packed as multiples of five on a pin. It is necessary to complete a count at the start of a procedure and repeat the count when the wound is being closed. It is the responsibility of the surgeon to make sure the count is correct. Babcock tissue forceps and a Morris retractor are part of a laparotomy set.

A1.31 When suturing any wound it is important to:

A achieve haemostasis
B close deeper tissues
C invert the skin edge
D to tie sutures tightly
E wipe the wound before closing to remove blood

A1.31 **A** = T **B** = T **C** = F **D** = F **E** = F

Surgical wounds should be made where possible along Langer's lines. Closure should achieve an acceptable cosmetic finish, with everted skin edges. Wounds may be closed immediately (primary closure), closed later when infection has resolved (delayed primary closure) or left to close by scarring (secondary intention). Wound closure may be achieved with sutures, clips or adhesive strips. Suture technique may be continuous or interrupted, simple or mattress or subcuticular. Principles of wound closure include: gentle tissue handling, removal of all devitalised tissue, dabbing (not rubbing) with a gauze swab to remove blood from the wound, closure of the deeper tissues to avoid a 'dead space', approximation of the wound edges and accurate placement of sutures. Sutures should be tied securely without excessive tension, as excessively tight sutures result in tissue ischaemia.

A1.32 A tourniquet during surgery is indicated:

A to create a bloodless surgical field
B to occlude inflow when creating a vascular anastomosis
C to prevent haematoma when reducing distal limb fractures
D to secure haemostasis in uncontrolled bleeding
E to isolate the distal limb for infusion of local anaesthetic

A1.32 **A** = T **B** = F **C** = F **D** = T **E** = T

Tourniquets are indicated for: creation of a bloodless field, haemostasis of uncontrolled distal bleeding and isolation of a distal limb for infusion of local anaesthetic, e.g. Biers block. Prior to inflating a tourniquet, it is necessary to elevate and exsanguinate the limb. The cuff is inflated to twice systolic blood pressure for the upper limb and three times systolic pressure for the lower limb. The cuff requires release every 90 min for at least 15 min. Patients with a Middle Eastern, Asian or African origin should be screened prior to application of a tourniquet for haemoglobinopathies (e.g. sickle cell, thalassemia) due to the risk of red cell sludging. The major complication of tourniquets is ischaemia due to prolonged application. Bruising may also occur due to a poorly fitted cuff.

Management and legal issues in surgery

A1.33 Regarding levels of evidence-based medicine:

A Ia – evidence from at least one randomised controlled trial
B Ib – evidence from a trial which is not randomised
C IIa – case control study results
D IIb – evidence from an expert committee
E III – evidence from a meta-analysis of randomised controlled trials

A1.33 **A** = F **B** = F **C** = F **D** = F **E** = F

Evidence based medicine is graded on its perceived scientific significance in order to best apply the findings in clinical practice. Evidence is graded as follows: Ia – evidence from a meta-analysis of several randomised controlled trails; Ib – evidence from at least one randomised control trial; IIa – evidence from at least one non-randomised study; IIb – evidence from at least one other type of study; III – evidence from descriptive studies, e.g. case reports; IV – evidence from expert committees. Each piece of evidence should be critically appraised for methodology and validity of results.

A1.34 The following statistical tests are for parametric data:

A Kruskal–Wallis
B Mann–Whitney U
C Pearson's correlation coefficient
D *t*-tests
E Wilcoxon signed rank test

A1.34 **A** = F **B** = F **C** = T **D** = T **E** = F

The choice of statistical test when analysing the statistical significance of data depends on, the type of data (nominal, ordinal, quantitative), certain assumptions about the distribution of the data, the way the different data sets relate to each other under the test conditions (independent or dependent) and the number of groups being compared. Usual assumptions about distribution include a normal distribution (Gaussian distribution, i.e. symmetrical bell-shaped curve); when the data are assumed to have a normal distribution then parametric tests may be employed. Parametric tests include *t*-tests (a significance test used to compare means of two different groups) and Pearson's correlation (assess the linear relationship between two sets of variables). Statistical analysis of data which does not have a normal distribution is assessed using non-parametric tests. Non-parametric tests include Mann–Whitney U (a non-parametric equivalent to the unpaired or independent *t*-test for comparing two groups of independent subjects or datasets), Kruskal–Wallis test (similar to the Mann–Whitney U test and used when there are more than 2 groups) and Wilcoxon signed rank test (takes into account the magnitude and the direction of differences when comparing groups in a repeated measures or matched pairs design).

A1.35 A clinical trial requires:
A a placebo control
B a protocol
C ethics committee approval
D patient matching within the trial
E randomisation

A1.35 **A** = F **B** = T **C** = T **D** = F **E** = T

A clinical trial is a prospective experimental study to assess the outcome of a new treatment (e.g. drug, surgical procedure) on human subjects. Investigation of a new drug requires pre-clinical phases before effects on human subjects can be assessed by a clinical trial. A clinical trial requires a comparator (control treatment) to ensure that any improvement is attributable to the new treatment, as long as there is tight control of preventable confounding variables and efforts to reduce bias. The control may be a standard treatment (positive control) or a placebo (negative control). Before seeking approval from the local ethics committee, it is necessary to write a protocol, which covers all aspects of the trial including the number of patients required, study methodology, inclusion and exclusion criteria, data collection methods, analysis including statistical methods, and data protection and patient confidentiality. Research carried out in the NHS requires local trust Research and Development approval. Any trial evaluating a drug therapy requires approval from the Medicines and Healthcare Products Regulatory Agency. To reduce bias, a patient admitted to a trial is allocated to a treatment group by means of randomisation, which the patient and researcher are usually blinded to (double-blinded). Patient matching may be performed, but is not always done or possible.

A1.36 The following are examples of audit projects:
A a study comparing the outcomes of a new laser surgery technique to the prostate with the gold standard of monopolar transurethral resection
B a study of the application of a new hospital guideline on the use of an intravenous cannula
C a study of the treatment pathway for a patient referred with rectal bleeding, from referral to definitive treatment
D a review of the management of patients with acute pancreatitis compared with the gold standard of the British Society of Gastroenterology guidelines
E a randomised study comparing patient's discomfort on insertion of an intravenous cannula with or without topical local anaesthetic

A1.36 **A** = F **B** = T **C** = T **D** = T **E** = F

Audit aims to tell us if we are doing what we should be doing in processes or outcomes as advised by guidelines or current best practice; research asks the question which is the better intervention in terms of efficacy, efficiency or effectiveness. Some statisticians describe audit as, 'whether the right thing has been done' and research as, 'what is the right thing to do?'. Projects comparing new treatments with accepted practice, when there is clinical equipoise between 'old' and 'new', are regarded as research, using the RCT. Many audit projects compare local practice with either locally or nationally produced guidelines. An important aspect of audit is to 'complete the loop'. After a project has been performed any deficiencies in practice should be identified, and changes put in place in order to correct these deficiencies. The same audit should then be repeated to ensure that the changes have resulted in a change in practice. Audits of process take into account many aspects of healthcare delivery and are important in identifying deficiencies and improving service delivery to patients.

A1.37 Clinical governance requires:
A clinical risk reduction programme to be in place
B consultants to be responsible for the clinical actions of their juniors
C evidence based practice should be employed in day-to-day practice
D poor clinical performance monitored and reviewed regularly
E participation in regular mortality and morbidity meetings

A1.37 **A** = T **B** = F **C** = T **D** = F **E** = T

Clinical governance is the system through which NHS organisations are accountable for continuously improving the quality of their services and safeguarding high standards of care, by creating an environment in which clinical excellence will flourish. Clinical governance requires: quality programmes to be in place (e.g. audit), leadership skill development at team level, evidence based practice, good practice dissemination, clinical risk reduction programmes, adverse events reporting, lessons learnt from complaints, professional development programmes, poor practice identified at an early stage and dealt with to prevent harm to patient. Junior doctors are responsible for their own clinical decision unless acting under supervision or direction of a consultant.

A1.38 The following methods are employed in theatre to avoid errors:
A on the operating list left and right are signified by 'L' and 'R', respectively
B patients are sent for by name
C the anaesthetist is responsible for checking the patient's identity
D the side to be operated is marked by the operating surgeon
E the surgeon sees the patient and reviews the notes following induction of anaesthesia

A1.38 **A** = F **B** = F **C** = F **D** = T **E** = F

Performing operations on the wrong patient or wrong side is indefensible in law. Therefore, safeguards are taken to avoid potential errors. All patients should wear identity bracelets stating their full name, address, date of birth and hospital number. When sending for a patient, it is necessary to have all of these details checked by both the ward nurse and theatre porter. When the patient arrives in theatre the patient identity should be checked by the nurse, the patient's identity should then be checked again by the anaesthetist when the patient is taken into the anaesthetic room. Prior to the induction of anaesthetic, the patient's identity, operation and side of operation should be checked by the operating surgeon. The operating surgeon is ultimately responsible for checking the patient's identity. The side of operation should only be marked by the operating surgeon after consulting the patient, notes and radiology. An operating list should be completed in full and should contain the patient's full name, address, date of birth and hospital number. Abbreviations are not acceptable.

Clinical microbiology

A1.39 The following patients should receive antibiotic prophylaxis prior to inserting a urethral catheter:
A a 72-year-old male who underwent a total hip replacement 2 months previously
B a 62-year-old female with rheumatic heart disease
C a 48-year-old male with a mechanical aortic valve
D a 56-year-old male who is being treated with steroids and azathioprine for retroperitoneal fibrosis
E a 33-year-old female receiving a bone marrow transplant

A1.39 **A** = T **B** = T **C** = T **D** = T **E** = T

Urethral catheterisation is associated with a risk of a transient bacteraemia, particularly when there is a co-existent urinary tract infection (which may not have been recognised). Prophylactic antibiotics should be used in patients in whom this may pose a significant risk. Patients with rheumatic heart disease and mechanical heart valves are at risk of bacterial endocarditis. Catheterisation after joint replacement is associated with higher rates of late prosthetic joint infection. Immunosuppressed patients are at significant risk from this transient bacteraemia. Oral ciprofloxacin or intravenous gentamicin/cefuroxime are recommended as prophylaxis immediately prior to catheterisation in these patients at high risk.

A1.40 The following bacteria are likely to be the causative organisms in the corresponding disease:
A *Escherichia coli* and urinary tract infection
B *Neisseria meningitidis* and post splenectomy sepsis
C *Pseudomonas aeruginosa* and a wound infection of an inguinal hernia repair
D *Staphylococcus aureus* and cholangitis
E *Streptococcus faecalis* and lower lobe pneumonia

A1.40 **A** = T **B** = T **C** = F **D** = F **E** = F

Almost all infections encountered in surgical practice come from an endogenous source. The causative organisms in peritonitis and postoperative abdominal infections are usually gut-derived; e.g. coliforms, *Bacteroides fragilis* and *Streptococcus faecalis*. Cholangitis is a specific infection of the bile ducts which is usually caused by gut-derived coliform bacteria. Surgical site infections are most commonly caused by *Staphylococcus aureus*, although coliforms, Bacteroides species and Streptococcus pyogenes are also implicated. There may be synergy between Gram-negative aerobes such as the coliforms and obligate anaerobes such as Bacteroides species. *Pseudomonas aeruginosa* is a ubiquitous Gram-negative organism which tends to cause opportunistic infections in immunosuppressed patients. The most commonly seen infections with this organism are in burns, tracheostomies and urinary catheter-related infection, particularly on ICU. Urinary tract infections are most commonly caused by gut-derived pathogens; *Escherichia coli* is the most commonly implicated organism but in patients who are catheterised, Pseudomonas and Proteus species may also be cultured. Respiratory tract infections presenting as postoperative pneumonias are commonly caused by *Streptococcus pneumoniae* and are seen more often in smokers. Ventilator associated pneumonia (VAP) is encountered on ICU and organisms such as Gram-negative aerobes may be cultured; there is increasing concern about the rise in incidence of glycopeptide resistant enterococci. Splenectomised patients are most at risk from sepsis caused by encapsulated organisms, e.g. *Streptococcus pneumoniae*, *Haemophilus influenzae* and *Neisseria meningitidis*.

A1.41 The following are proven to reduce the risk of surgical infection:

A admission to hospital on the day of surgery
B early mobilisation and physiotherapy
C removal of all indwelling lines and catheters at the earliest opportunity
D shaving of the operation site by the patient prior to admission to hospital
E use of appropriate antibiotic prophylaxis

A1.41 **A** = F **B** = T **C** = T **D** = F **E** = T

Shaving of the operation site by the patient often results in minor skin abrasions and where done 24 hours prior to surgery, results in proliferation of skin commensals and a higher rate of surgical site infections. Where necessary, shaving should be performed by the surgeon in the operating theatre immediately prior to surgery. Rates of antibiotic resistant bacterial (e.g. MRSA) skin colonisation are proportional to length of stay in hospital. Admission on the day of surgery reduces the risk of this colonisation and is of particular relevance in orthopaedic and vascular surgery. Antibiotic prophylaxis where indicated significantly reduces the risk of infection. The use of prophylaxis in clean, non-implant surgery is controversial. Prophylaxis should not exceed 24 hours (three shot prophylaxis is appropriate in prosthetic joint and vascular surgery); if it is extended beyond this, it is classified as treatment and adds to the risk of emergence (e.g. *Clostridium difficile enteritis*) and resistance (e.g. MRSA). All indwelling lines and catheters (intravascular lines are at greatest risk of infection with resultant bacteraemia) should be removed as soon as they are not necessary; urinary catheters are associated with a rate of urinary tract infection of 6% per day of catheterisation. Early mobilisation and physiotherapy not only results in a reduced hospital stay but also improves ventilation and reduces the risk of atelectasis and chest infections.

A1.42 The response to infection and the development of the systemic inflammatory response syndrome (SIRS):

A during phase 1 there is commonly a tachycardia and pyrexia >38°C

B in phase 3 the release of inflammatory mediators becomes destructive, resulting in dysfunction of various end organs

C normal resolution occurs without progression beyond phase 2

D the earliest response involves the local production of cytokines and recruitment of monocytes and macrophages to the site of injury

E this acute phase response is kept in check by the simultaneous release of pro-inflammatory mediators and endogenous antagonists

A1.42 **A** = F **B** = T **C** = T **D** = T **E** = T

The pathophysiological response to sepsis occurs in three phases: (1) local response involves release of pro-inflammatory cytokines (e.g. TNFα, IL-6) following recruitment of monocytes to the site of injury with a localised inflammatory response; (2) following the release of these small quantities of cytokines into the systemic circulation there is enhancement of the local response with further macrophage and platelet recruitment, and growth factor production (e.g. PDGF, IGF). The acute phase response is kept in check by the simultaneous release of endogenous antagonists. This process continues until the infection has resolved and homeostasis restored. If homeostasis is not restored SIRS (phase 3) develops, signs of which include tachycardia and pyrexia, with a massive systemic reaction which may result if not treated in loss of integrity of the microcirculation and dysfunction of various distant end-organs.

A1.43 When preparing a patient's skin for surgery:

A a preoperative shower with chlorhexidine reduces wound infections

B pre-existing skin infections should be pre-treated

C preoperative shaving should be performed the night before surgery

D the patient's skin should be prepared using an antiseptic solution which is rubbed onto the skin and then immediately wiped dry with a clean swab

E the use of incisional plastic drapes over the operative site results in significantly reduced wound infection rates

A1.43 **A** = F **B** = T **C** = F **D** = F **E** = F

Patients undergoing surgery should be encouraged to shower preoperatively, ideally using an antiseptic such as chlorhexidine. However, the results of clinical trials have shown mixed results and there is no definite evidence that surgical site infection is reduced by an antiseptic shower. It is common sense that patients should be presented for surgery with optimal hygiene and excluded if they have an unrelated infection (e.g. a skin abscess). These pre-existing skin infections should be treated. If urgent or emergency surgery is required, such skin lesions can be covered and isolated using an adhesive, waterproof polyurethane skin dressing. Shaving results in higher wound infection rates and where necessary, should be performed as near to the time of surgery as possible, ideally by the surgeon, in theatre just prior to patient's antiseptic skin preparation. In the UK, the patient's skin is not scrubbed first with a sponge or swab impregnated with detergent to degrease the skin; but application of an alcoholic antiseptic solution, such as povidone-iodine or chlorhexidine, which reduces the surface organisms count by >95%, is considered to be sufficient. Care must be taken not to allow pooling of the solution where diathermy is to be used, and the skin should be allowed to dry before application of skin drapes. Cultures from postoperative wound infections often suggest that the organisms are transferred from other areas of the patient to the operative site. Incisional plastic drapes and wound guards do not result in any reduction in wound infection rates.

A1.44 Surgical practice sterilisation:

A is achieved using dry heat at 160°C for 1 hour
B of flexible endoscopes is achieved with glutaraldehyde (2%)
C of reusable instruments is achieved with gamma radiation
D of the skin is commonly achieved using an alcoholic solution of chlorhexidine
E using autoclaves is achieved by the utilisation of steam at pressure

A1.44 **A** = F **B** = F **C** = F **D** = F **E** = T

Sterilisation is defined as the complete destruction of all viable microorganisms including spores, viruses and mycobacteria. It may be achieved using steam under pressure, ethylene oxide and chemical agents or gamma-irradiation. Disinfection using low temperature steam, boiling water, formaldehyde or other chemical disinfectants (such as glutaraldehyde 2%) reduces the number of viable microorganisms to an acceptable level but may not in-activate some viruses or spores. The skin cannot be sterilised and only antisepsis can be achieved. Steam under pressure (134°C, 2 atmospheres, 3 minute hold time) is used in autoclaves. Hot air (dry heat) can be used but requires a higher temperature and a longer hold time (160°C, 2 hours hold time). Ethylene oxide is mainly used industrially in the manufacture of single use medical devices as it is expensive and dangerous. Low-temperature steam and formaldehyde achieve sterilisation at a low temperature (73°C) so can be used on heat sensitive equipment. They cannot be used on endoscopes as the condensed water and formaldehyde may become trapped in narrow bore tubing and be hazardous to patients. Irradiation with gamma-irradiation or accelerated electrons is an industrial process used for the sterilisation of large batches of similar products.

A1.45 Antibiotic prophylaxis:

A should be used in all elective and emergency surgical procedures

B administered topically at wound closure reduces the rate of deep surgical site infection (SSI)

C should be administered parenterally immediately prior to surgery (at induction of anaesthesia)

D should be appropriate to the procedure being undertaken

E is more effective if prescribed for 5 days

A1.45 **A** = F **B** = F **C** = T **D** = T **E** = F

Antibiotic prophylaxis should be given when contamination of the wound is expected or when operations may lead to bacteraemia. Generally, it is required in all clean-contaminated and contaminated wound procedures (in dirty procedures, antibiotics should be given as treatment), and the choice of antibiotics should be guided by the likely source of infection (e.g. anaerobic and Gram-negative cover in bowel surgery). They are not required in clean wound procedures unless an implant or graft is being inserted. They are required in the presence of valvular heart disease, during emergency surgery in a patient with pre-existing or recently active infection, and where an infection would be severe or have life-threatening consequences. Antibiotic powders placed in the wound at closure have been shown to reduce the risk of superficial surgical site infections but are ineffective in prophylaxis of deep or organ space infections. Prophylaxis should be given immediately before surgery (at induction of anaesthesia) to ensure effective tissue levels. In general, single dose, intravenous prophylaxis is adequate. When a prosthetic joint or vascular prosthesis is being placed, when surgery exceeds 3–4 hours, or when there is excessive blood loss, a further 1–2 doses should be given. There is no evidence to suggest that a prolonged course of antibiotics (>24 hours) is more effective than a single or a short course.

A1.46 Antibiotic resistance by bacteria may be developed by the following mechanisms:

A β-lactamase producing organisms are resistant to quinolones as the enzyme inactivates the antibiotic

B partial treatment of an infection may select out a resistant subpopulation which then proliferates

C plasmids encoding genes conferring resistance may be transferred from one organism to another by conjugation

D tetracycline resistance occurs by changes in the cell membrane becoming impermeable to the drug

E trimethoprim resistance is acquired through the production of an alternative form of dihydrofolate reductase which has no affinity for the drug

A1.46 **A** = F **B** = T **C** = T **D** = T **E** = T

Antibiotic resistance can occur by:

1. production of inactivating enzymes that destroy the drug (β-lactamase destroys penicillins and cephalosporins)

2. decreased drug accumulation (tetracycline resistance is the result of changes in the permeability of the cell membrane)

3. alteration of binding sites (gentamicin binds to bacterial ribosomes, in resistant organisms this binding site is altered so they no longer have affinity for the drug)

4. development of alternative metabolic pathways (trimethoprim resistance is the result of the production of an alternative form of dihydrofolate reductase which has a reduced affinity for the drug).

Antibiotic resistant populations may be the result of selection (antibiotic treatment selects out a resistant sub-population which then proliferates), or transferred resistance (genes encoding for resistance contained on plasmids are transferred from one organism to another by conjugation or by transduction).

A1.47 When operating on a high-risk surgical patient:

A an additional assistant is required to improve exposure

B disposable protective clothing (impervious gowns, eye protectors etc.) should be worn

C gloves offer some protection from needle stick injury

D scalpels should be passed hand to hand to avoid risk of injury to the surgeon

E solid needles have a higher rate of blood transfer than hollow needles

A1.47 **A** = F **B** = T **C** = T **D** = F **E** = F

Since it is not possible or practical to screen all surgical patients for the presence of blood-borne viral infections, universal precautions should be prastised when undertaking surgery in high risk patients. Where possible a 'no touch' surgical technique should be employed, using retractors instead of hands, instrument ties, and only one person working in the open wound at any time. Where a single pair of gloves is worn there is a perforation rate of 11–54%, but this is reduced to 2% by double gloving. In addition, penetration of the glove material by the instrument has a significant wiping effect and this reduces the volume of blood transferred. Hollow needles carry a higher rate of blood transfer and this is also proportional to the gauge of the needle.

A1.48 The following statements regarding universal precautions are true:

A intraoperatively-fixed retraction devices reduce the risk of sharps injuries

B masks and water repellent clothing should be worn during all surgical procedures

C needles should be re-sheathed before handing back to the scrub nurse

D scalpels should be passed in a kidney bowl

E wearing rubber gloves protects against sharps injury

A1.48 **A** = T **B** = T **C** = F **D** = T **E** = F

Universal precautions should be practised to minimise the risk to the operator and others of the transmission of blood-borne disease while performing the procedure. The precautions for each procedure vary according to the risk of contact with each procedure. In the operating theatre, protective clothing should include double gloving, water repellent gown and apron, protective headwear, masks, protective eyewear and shoe wear. Rubber gloves do not protect against sharps injury but do have a wiping effect and reduce the risk of disease transmission. Needles should never be re-sheathed, and sharp objects should be passed in an appropriate container. Assistants should be kept to the minimum necessary; fixed retraction devices reduce the number of assistants required.

A1.49 After sustaining a sharps injury during a surgical procedure:

A an incident report should be completed and filed

B blood tests for HIV and Hepatitis should be obtained from the patient while still in theatre

C post-exposure prophylaxis for HIV should be administered ideally within 1 hour of the injury if the patient is in a high risk group

D the healthcare worker who has failed to respond to a Hepatitis B vaccination should receive a booster vaccination soon after

E the wound should be washed liberally with soap and water once the case is finished

A1.49 **A** = T **B** = F **C** = T **D** = F **E** = F

After sustaining a sharps injury, the wound should be washed liberally with soap and water as soon as possible (i.e. as soon as the patient is stable and can be left in the care of others). An incident report should be filed and the occupational health department contacted. It is normal practice for a blood sample to be obtained from the injured party and the patient after obtaining fully informed consent. If the patient is considered to be a high risk for Hepatitis B carriage, the next step is dependent on the immunisation status of the injured person. Non-responders or those who have not been immunised should receive Hepatitis B immunoglobulin within 48 hours of the injury. If post-exposure HIV prophylaxis is to be considered, it should be commenced ideally within 1 hour of exposure.

Emergency medicine and management of trauma

A1.50 Class II hypovolaemic shock in a fit young man results in:
A a pulse rate >140 bpm
B a raised diastolic pressure but normal systolic blood pressure
C a urine output of 10 ml/hour
D confusion
E widened pulse pressure

A1.50 **A** = F **B** = T **C** = F **D** = F **E** = F

Shock is defined as inadequate organ perfusion and tissue oxygenation. Haemorrhage is the most common cause of shock in trauma patients. Septic shock may occur in trauma patients from grossly contaminated wounds and when the treatment is delayed. The other types of shock include: cardiogenic, neurogenic and anaphylactic. Hypovolaemic shock is classified into four classes (I–IV) depending on the amount of blood loss (Class I: <750 ml; Class II: 750–1500 ml; Class III: 1500–2000 ml; Class IV: >2000 ml). In a fit, young adult, Class II shock (a blood loss of 750–1500 ml) results in a pulse rate of around 120 bpm; if the pulse rate is >140 bpm, then it denotes a Class III shock. Class II shock results in a normal systolic blood pressure and a raised diastolic pressure. The pulse pressure becomes increasingly narrowed as the degree of blood loss increases. The urine output is 20–30 ml in patients with Class II shock (>30 ml in Class I; 5–15 ml in Class III and; it is negligible in Class IV). Increasing blood loss results in a decrease in the cerebral perfusion. This causes the patient to be anxious or aggressive in the early stages (Class II), but may become confused or unconscious with continued blood loss (Classes III or IV). The diastolic pressure is usually unobtainable in patients with Class IV. The other signs and symptoms of Class IV shock include a pale and cold skin, marked tachycardia and a significant reduction in the systolic blood pressure.

A1.51 The following are definitive airways:
A nasopharyngeal
B nasotracheal
C oropharyngeal
D orotracheal
E tracheostomy

A1.51 **A** = F **B** = T **C** = F **D** = T **E** = T

Oropharyngeal or nasopharyngeal tubes (airways) are not forms of definitive airways. A definitive airway requires a tube to be placed in the trachea with the cuff inflated (although uncuffed for young children) and the tube connected to oxygen-enriched assisted ventilation. Definitive airways are of three varieties: orotracheal tube, nasotracheal tube and surgical airway (cricothyroidotomy or tracheostomy). Rapid sequence induction of anaesthesia with orotracheal intubation is preferred by most anaesthetists as the primary method of securing a definitive airway. The decision to provide a definitive airway is based on clinical findings including: apnoea, inability to maintain a patent airway, need to protect the lower airway from aspiration, impending or potential compromise of the airway (e.g. facial fractures, major facial burns), extrinsic tracheal compression (e.g. post-thyroidectomy haematoma), upper airway haemorrhage, head injury associated with a decreasing GCS and inability to maintain adequate oxygenation by face mask oxygen supplementation. See 3.36 Endotracheal intubation and tracheostomy.

A1.52 Myocardial contusions from blunt trauma:

A are associated with valvular disruption
B are diagnosed on echocardiogram
C result in cardiogenic shock
D require early surgical intervention
E require monitoring by serial cardiac enzymes

A1.52 **A** = T **B** = F **C** = F **D** = F **E** = F

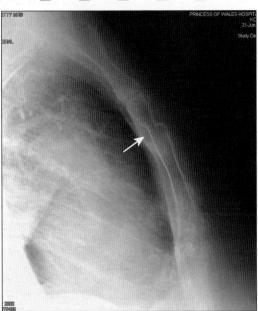

Fig. 1.52.1 A lateral chest radiograph showing a sternal fracture where both cortices have been displaced.

Blunt cardiac injury results most frequently from deceleration trauma as in road traffic accidents. Trauma to the central chest may result in a sternal fracture (Fig. 1.52.1), increasing the risk of cardiac injury. The trauma results in myocardial contusion (bruising) and, if severe, may cause a pericardial effusion, valvular disruption or cardiac chamber rupture. Patients with myocardial contusion usually report central chest pain and may be hypotensive. However, cardiogenic shock is rarely seen with myocardial contusion alone. Myocardial contusion is not detectable on transthoracic or transoesophageal echocardiography and can only truly be diagnosed by direct inspection at operation. Electrocardiographic changes associated with myocardial contusion include: multiple premature ventricular contractions, unexplained sinus tachycardia, atrial fibrillation, bundle branch block (usually right), non-specific ST and T wave changes, and features suggestive of frank myocardial infarction. Serial cardiac enzymes have no role in the evaluation and management of patients with myocardial contusion. Appropriate monitoring for 24 hours is sufficient in patients with myocardial contusion diagnosed by conduction abnormalities (since they are at an increased risk for sudden dysrhythmias during this period). Surgical intervention is indicated in patients with acute or delayed cardiac rupture, ventricular septal rupture or valvular disruption.

A1.53 Regarding cervical spine fractures:

A a Jefferson fracture affects the axis
B atlantoaxial fracture dislocation is associated with sudden death
C the odontoid process is affected in 60% of axis fractures
D type I odontoid fractures occur through the base of the dens
E type II odontoid fractures require surgical fixation

A1.53 **A** = F **B** = T **C** = T **D** = F **E** = T

A Jefferson fracture is a fracture of the atlas vertebra. It is a 'bursting type' of fracture involving the anterior and posterior arches, and causes the lateral masses to be displaced laterally. This type of injury does not produce neurological injury, as there is no encroachment on the neural canal. Atlantoaxial fracture dislocation resulting in a posterior dislocation of the axis causes the odontoid process to compress the spinal cord producing sudden death. Acute fractures of the axis (C2) vertebra represent about 18% of all cervical-spine injuries and approximately 60% of axis fractures involve the odontoid process. Type I odontoid fractures involve the tip of the odontoid process; type II fractures are through the base of the dens (involving the junction of the odontoid peg with the body) and; type III fractures occur at the base of the dens and extend obliquely into the body of the axis. Odontoid fractures are initially identified by a lateral cervical-spine film or open-mouth odontoid views. A CT scan is frequently required to further delineate the type and extent of the fracture. Type II is the most common type of odontoid fracture. The posterior elements of the axis, i.e. the pars interarticularis may be fractured (a hangman's fracture) by a hyperextension injury. Patients with this fracture should be maintained in external immobilisation until specialised care is available.

A1.54 Cerebral blood flow is:

A approximately 250 ml/100 g of brain tissue/min in an adult

B higher in adults compared with children

C autoregulated in response to mean systolic blood pressure

D autoregulated in response to changes in PaO_2

E reduced by <10% if a brain injury is severe enough to cause unconsciousness

A1.54 **A** = F **B** = F **C** = T **D** = T **E** = F

The cerebral blood flow in normal adults is approximately 50–55 ml/100 g of brain tissue/min, with the flow being higher in children (at 5 years of age, it is approximately 90 ml/100 g per minute, with levels declining until young adulthood). In normal physiological conditions, the cerebral blood flow is usually maintained by both pressure and chemical autoregulation. The pressure autoregulation is facilitated by reflex constriction or dilatation of the precapillary cerebral vasculature in response to mean systolic blood pressures between 50 and 160 mmHg. Chemical autoregulation is maintained by constriction or dilatation of the precapillary vessels in response to changes in the PaO_2 or $PaCO_2$. Severe traumatic brain injury causes disruption of both these autoregulatory mechanisms. Brain injury severe enough to cause coma can cause a 50% reduction in the cerebral blood flow during the first 6–12 hours after injury. It usually recovers over the next few days, but may remain below normal for days or even weeks after injury.

A1.55 Early management of partial thickness burns affecting 5% of the total body surface require:

A clothing to be left intact until the patient is transferred to the operating theatre

B aggressive intravenous fluid management

C application of icy cold water to burnt areas

D intravenous antibiotics

E transfer to the specialised burns unit

A1.55 **A** = F **B** = F **C** = F **D** = F **E** = F

Clothing should be removed as soon as possible; any skin that is adherent and peels off with the clothing is 'dead'. All devitalised tissue should be removed. Those in whom clothing is alight should 'drop and roll'. The use of a wet blanket may facilitate extinguishing the burning clothing. Following the removal of clothing, an estimate should be made of the extent (rule of nines) and depth of the burn(s). Partial thickness burns may extend as deep as the dermis and can be distinguished from full thickness burns as pain perception is retained. Early burns management requires cooling with luke-warm running water for at least 20 min. Icy cold water should be avoided, as blood flow to the affected area will be reduced. This may lead to hypothermia, which is a particular risk in infants and the elderly. Partial thickness burns affecting 15% of the total body surface in an adult are managed with oral fluids and oral antibiotics. The wound is managed dry as this provides an inhospitable environment for bacteria. Full-thickness burns affecting 5% of the total body surface area is an indication for transfer to the specialised burns unit.

Principles of surgical oncology

A1.56 The phases of the normal cell cycle include:
A G_2
B M
C R
D S
E T

A1.56 **A** = T **B** = T **C** = F **D** = T **E** = F

The cell cycle is the period of time taken for a single cell to divide into two daughter cells. Cell division is central to the development tissues and organs. Certain cells, such as the neurons, mature (differentiate) and lose their ability to divide further. They are known as stable cells. Other cells retain their ability to divide (stem-cells) throughout the individual's lifetime. Stem-cells do not differentiate but instead give rise to daughter cells, which will eventually differentiate and ultimately die and be replaced by other cells derived from the adult stem-cell. The cell cycle varies in duration depending on the cell type but is divided into four distinct phases (G_1, S, G_2, M). G_1 is the initial phase, which is under the influence of growth factors. DNA replication occurs in the S-phase while G_2 relates to the condensation of chromosomes and the division of the nuclear membrane. M is the mitotic phase (production of two identical copies of the parental genome). G_0 phase, also known as the resting phase, is characterised by cellular quiescence. The cells in this phase are 'outside' the cell cycle but have the ability to enter the cell cycle on appropriate stimulus. See 3.18 Cell cycle.

A1.57 Disordered cell replication results from the presence of:
A CDKs
B E2F
C p53
D RB1
E R points

A1.57 **A** = F **B** = F **C** = F **D** = F **E** = F

Cancer is fundamentally linked to disordered cell replication. To prevent replication of abnormal cells, restriction (R) points are placed at gap phases. R points act as a checkpoint to ensure that the cell is competent to undergo DNA replication. The major control of the cell cycle is protein phosphorylation, which is catalysed by cyclin-dependent kinases (CDKs). The transcription factor E2F controls the progression through G_1. The RB1 and p53 genes are both tumour suppressor genes, which regulate the cell cycle. Tumour suppressor genes may become oncogenic as the result of mutations inhibiting their normal functions.

A1.58 In a neoplasm the:
A cell cycle time is increased
B cell differentiation is increased
C cell loss coefficient is reduced
D growth fraction is reduced
E total cell number is increased

A1.58 **A** = F **B** = F **C** = T **D** = F **E** = T

In healthy tissue, a normal cell divides only to replace a lost one, therefore the total cell number remains constant. In a neoplasm, the normal control mechanisms are lost and cells divide continually, therefore increasing the total cell number. The growth fraction is the ratio of actively dividing cells to resting cells. Due to the loss of the normal ordered and regulated cell cycle in neoplasia the cell cycle time decreases. The cell loss coefficient is the ratio of cells lost to cells produced and is one in normal tissues. In neoplasia the coefficient is <1 as the number of cells lost is less than that produced. Rapid cell cycling in neoplasia results in further division before the cell is fully mature (differentiated).

A1.59 Which of the following associations between a cancer and gene are true:
A breast – BRCA1
B familial adenomatosis polyposis – FAA
C gastric cancer – TP53
D multiple endocrine neoplasia 2 (MEN II) – RET
E papillary renal cell cancer – MET

A1.59 **A** = T **B** = F **C** = F **D** = T **E** = T

Certain cancers result from an inherited abnormal gene. This is important, as individuals at risk of inheriting a gene may benefit from screening. Approximately 15% of breast cancers are inherited. Mutations to two genes – BRCA1 (chromosome 17) and BRCA2 (chromosome 13) – results in familial breast cancer. Transmission is autosomal dominant. Familial adenomatosis polyposis is a rare form of inherited colonic cancer caused by a mutation to the APC gene (chromosome 5). There is an association between diffuse-type gastric cancer (ill-defined with signet ring cells) and the gene CDH1 (chromosome 16). Multiple endocrine neoplasia I (MEN I) causes gastrointestinal endocrine tumours, anterior pituitary tumours and insulinomas and is due to a mutation of the MEN I gene found on chromosome 16. MEN II causes medullary thyroid cancers, parathyroid hyperplasia and phaeochromocytomas and is due to mutations of the RET proto-oncogene found on chromosome 10. Familial renal cell cancers are classified as either papillary on non-papillary. Papillary cancers results from a mutation of the MET proto-oncogene found on chromosome 7. See 3.23 Tumour markers.

A1.60 DNA mutations are:
A heritable
B permanent
C repairable
D silent
E spontaneous

A1.60 **A** = T **B** = T **C** = T **D** = T **E** = T

Mutations are permanent alterations in the base sequence of DNA. Mutations in a viable cell are heritable, i.e. passed on to daughter cells by replication. They result from spontaneous errors in DNA replication or as the result of damaging effects, e.g. radiation. The most common mutation is a point mutation where a single base pair is replaced by another, i.e. a purine for a purine (transition) or a purine for a pyrimidine (transversion). The phenotypes of these changes may be silent (have no affect), missense (i.e. altered amino-acid with a spectrum of effects from none to lethal) or a nonsense (i.e. introduce new stop codons producing truncated proteins). Mutations can affect any part of the cell cycle resulting in abnormal cell growth, cell death and tumorigenesis (cancer forming). Mutations identified by the cell can be repaired by excision (nucleotide or base excision) repair. Disorders of the repair mechanism predisposes to tumorigenesis.

A1.61 The association between the following tumour markers and tumours are recognised:
A α-fetoprotein (AFP) – hepatoma
B CA125 – gastric carcinoma
C CA19-9 – pancreatic carcinoma
D CA15-3 – breast carcinoma
E CA27.29 – bronchial carcinoma

A1.61 **A** = T **B** = F **C** = T **D** = T **E** = F

Tumours produce metabolically active products, which are either tumour-derived or tumour associated, but not necessarily tumour specific. These products are secreted (e.g. blood, urine) in quantities greater than in normal tissues. They can be used to help make the diagnosis but more often, they are used to detect recurrence of a tumour following treatment. AFP is a protein produced in the fetus. In the adult, levels are usually very low, raised levels are associated with non-seminomatous germ cell tumours of the testes and with hepatomas. AFP is also raised to a lesser degree in seminomas of the testis. Other causes of an elevated AFP include germ cell tumours of the ovary, lymphoma, renal cell carcinoma and liver cirrhosis. CA125 has a high degree of sensitivity and specificity for ovarian cancer, although it is not specific enough for diagnosis on its own. Other conditions associated with an elevated CA125 include pancreatitis, pelvic inflammatory disease, liver cirrhosis, ascites, as well as cancers of the female genital tract, pancreas, colon, lung and breast. CA19-9 is primarily used to aid the diagnosis of pancreatic and hepatobiliary cancers. Other conditions associated with an elevated CA19-9 include pancreatitis, biliary calculi, liver cirrhosis, inflammatory bowel disease as well as cancers of the stomach, colon and liver. CA15-3 and CA27.29 are tumour markers used to monitor the response of metastatic breast cancer to treatment.

A1.62 Prerequisites for a tumour to metastasise include:
A angiogenesis
B cell adhesion
C dismantle cell–cell adhesions
D extra-cellular matrix degradation
E motogenesis

A1.62 **A** = T **B** = T **C** = T **D** = T **E** = T

The formation of metastasis is composed of a number of essential steps. The first step is the loss of cell–cell adhesions at the site of the primary tumour. This is followed by the adhesion and the invasion of the tumour through the basement membrane and extra-cellular matrix, entry of the tumour cells into blood stream or lymphatic system, and adhesion to the blood vessel or lymphatic vessel wall to enable the cells to implant in distant tissues. The cancerous cells then require the formation of a new blood supply (angiogenesis) to enable its survival. The process of invasion is controlled by a number of different growth factors such as the hepatocyte growth factor, which help in mitogenesis and motogenesis.

A1.63 The main functions of Cancer Registries are:
A distributing information on palliative care
B evaluation of the impact of treatment
C investigations of links between environmental factors and cancer formation
D monitoring trends in cancer
E organisation and funding screening programmes

A1.63 **A** = F **B** = T **C** = T **D** = T **E** = F

Cancer Registries are responsible for the collection, analysis and dissemination of cancer data. The information recorded must be uniform to enable the accurate analysis of data. These registries have been in place since the 1960s, with the data being submitted to the Office of National Statistics for analysis. Functions of cancer registries include monitoring trends in cancer, evaluation of screening programmes and outcomes of treatments. To achieve these, the registries need to collate data on individual patients from multiple sources over long time periods. Information on individual patients is protected under the data protection legislation.

A1.64 The 5-year survival rates of:
A breast cancer is 86%
B Duke's B colonic cancer is 67%
C Stage I gastric cancer is 22%
D oesophageal cancer is 45%
E prostatic cancer is 41%

A1.64 **A** = F **B** = T **C** = F **D** = F **E** = T

Breast cancer is the most common malignancy affecting women, with approximately 35000 new cases being diagnosed in the UK every year. The incidence of breast cancer is increasing, while the mortality rate is decreasing, with a 5-year standardised survival of 66%. Approximately 28000 new cases of colorectal cancer are diagnosed annually and is the second most common cause of cancer death. After curative resection, the age-adjusted 5-year survival for Duke's A, B and C is 85%, 67% and 37%, respectively. The incidence of gastric adenocarcinoma has a widespread variation around the world. The overall incidence has fallen over the last 50 years in the UK. Following curative resection, the age-adjusted 5-year survival for Stages I–IV is 72%, 32%, 10% and 1%, respectively. As with gastric carcinoma, there is a widespread variation around the world of oesophageal adenocarcinoma. The overall 5-year age-standardised survival is 21% following curative resection. Approximately 21000 new cases of prostate cancer are diagnosed annually. The 5-year age-standardised survival is 41%.

A1.65 NHS screening programmes exist for:
A breast
B cervix
C colon
D oesophagus
E prostate

A1.65 **A** = T **B** = T **C** = T **D** = F **E** = F

Cancer screening aims to identify the disease in the population at an early curable stage to reduce mortality by early treatment. The NHS Breast Screening Programme was introduced in 1988 and is nationally coordinated. Women between the ages of 50 and 70 years are invited to attend for two-view mammography every 3 years. Women in whom abnormalities are detected on mammography are recalled to regional assessments where further investigations are performed. The NHS cervical screening programme invites women between the ages of 25 and 64 for a cervical smear test every 3–5 years. The smear is then assessed for abnormal cytology. A national Bowel Cancer Screening Programme will be phased in from April 2006. Men and women aged 60 and 69 years will be invited to take part in screening every 2 years by means of faecal occult blood test (FOBt). There is no organised NHS screening programme for oesophageal cancer. However, patients with Barrett's oesophagus (columnar lined oesophagus) should undergo surveillance endoscopy approximately every year due to the increased risk of developing oesophageal cancer with this condition. There is presently no NHS screening programme for prostate cancer, although annual prostate specific antigen (PSA) assessment in older men is practiced by many general practitioners.

A1.66 The following statements regarding chemotherapeutic agents are true:

A Cisplatin is used in bladder and lung cancers and the dosage used is dependent upon renal function

B Cyclophosphamide, used to treat haematological malignancies, may cause significant haematuria

C Docetaxel is used in breast cancer and works by linking the alkyl group to chemical groups in proteins and nucleic acids

D Doxorubicin inhibits topoisomerase II and is used in breast cancer chemotherapy

E 5-Fluorouracil blocks DNA synthesis/replication and is used in colorectal cancer

A1.66 **A** = F **B** = T **C** = F **D** = F **E** = T

There are a number of different groups of chemotherapeutic agents with specific mechanisms of action and adverse-effects. In addition, some drugs have very specific side-effects, e.g. cyclophosphamide which can cause life-threatening haemorrhagic cystitis, or cisplatin which can cause irreversible renal damage and deafness. Cisplatin dosage is based on body surface area (as nearly all chemotherapy is), rather than renal function. It requires adequate renal function to be given (GFR >50 ml/min). Alkylating agents (e.g. cyclophosphamide and cisplatin) work by linking the alkyl group to chemical groups in proteins and nucleic acids. Anti-metabolites (e.g. 5-fluorouracil, methotrexate) resemble DNA precursors and block DNA synthesis or replication. Vinca alkaloids (e.g. vincristine, vinblastine) bind to tubulin and inhibit assembly of the mitotic spindle. Taxanes (e.g. paclitaxel, docetaxel) bind to tubulin and stop disassembly of the mitotic spindle. Epipodophyllotoxins (etoposide) inhibit topoisomerase II, camptothecins (Irinotecan, topotecan) inhibit topoisomerase I. Anti-tumour antibiotics have a variety of modes of action, doxorubicin binds to DNA and intercalates between base pairs, epirubicin inhibits topoisomerase II and bleomycin causes single and double stranded DNA breaks.

A1.67 With regard to hormone therapy in prostate cancer:

A adverse effects of hormone treatment are minimal

B chemical castration, in the form of LHRH analogues, causes an initial rise in serum testosterone levels

C oestrogen therapy (oestradiol) is effective at controlling prostate cancer

D prostate cancers do not grow in the absence of testosterone and hormone treatment offers patients a long-term cure

E surgical and chemical castration have similar long-term outcomes in terms of disease control

A1.67 **A** = F **B** = T **C** = T **D** = F **E** = T

Prostatic epithelium and cancer cell growth is stimulated by testosterone, and in the absence of testosterone, the disease is controlled for long periods, but this treatment does not offer a cure. Early hormonal treatment was surgical castration and oestrogen therapy. Oestrogen therapy is effective in controlling disease but has a high incidence of thromboembolic complications. It may be used in combination with aspirin with similar disease control to standard therapies, while the anti-platelet action of aspirin reduces thromboembolic complications. LHRH analogues have an effect equal to surgical castration and are the most commonly used form of hormonal treatment in prostate cancer, as they mimic LHRH released by the hypothalamus. Initial treatment results in a rise in serum testosterone, which may result in a sudden surge in prostatic cancer growth resulting in ureteric obstruction, renal failure and spinal cord compression. These complications are limited now by the administration of anti-androgens such as cyproterone acetate before and after administration of the first dose of an LHRH analogue. Hormonal therapy does have a number of significant adverse-effects including lack of libido, impotence, hot flushes, mood changes, lethargy, loss of bone density and risk of fracture with long-term therapy.

EMQs

Clinical problem solving

QUESTIONS

Cardiothoracic surgery

Q2.1 Haemodynamic control

A Adenosine
B Atropine
C Digoxin
D Dobutamine
E Lidocaine hydrochloride
F Sodium nitroprusside
G Noradrenaline
H Phenylephrine
I Propanolol

For each of the situations below, select the single most likely drug from the list of options above. Each option may be used once, more than once or not at all.

1. *Following administration* there is vasodilatation due to a direct effect on arterial and venous smooth muscle, with no effect on uterine or duodenal smooth muscle or on myocardial contractility. The peripheral resistance is reduced, which has a variable effect on cardiac output.

2. *Following administration* there is an increase in heart rate, dry mouth and relaxation of smooth muscle in the gut, urinary tract and biliary tree.

3. *Following administration* there is a slowing of conduction time through the atrioventricular node.

Answer found on p. 124.

Q2.2 **Surgical disorders of the heart vessels and heart valves**

A Aortic regurgitation
B Aortic stenosis
C Mitral regurgitation
D Mitral stenosis
E Pulmonary regurgitation
F Pulmonary stenosis
G Tricuspid regurgitation
H Tricuspid stenosis

For each of the situations below, select the single most likely heart valve pathology from the list of options above. Each option may be used once, more than once or not at all.

1. A 54-year-old male with known ischaemic heart disease presents with acute onset of dyspnoea. On examination, he has a soft first heart sound, loud second heart sound and a pansystolic murmur. A third heart sound is also heard.

2. A 62-year-old female presents with worsening dyspnoea and angina. On examination, she has a collapsing pulse and prominent carotid arterial pulsations. On auscultation, she has a soft second heart sound and a high-pitched early diastolic murmur heard best at the lower left sternal edge.

3. A 68-year-old male with angina presents with fainting following exertion. On examination, he has a harsh ejection systolic murmur.

Answer found on pp. 124-125.

Q2.3 Cardiopulmonary bypass and cardiac devices

A Axial-flow pump
B Cardioplegia
C Cardiopulmonary bypass
D Extracorporeal membrane oxygenation
E Intra-aortic balloon pump
F Pulsatile intracorporeal pump

For each of the situations below, select the single most likely cardiac device from the list of options above. Each option may be used once, more than once or not at all.

1. A 62-year-old male with severe angina pectoris is undergoing a coronary artery bypass grafting for 3-vessel disease.

2. A 58-year-old male is undergoing a combined aortic valve replacement and coronary artery bypass graft. The surgeon places the patient on cardiopulmonary bypass, cross clamps the aorta and injects a cold crystalloid solution into the aortic root.

3. A 56-year-old male has been admitted to the intensive care unit following a large myocardial infarction, which resulted in papillary muscle rupture. He has developed severe heart failure with an ejection fraction of 20%. He is on a maximal dose of inotropes and is awaiting coronary artery bypass grafting and mitral valve replacement.

Q2.4 **Pathophysiology of thoracic trauma**
- **A** Cardiac tamponade
- **B** Diaphragmatic rupture
- **C** Flail chest
- **D** Massive haemothorax
- **E** Myocardial contusion
- **F** Oesophageal rupture
- **G** Open pneumothorax
- **H** Pulmonary contusion
- **I** Ruptured aorta
- **J** Tension pneumothorax

For each of the situations below, select the single most likely diagnosis from the list of options above. Each option may be used once, more than once or not at all.

1. A 32-year-old male presents with an acute shortness of breath after falling from a first floor window. On examination, he has reduced breath sounds on the right side. The trachea deviates to the left.

2. A 42-year-old male presents with shortness of breath 6 hours following a motorcycle accident in which he was ejected from the motorcycle. On examination, there are reduced breath sounds on the right. There is no tracheal deviation.

3. A 27-year-old male presents with increasing shortness of breath. On examination, there are reduced breath sounds on the left. Chest radiograph reveals an abnormal gas pattern on the left chest.

Answer found on pp. 126-128.   **61**

Q2.5 **Thoracotomy**

A Axillary
B Bilateral trans-sternal anterior
C Left anterolateral
D Left posterolateral
E Median sternotomy
F Right anterolateral
G Right posterolateral
H Transverse thoracosternotomy
I Trap door

For each of the situations below, select the single most likely approach from the list of options above. Each option may be used once, more than once or not at all.

1. A 67-year-old female undergoing an elective mitral valve replacement.

2. A 63-year-old male undergoing an elective right upper lobectomy for a localised squamous cell carcinoma of the lung.

3. A 28-year-old male with cystic fibrosis undergoing an elective heart–lung transplant for end-stage disease.

Answer found on p. 128.

Q2.6   **Surgical disorders of the lung**
A   Bronchiectasis
B   Carcinoma of the lung
C   Congenital bronchogenic cysts
D   Hamartoma
E   Lung abscess
F   Lung hydatid
G   Lung trauma
H   Pulmonary embolism
I   Pulmonary metastases
J   Tuberculosis

For each of the situations below, select the single most likely diagnosis from the list of options above. Each option may be used once, more than once or not at all.

1. A 29-year-old female presents with left chest pain, cough and dyspnoea. On examination, she is anxious and tachycardic, there is a left pleural rub on auscultation.

2. The chest radiograph of a 51-year-old female reveals bilateral cystic changes with 'tram-line' shadows. She has suffered repeat severe chest infections since childhood. Recently she has developed haemoptysis.

3. A 55-year-old male presents with a 2 month history of a bovine cough and intermittent haemoptysis. On examination, he is noted to have lost weight and has finger clubbing. Chest radiograph reveals a collapse of the left lower lobe.

Q2.7   Complications of thoracic operations

A Chylothorax
B Consolidation
C Diaphragmatic paresis
D Empyema
E Haemothorax
F Mediastinitis
G Pleural effusion
H Pneumothorax

For each of the situations below, select the single most likely complications from the list of options above. Each option may be used once, more than once or not at all.

1. A 68-year-old male undergoes insertion of a central venous cannula to provide parenteral nutrition. Shortly after the procedure he becomes increasingly tachycardic, tachypnoeic and hypotensive but with only minimal respiratory distress.

2. A 71-year-old female is 1 week post-mitral valve replacement. She is pyrexial and complains of rigors. The chest radiograph reveals a widening of the mediastinum, with a fluid level seen in the posterior mediastinum.

3. A 58-year-old male has undergone a two stage Ivor–Lewis oeso-phagectomy. Postoperatively he has a persistent white fluid discharge from the chest drain.

Answer found on pp. 129-130.

Q2.8 **Thoracic procedures**
 A Chest drain
 B Fibrinolysis
 C Guided needle aspiration
 D Pleurodesis
 E Thoracoplasty
 F Thoracoscopy
 G Thoracotomy

For each of the situations below, select the single most likely procedure from the list of options above. Each option may be used once, more than once or not at all.

1. A 24-year-old male who has previously been fit and well presents with a 1-day history of breathlessness. On examination, he is mildly tachypnoeic with decreased breath sounds and hyper-resonance on the right side. The trachea is central.

2. A 28-year-old female with cystic fibrosis has developed an empyema, which has failed to resolve with antibiotics and guided needle aspiration. Chest radiograph reveals a multiloculated empyema.

3. A 65-year-old male presents with symptoms of malignant pleural effusions secondary to breast cancer.

Answer found on pp. 131-132.

General surgery

Q2.9 Causes of abdominal pain

A Acute appendicitis
B Biliary disease
C Colonic diverticular disease
D Intestinal obstruction
E Mesenteric ischaemia
F Non-specific abdominal pain
G Pancreatitis
H Perforated peptic ulcer
I Ruptured abdominal aortic aneurysm
J Urinary tract infection

For each of the situations below, select the single most likely diagnosis from the list of options above. Each option may be used once, more than once or not at all.

1. A 36-year-old male presents with epigastric and right upper quadrant pain radiating through to his back. The pain was preceded by a heavy meal. On examination, he has epigastric and right upper quadrant tenderness with no signs of peritoneal irritation. All blood variables are within normal limits.

2. A 36-year-old male presents with an acute onset of severe upper abdominal pain. He admits to drinking excessive amounts of alcohol and is taking non-steroidal anti-inflammatory drugs for a recent ankle fracture. On examination, he is exquisitely tender all over the abdomen, with abdominal wall rigidity.

3. A 36-year-old male presents with an increasingly severe epigastric and central abdominal pain radiating through to his back. He also complains of vomiting and retching. He admits to drinking excessive amounts of alcohol and has experienced similar less severe pain in the past. On examination, the upper abdomen is tender with no signs of peritoneal irritation.

Q2.10 Abdominal masses

A Acute urinary retention
B Abdominal aortic aneurysm
C Appendix mass
D Colonic diverticular mass
E Colonic malignancy
F Empyema of gallbladder
G Gravid uterus
H Ovarian cyst
I Pancreatic pseudocyst

For each of the situations below, select the single most likely diagnosis from the list of options above. Each option may be used once, more than once or not at all.

1. A 72-year-old female presents to the accident and emergency department with lower abdominal pain. She denies any weight loss or change in bowel habit. On examination, she has a temperature of 37.8°C and has a tender immobile mass in the left iliac fossa.

2. A 76-year-old male presents to his general practitioner with increasing urinary frequency and nocturia. On examination, he is obese with nicotine staining of his right index and middle fingers. Abdominal examination reveals a pulsatile mass in the central abdomen.

3. A 69-year-old female presents to her general practitioner with tiredness, she denies weight loss or change in bowel habit. On examination, she appears pale and thin, abdominal examination reveals a mass in the right iliac fossa.

Answer found on pp. 133-134.

Q2.11 The acute abdomen

A Acute appendicitis
B Acute colonic diverticulitis
C Crohn's disease
D Malignant large bowel obstruction
E Pyelonephritis
F Ruptured ectopic pregnancy
G Salpingitis
H Sigmoid volvulus
I Ulcerative colitis

For each of the situations below, select the single most likely diagnosis from the list of options above. Each option may be used once, more than once or not at all.

1. A 23-year-old female presents to the accident and emergency department with supra-pubic and right iliac fossa pain. Initially the pain was colicky in nature and is now constant. She reports fainting at home and is presently menstruating. On examination, she is tachycardic and has signs of peritoneal irritation in the supra-pubic and right iliac fossa.

2. A 23-year-old female presents to the accident and emergency department with a 24 hour history of right iliac fossa pain. She complains of nausea having vomited earlier, she does not report diarrhoea. On examination, she has a temperature of 37.5°C with focal peritoneal irritation in the right iliac fossa. Percussion tenderness is also elicited in the right iliac fossa.

3. A 23-year-old female presents to the accident and emergency department with a 1-week history of worsening lower abdominal pain and profuse watery diarrhoea. She has experienced three similar episodes to this in the last year and has lost 10 kg in weight. On examination, she has a temperature of 37.4°C, abdominal examination reveals a tender mass in the right iliac fossa. There are no signs of peritoneal irritation. Blood analysis reveals an elevated white cell count, platelet count, alkaline phosphatase and eosinophil sedimentation rate.

Q2.12 Intestinal obstruction

A Acute colonic pseudo-obstruction
B Adhesional small bowel obstruction
C Colonic carcinoma
D Crohn's disease
E Gallstone ileus
F Incisional hernia
G Lymphoma
H Radiation enteritis
I Sigmoid volvulus

For each of the situations below, select the single most likely diagnosis from the list of options above. Each option may be used once, more than once or not at all.

1. A 46-year-old female has presented on the surgical take with central abdominal colicky pain and vomiting. A subtotal colectomy and formation of an end ileostomy for ulcerative colitis had been performed previously. Her ileostomy has not functioned for 2 days. On examination, she is tender in the upper abdomen, but with minimal abdominal distension. There are a number of small loops on the plain abdominal radiograph.

2. A 62-year-old male presents on the surgical take with generalised abdominal pain and distension. He reports increasing constipation over the previous 2 months with occasional fresh blood mixed with the stool. On examination, he has no abdominal scars with moderate distension. He is also tender in the right iliac fossa with no signs of peritoneal irritation. The colon is markedly dilated on the plain abdominal radiograph with no small bowel loops seen.

3. A 79-year-old female presents on the surgical take with increasing abdominal distension. This episode of distension was preceded by right upper abdominal pain for approximately 1 week. On examination, she has a markedly distended abdomen that is soft and non-tender. There are multiple loops of small bowel on the plain abdominal radiograph, with an abnormal gas marking in the right upper quadrant.

Answer found on p. 135. **69**

Q2.13 Abdominal and pelvic abscess

A Anastomotic dehiscence
B Crohn's disease
C Pancreatitis
D Pelvic abscess
E Perforated duodenal ulcer
F Perforated sigmoid diverticular disease
G Pyonephrosis
H Pyosalpingitis
I Subphrenic abscess

For each of the situations below, select the single most likely diagnosis from the list of options above. Each option may be used once, more than once or not at all.

1. A 42-year-old female is re-admitted to the surgical ward 8 days after a laparoscopic cholecystectomy. She complains of hiccoughs, nausea, sweats and rigors over the 3 days prior to admission. On examination, she is pale and sweating with a temperature of 38.1°C, examination of her abdomen is unremarkable. Her white cell count is 19×10^9/L and there is a right pleural effusion on the chest radiograph.

2. A 62-year-old male is 6 days post anterior resection for a Dukes' C1 adenocarcinoma of the rectum. He complains of diarrhoea and 'flu-like symptoms'. He has a persistent low-grade pyrexia. Examination reveals mild tenderness in the lower abdomen.

3. A 12-year-old female is 4 days post-open appendicectomy. At the time of operation the appendix had perforated, the surgeon performed a thorough peritoneal lavage and prescribed a 5-day course of intravenous antibiotics. She has had a swinging pyrexia since the surgery. On examination, the wound appears healthy with no fluctuation to suggest suppuration, with only minimal tenderness in the lower abdomen. Rectal examination reveals a soft boggy mass laterally.

Answer found on pp. 135-136.

Q2.14 Gastrointestinal haemorrhage

A Aorto-enteric fistula
B Barrett's ulcer
C Crohn's disease
D Diverticular disease
E Meckel's diverticulum
F Oesophageal varices
G Oesophagitis
H Peptic ulcer
I Tumour of the small bowel
J Vascular malformation

For each of the situations below, select the single most likely diagnosis from the list of options above. Each option may be used once, more than once or not at all.

1. A 73-year-old male presents with acute onset of fresh rectal bleeding. He suffers with intermittent constipation and has recently undergone a colonoscopy, which revealed moderate sigmoid diverticular disease, with an otherwise normal colonic mucosa. On examination, he is pale with a pulse of 100 bpm, abdominal examination reveals a soft non-tender abdomen. Altered blood is noted on rectal examination.

2. A 43-year-old male presents with haematemesis and the passage of a moderate amount of melaena. He denies excessive alcohol and was recently prescribed diclofenac for a knee injury. On examination, he is pale and tachycardic and normotensive, he has upper abdominal tenderness with no signs of peritoneal irritation. Rectal examination confirms melaena.

3. A 29-year-old male is admitted with frank haematemesis. He admits to drinking in excess of 80 units of alcohol a week for the previous 12 months. On examination, he is pale, tachycardic and hypotensive. Abdominal examination reveals a distended non-tender abdomen with prominent periumbilical blood vessels.

Answer found on pp. 136-137.

Q2.15 Groin hernia repair

A Darn repair
B Herniotomy
C High approach
D Laparoscopic transabdominal preperitoneal prosthetic repair
E Low approach
F Shouldice repair
G Tension-free prosthetic mesh repair
H Trans-inguinal approach

For each of the situations below, select the single most suitable procedure from the list of options above. Each option may be used once, more than once or not at all.

1. A 32-year-old male builder presents with a right groin lump which appears when lifting heavy weights and which disappears on lying down. The lump when present causes discomfort. On examination, a reducible lump is palpable in the right groin when the patient strains and returns in an upward and lateral direction on relaxing. Control is achieved over the mid-inguinal point.

2. A 71-year-old female presents with a 2-day history of vomiting and colicky mild abdominal pain. On examination, she has a moderately distended abdomen with a hard tender palpable lump below and lateral to the pubic tubercle. There are multiple small bowel loops on the plain abdominal radiograph.

3. A 3-month-old infant male presents to the paediatric surgical clinic with a history of a left groin lump that appears when he cries. On examination, when the child cries an obvious bulge is seen at the site of the external inguinal ring, both testes are noted to be lying normally in the scrotum.

Answer found on pp. 137-138.

Q2.16 Intestinal fistulas

A Aorto-enteric
B Colocutaneous
C Enterocutaneous
D Enterocolic
E Enteroperineal
F Pancreatic
G Recto-vaginal
H Vesicocolic

For each of the situations below, select the single most likely diagnosis from the list of options above. Each option may be used once, more than once or not at all.

1. A 68-year-old male presents to the urology outpatients clinic. He reports urinary frequency and burning, and on further questioning he also reports passing debris and bubbles in his urine.

2. A 47-year-old female is 8 days post emergency para-umbilical hernia repair. At the time of surgery, strangulated small bowel was resected and anastomosed end-to-end. Postoperatively she has had a swinging pyrexia and developed a wound infection. Now offensive effluent is discharging from the wound.

3. A 22-year-old female presents with a 3-week history of worsening diarrhoea. She reports being unwell for the preceding 3 months, having lost approximately 10 kg in weight.

Answer found on pp. 138-139.

Q2.17 Gastrointestinal stomas

A Caecostomy
B Jejunostomy
C Loop ileostomy
D Mucous fistula
E End colostomy
F Percutaneous endoscopic gastrostomy
G End ileostomy

For each of the situations below, select the single most likely diagnosis from the list of options above. Each option may be used once, more than once or not at all.

1. The distal end of the sigmoid colon is taken out on to the skin at laparotomy.

2. A proximal stoma is formed to protect a low rectal anastomosis following anterior resection for rectal carcinoma.

3. A 73-year-old male has suffered a debilitating stroke resulting in marked dysphagia and right hemiplegia. He requires access for long-term enteral nutrition.

Q2.18 Oesophageal disorders

A Achalasia
B Gastro-oesophageal reflux disease
C Oesophageal carcinoma
D Oesophageal diverticulum
E Oesophageal foreign body

For each of the situations below, select the single most likely condition from the list of options above. Each option may be used once, more than once or not at all.

1. A 52-year-old male presents with retrosternal chest pain. He also reports worsening heartburn especially on bending or lying flat. Electrocardiogram and cardiac enzymes are considered normal.

2. A 45-year-old male presents with worsening dysphagia and is now unable to swallow solids or liquids. He also reports regurgitating food when lying flat. There is an air-fluid level in the thorax and an absence of the gastric air bubble on the plain chest radiograph.

3. A 68-year-old female presents to the surgical outpatients clinic complaining of increasing dysphagia. She also reports a weight loss of 5 kg in 3 months.

Answer found on pp. 140-141.

Q2.19 Carcinoma of the stomach

A Billroth-I gastrectomy
B Distal gastrectomy and gastrojejunostomy
C Gastroenteric bypass
D Oesophagogastrectomy
E Total gastrectomy and lymphadenectomy

For each of the situations below, select the single most likely procedure from the list of options above. Each option may be used once, more than once or not at all.

1. A 62-year-old male presents with upper abdominal discomfort and a 5 kg weight loss over the prior 3 months. At gastroscopy, a 10 cm pedunculated lesion on the greater curve is biopsied, histology confirmed the lesion to be an adenocarcinoma. A CT scan of the thorax and abdomen shows no signs of local or regional spread.

2. A 68-year-old male presents with increasing dysphagia and weight loss. At gastroscopy a 2 cm ulcer is biopsied. Histology confirmed an adenocarcinoma. A CT scan of the thorax and abdomen shows no signs of local or regional spread. A diagnostic laparoscopy showed no evidence of serosal disease.

3. An 88-year-old female presents with a 1-week history of vomiting. She reports a 10 kg weight loss over the prior 6 months. On examination, she is pale and frail. Abdominal examination reveals a non-tender moderately distended upper abdomen. A succussion splash is present.

Answer found on pp. 141-142.

Q2.20 Jaundice

A Disturbed bilirubin excretion
B Disturbed bilirubin uptake
C Increased bilirubin conjugation
D Increased bilirubin load

For each of the situations below, select the single most likely diagnosis from the list of options above. Each option may be used once, more than once or not at all.

1. A 72-year-old female has received an incompatible blood transfusion; initially she developed a pyrexia and tachycardia, which settled soon after stopping the transfusion but now she has developed mild jaundice.

2. A 42-year-old male presents with increasing jaundice. He reports drinking in excess of 80 units of alcohol per week for a prolonged period. On examination, he has moderate ascites.

3. A 53-year-old female presents with an exacerbation of right upper quadrant pain. She is known to suffer with biliary calculi and is awaiting cholecystectomy. On examination, she is moderately jaundiced, with abdominal examination revealing tenderness in the right upper quadrant.

Q2.21 Acute pancreatitis

A Glasgow–Imrie score = 0
B Glasgow–Imrie score = 1
C Glasgow–Imrie score = 2
D Glasgow–Imrie score = 3
E Glasgow–Imrie score = 4

For each of the situations below, select the single most likely score from the list of options above. Each option may be used once, more than once or not at all.

1. A 24-year-old female is admitted with acute onset of upper abdominal pain radiating through to her back. She normally drinks alcohol in moderation but admits to a recent binge. On examination, she is tender across the upper abdomen with no signs of peritoneal irritation. Her serum amylase is 2034 U/litre, white blood cell count 10×10^9/litre, glucose 8 mmol/litre, urea 9.6 mmol/litre, PaO_2 15.6 kPa Hg, calcium 2.27 mmol/litre, albumin 45 g/litre, lactate dehydrogenase 320 U/litre, aspartate aminotransferase 81 U/litre.

2. A 48-year-old female has undergone an elective endoscopic retrograde cholangiopancreatography to remove a common bile duct calculus. The procedure was difficult. Following the procedure, she developed upper abdominal pain. Blood tests obtained at 6 hours following the procedure showed a serum amylase of 1540 U/litre, white blood cell count 17×10^9/litre, glucose 16 mmol/litre, urea 2.5 mmol/litre, PaO_2 9.0 kPa, calcium 2.36 mmol/litre, albumin 33 g/litre, lactate dehydrogenase 470 U/litre, aspartate aminotransferase 60 U/litre.

3. A 65-year-old female is admitted to the Emergency department following a collapse. She complained of a 2-day history of upper abdominal pain and is known to have biliary calculi. On examination, she is distressed and pale with tachycardia and hypotension; abdominal examination reveals upper abdominal tenderness with no signs of peritoneal irritation. 15 ml of residual urine are obtained on catheterisation. Blood tests on admission were as follows: serum amylase 1722 U/litre, white blood cell count 21×10^9/litre, glucose 8 mmol/litre, urea 14 mmol/litre, PaO_2 7.1 kPa, calcium 2.21 mmol/litre, albumin 37 g/litre, lactate dehydrogenase 580 U/litre, aspartate aminotransferase 94 U/litre.

Q2.22 Chronic pancreatitis

A Ascites
B Common bile duct obstruction
C Duodenal obstruction
D Endocrine insufficiency
E Exocrine insufficiency
F Pancreatic adenocarcinoma
G Pancreatic pseudocyst
H Splenic venous thrombosis

For each of the situations below, select the single most likely diagnosis from the list of options above. Each option may be used once, more than once or not at all.

1. A 42-year-old male presents to the surgical outpatients clinic complaining of an exacerbation of upper abdominal pain radiating through to his back. He has had multiple admissions to hospital with alcohol-induced, acute pancreatitis. He also reports weight loss of approximately 5 kg, despite having a good appetite and bulky, frothy, loose stools. On examination, his abdomen is soft with no palpable masses.

2. A 38-year-old male with known chronic pancreatitis was recently admitted to hospital with an episode of acute pancreatitis. The episode was slow to resolve with episodes of hyperamylasaemia following the initial episode. On examination, he has a non-tender fullness in the upper/central abdomen.

3. A 45-year-old male with known chronic pancreatitis presents with a 1-week history of vomiting after every meal. On examination, he is pale but not jaundiced, with tenderness in the upper abdomen but with no signs of peritoneal irritation. He has an obvious succussion splash.

Q2.23 Diseases of the biliary tract

A Adenomyomatosis
B Biliary atresia
C Carcinoma of the head of the pancreas
D Cholangiocarcinoma
E Choledochal cyst
F Iatrogenic
G Mirizzi syndrome
H Sclerosing cholangitis
I Solitary benign tumour

For each of the situations below, select the single most likely diagnosis from the list of options above. Each option may be used once, more than once or not at all.

1. A 59-year-old female presents with a 2-day history of acute abdominal pain. She also complains of pale stools and dark urine and is clinically jaundiced. On abdominal examination, she is tender in the right upper quadrant with no palpable masses. An ultrasound confirms a dilated proximal common bile duct with intrahepatic duct dilatation. A MR cholangiopancreatogram confirms a fistula between the gallbladder and the common bile duct with large calculi present in the common bile duct just distal to the fistula.

2. A 38-year-old female attends the Emergency unit 7 days following a laparoscopic cholecystectomy. She complains of right upper quadrant pain and is clinically jaundiced.

3. A 73-year-old female has presented with progressive painless jaundice. There is proximal common bile duct dilatation on the ultrasound scan. On examination, she is pale with obvious signs of weight loss, abdominal examination reveals moderate ascites. A MR cholangiopancreatogram confirms an irregular stenosing lesion in the mid common bile duct.

Q2.24 Portal hypertension and ascites

A Chylous ascites
B Extrahepatic portal hypertension
C Exudative ascites
D Increased flow portal hypertension
E Intrahepatic portal hypertension
F Portal vein thrombosis
G Transudative ascites

For each of the situations below, select the single most likely diagnosis from the list of options above. Each option may be used once, more than once or not at all.

1. A 44-year-old male presents with an episode of haematemesis with the bleeding stopping spontaneously. He admits to drinking in excess of 60 units of alcohol per week. On examination, he has a pulse of 72 bpm and is normotensive, examination of his abdomen reveals several spider naevi and a caput medusae; on palpation there is a large spleen and a small nodular liver.

2. An 8-year-old male presents with haematemesis. He was born at 28 weeks' gestation and developed necrotising enterocolitis and underwent a laparotomy and small bowel resection at 10 days and venous access was achieved by catheterisation of the umbilical vein. On examination, he is pale and has an enlarged spleen. Liver function tests are within normal limits. Oesophagoscopy confirms oesophageal varices.

3. A 35-year-old male with known alcohol liver cirrhosis presents to the clinic with worsening abdominal distension. On examination, he is jaundiced with multiple spider naevi, abdominal examination reveals a tensely distended abdomen, tightly stretched skin, bulging flanks and an everted umbilicus.

Answer found on pp. 145-146.

Q2.25 Surgical disorders of the colon and rectum

A Extended right hemicolectomy
B Left hemicolectomy
C Sigmoid colectomy
D Subtotal colectomy
E Total colectomy
F Total mesorectal excision
G Transverse colectomy

For each of the situations below, select the single most likely operation from the list of options above. Each option may be used once, more than once or not at all.

1. A 72-year-old male undergoes resection of a hepatic flexure tumour.
2. A 52-year-old female undergoes surgical resection of a sigmoid tumour.
3. A 62-year-old female undergoes surgical resection of a mid-rectal tumour, which has advanced through the bowel wall on MR imaging.

Answer found on pp. 146-147.

Q2.26 Perianal disorders

A Anal carcinoma
B Anal fissure
C Anal fistula
D Coccydynia
E Haemorrhoids
F Hydradenitis suppurativa
G Inflammatory bowel disease
H Proctalgia fugax
I Proctitis

For each of the situations below, select the single most likely diagnosis from the list of options above. Each option may be used once, more than once or not at all.

1. A 35-year-old male presents to the surgical clinic complaining of passing fresh blood at stool. He also complains of perianal itching, occasional faecal soiling and an intermittent perianal swelling. Examination reveals prominent anal skin tags with fresh blood noted on the finger.

2. A 23-year-old female presents to the surgical clinic complaining of pain on defecation, with a burning sensation persisting for several hours following evacuation, with fresh blood on wiping. She is 6 months post-partum. On examination, there is a prominent skin tag at the '12 o'clock position'; she is unable to tolerate a digital examination.

3. A 38-year-old male presents to the surgical clinic complaining of persistent anal bleeding. He admits to being homosexual and frequent anoreceptive intercourse. Inguinal lymphadenopathy is palpable on abdominal examination. Anal digital examination is painful with an ulcer apparent just distal to the anal verge.

Answer found on pp. 147-148.

Q2.27 Common breast disorders

A Carcinoma
B Cystosarcoma phyllodes
C Duct ectasia
D Fibroadenoma
E Fibrocystic disease
F Mondor's disease
G Paget's disease

For each of the situations below, select the single most likely diagnosis from the list of options above. Each option may be used once, more than once or not at all.

1. A 47-year-old female is referred to the rapid access breast clinic with a lump, which she has recently noted in her right breast. There is no family history of breast cancer. On examination, there is a 3 cm smooth edged, mobile lump in the right upper quadrant. There is no palpable axillary lymphadenopathy.

2. A 24-year-old female is referred to the rapid access breast clinic with a lump in her left breast, which she has recently noticed. Her paternal aunt died aged 56 years from breast cancer. On examination, there is a 2 cm firm mobile, smooth lump in the left inner quadrant. There is no palpable axillary lymphadenopathy.

3. A 56-year-old female is referred to the rapid access breast clinic with a recently noticed right breast lump. There is no family history of breast cancer. On examination, there is a 3 cm irregular fixed lump in the upper outer quadrant of the right breast. There are fixed palpable axillary lymph nodes in the right axilla.

Answer found on pp. 148-149.

Q2.28 Surgery of the thyroid gland

A Isthmusectomy
B Selective nodal dissection
C Subtotal thyroidectomy
D Total thyroidectomy
E Thyroid lobectomy

For each of the situations below, select the single most likely procedure from the list of options above. Each option may be used once, more than once or not at all.

1. A 38-year-old male presents with a palpable lump in the right neck. On examination, there is a solitary nodule in the right lobe of the thyroid gland, no lymph nodes are palpable. Fine needle aspiration cytology and ultrasound scanning confirm this nodule to a solitary 1 cm papillary cancer.

2. A 72-year-old male presents with stridor. On examination, he is frail and has a hard fixed irregular thyroid. Ultrasonography and cytology confirm an anaplastic carcinoma.

3. A 36-year-old female presents with an exacerbation of her Graves' disease. She has previously been treated with carbimazole, which rendered her euthyroid for a short period of time. On examination, she is thyrotoxic and has a moderate-sized, smooth thyroid.

Answer found on pp. 149-150.

Q2.29 Parathyroid disorders

A Multiple Endocrine Neoplasia I
B Multiple Endocrine Neoplasia IIa
C Multiple Endocrine Neoplasia IIb
D Parathyroid carcinoma
E Primary hyperparathyroidism
F Secondary hyperparathyroidism
G Tertiary hyperparathyroidism

For each of the situations below, select the single most likely diagnosis from the list of options above. Each option may be used once, more than once or not at all.

1. A 53-year-old female presents with an acute onset of colicky right loin pain. She also complains of increasing fatigue, constipation and weight loss. An intravenous urogram confirms a ureteric calculus. Her corrected serum calcium is 2.99 mmol/litre with a parathyroid hormone (PTH) level of 82 ng/litre.

2. A 22-year-old male presents with increasing abdominal pain, constipation and weight loss, despite a good appetite. He is found to have a corrected serum calcium of 3.14 mmol/litre and a PTH of 87 ng/litre. Radiological imaging confirms pituitary hyperplasia. He is subsequently found to have a pancreatic islet cell tumour and a pituitary adenoma.

3. A 32-year-old female presents with sweating, headache and is found to be hypertensive. Twenty-four hour urinary catecholamines, metanephrines and vanillylmandelic acid are elevated. A CT and a ^{131}I-meta-iodo-benzyl-guanidine scan confirms a phaeochromocytoma. She is subsequently found to have a medullary thyroid carcinoma.

Q2.30 Adrenal disorders and secondary hypertension

A Adrenocortical adenoma
B Adrenocortical hyperfunction
C Congenital adrenal hyperplasia
D Congenital hypoplasia
E Incidentalomas
F Phaeochromocytoma
G Primary adrenal insufficiency
H Primary aldosteronism
I Secondary adrenal insufficiency

For each of the situations below, select the single most likely diagnosis from the list of options above. Each option may be used once, more than once or not at all.

1. A 49-year-old female presents complaining of progressive muscular weakness, acne and facial hair. On examination, she has thin skin with multiple purpura, abdominal striae and truncal obesity. Her 24-h urinary free cortisol is raised.

2. A 53-year-old male presents with muscle cramps and weakness, he also reports polydipsia and polyuria. On examination, he is hypertensive. Blood biochemistry shows a potassium of 2.7 mmol/litre and sodium of 149 mmol/litre.

3. A 38-year-old female presents with episodic attacks of tremor, palpitations and chest pain, with associated facial pallor lasting for approximately 30 min. She is found to be hypertensive. Twenty-four hour urinary catecholamines, metanephrines and vanillylmandelic acid are elevated.

Answer found on pp. 151-152.

Q2.31 Endocrine disorders of the pancreas

A ACTH secreting
B Carcinoid
C Gastrinoma
D Glucagonoma
E Insulinoma
F Non-functioning islet cell tumour
G Somatostatinoma
H Vasoactive intestinal peptide tumour

For each of the situations below, select the single most likely diagnosis from the list of options above. Each option may be used once, more than once or not at all.

1. A 42-year-old female presents following a seizure. She reports recent morning episodes of visual disturbances, confusion, lethargy and weakness, with the episodes followed by sweating, anxiety and palpitations. Eating appears to improve the symptoms.

2. A 29-year-old male presents with increasing coffee ground vomits, upper abdominal pain, dysphagia and diarrhoea. Upper gastrointestinal endoscopy confirms multiple ulcers in the stomach and duodenum.

3. A 52-year-old female presents with weight loss, muscle wasting and cachexia. She has recently been diagnosed with type II diabetes. On examination, she has a raised, red, itchy rash on the lower limbs, groins and perioral area.

Q2.32 Arterial surgery

A Aortobifemoral bypass
B Aorto-iliac
C Axillobifemoral bypass
D Disobliteration
E Embolectomy
F Endoluminal aortic stent
G Endarterectomy
H Femoro-distal bypass graft
I Femoro-femoral bypass
J Femoro-popliteal bypass

For each of the situations below, select the single most likely procedure from the list of options above. Each option may be used once, more than once or not at all.

1. A 62-year-old male presents to the vascular clinic complaining of short distance intermittent claudication of <50m. The pain is confined to his left calf. His left ankle-brachial pressure index is 0.62. A duplex and arteriogram confirm a 12cm occlusion of the left superficial femoral artery with good run-off.

2. An 82-year-old female presents with an acutely cold, painful right leg. On examination, she has an irregularly-irregular pulse. The right lower limb appears marble white with no mottling and no pulses palpable. She is unable to dorsi- or plantar flex her right foot.

3. A 74-year-old male with moderate chronic obstructive pulmonary disease presents with left buttock and thigh claudication which prevents him walking more than 100m. On examination, the left femoral pulse is absent. An arteriogram confirms a 5cm occlusion of the left common iliac and a disease-free right common iliac artery. The aorta, both external iliac arteries and femoral arteries are also disease free.

Answer found on pp. 153-154. **89**

Q2.33 Venous disorders of the lower limb

A Abnormal calf vein pump
B Deep venous occlusion
C Long saphenous vein reflux
D Perforator vein reflux
E Post-thrombotic syndrome
F Primary deep venous incompetence
G Short saphenous vein reflux

For each of the situations below, select the single most likely diagnosis from the list of options above. Each option may be used once, more than once or not at all.

1. A 37-year-old female presents with unsightly bilateral lower leg varicosities. On examination, a prograde and retrograde signal with a hand-held Doppler is heard on squeezing and releasing the calf muscle, the signal is abolished by mid-thigh compression.

2. A 63-year-old female presents with a pale, swollen and painful left leg. On examination, distal pulses are palpable but the limb is very painful throughout. She has recently been diagnosed with disseminated colonic cancer.

3. A 67-year-old female has presented with an ulcer over the medial aspect of the right lower leg. She also reports pain and heaviness in the leg with swelling, which is aggravated by standing or walking. On examination, the ulcer is classically venous with hyperpigmentation of the surrounding skin and lipodermatosclerosis.

Answer found on p. 155.

Q2.34 Swollen limb

A Deep vein thrombosis
B Elephantiasis
C Klippel–Trenaunay syndrome
D Lymphoedema artefacta
E Lymphoedema praecox
F Lymphoedema tarda
G Milroy's disease
H Pedal oedema
I Post radiotherapy

For each of the situations below, select the single most likely diagnosis from the list of options above. Each option may be used once, more than once or not at all.

1. A 72-year-old male presents with a short history of increasing bilateral swelling of the lower limbs. On examination, the oedema is pitting.

2. A 17-year-old female presents with a slowly progressive, non-painful swelling of the right lower limb. The swelling was initially distal and has now progressed proximally and becomes exacerbated by prolonged standing. On examination, the swelling is non-pitting and the skin has a 'peau d'orange appearance'. The deep leg veins are patent on duplex scanning.

3. A 56-year-old male presents to the clinic with a swollen right lower limb 1 year following a resection of a right thigh soft tissue sarcoma. The deep leg veins are patent on duplex scanning.

Answer found on p. 156.

Q2.35 Renal transplantation complications

A Accelerated rejection
B Acute rejection
C Acute tubular necrosis
D Chronic rejection
E Hyperacute rejection
F Renal artery stenosis
G Renal vein thrombosis
H Ureteric obstruction
I Urine leak

For each of the situations below, select the single most likely diagnosis from the list of options above. Each option may be used once, more than once or not at all.

1. A 38-year-old male underwent a cadaveric renal transplantation. There was a delay of 24 hours from removal from the donor to implantation. Following anastomosis, no urine was produced. The patient was supported with dialysis and produced a urine diuresis on the third postoperative day.

2. A 47-year-old female underwent a living related donor renal transplantation. Following implantation, she produced good volumes of urine. On the third postoperative day, she developed anuria and an acute rise in serum creatinine. On examination, she is acutely tender over the graft.

3. A 55-year-old male underwent a re-graft cadaveric renal transplant. Initially the graft produced urine but within 12 hours, this has ceased.

Answer found on p. 157.

Otorhinolaryngology, head and neck surgery

Q2.36 Ear, nose and throat disorders

A Acute otitis media
B Acute tonsillitis
C Infectious rhinosinusitis
D Laryngotracheobronchitis
E Mastoiditis
F Peritonsillar abscess
G Pharyngeal pouch
H Pharyngeal web
I Sialadenitis

For each of the situations below, select the single most likely diagnosis from the list of options above. Each option may be used once, more than once or not at all.

1. A 5-year-old male presents with blood and purulent discharge from his right ear. He has recently suffered from an upper respiratory viral infection, generalised malaise, pyrexia and gastrointestinal upset.

2. A 72-year-old male presents with dysphagia localised to the cervical region and regurgitation of food. He also complains of recurrent chest infections and weight loss. On examination, a soft mass is palpable in the right anterior triangle of the neck.

3. A 12-year-old female presents with increasing throat pain and excessive salivation. Her speech is thick and muffled. On oral examination, there is erythema and swelling of the space between the tonsil capsule and the superior constrictor muscle. The soft palate and tonsil are bulging medially.

Answer found on p. 158.   **93**

Q2.37 Common neck swellings

A Branchial cyst
B Carotid body tumour
C Cervical lymphadenopathy
D Cystic hygroma
E Laryngocele
F Papillary thyroid carcinoma
G Submandibular sialolithiasis
H Thyroglossal cyst

For each of the situations below, select the single most likely diagnosis from the list of options above. Each option may be used once, more than once or not at all.

1. A 10-year-old female presents with a 3 cm lump in the posterior triangle of the left neck. On examination, the lump is soft and is brilliantly transilluminable.

2. A 22-year-old male presents with a 3 cm erythematous, tender lump in the upper neck. On examination, the lump protrudes into the anterior triangle of the neck and partially lies behind the sternocleidomastoid muscle. It is tender, fluctuant and reveals pus-like fluid on aspiration.

3. A 54-year-old female presents with a lump on the left side of her neck. On examination, the lump lies at the level of the thyroid cartilage in the anterior triangle of the neck and is ovoid, firm, painless and pulsatile.

Q2.38 Salivary gland disorders

A Acute sialadenitis
B Salivary gland tumour
C Sarcoidosis
D Sialadenosis
E Sialectasis
F Sialocele
G Sialolithiasis
H Sicca syndrome

For each of the situations below, select the single most likely diagnosis from the list of options above. Each option may be used once, more than once or not at all.

1. A 45-year-old female presents with intermittent swelling and pain in the floor of her mouth around mealtimes. On bimanual palpation of the floor of the mouth, there is a hard lump within the right submandibular duct.

2. A 16-year-old male presents with bilateral painful cheek swellings, low-grade fever, arthralgia, malaise and headaches.

3. A 65-year-old female presents with a slow-growing mass in the right parotid gland. On examination, the lump is firm, elastic and slightly lobulated. Intra-oral examination is normal.

Answer found on pp. 159-160.   **95**

Oral and maxillo-facial surgery

Q2.39 Maxillo-facial trauma

A Le Fort I
B Le Fort II
C Le Fort III
D Mandibular dentoalveolar
E Mandibular symphyseal
F Mandibular body
G Mandibular angle
H Mandibular ramus
I Mandibular condylar
J Nasal
K Zygomatic

For each of the situations below, select the single most likely fracture from the list of options above. Each option may be used once, more than once or not at all.

1. A 38-year-old male presents following a fight, with pain and swelling of the right side of his face. The orthopantomograph reveals a fracture passing infero-posteriorly from the right mandibular notch.

2. A 22-year-old male presents following an assault with facial injuries. Plain radiographs (Waters' view) and CT scanning reveal a fracture passing from dorsum of the nose passing backwards across the medial wall of the orbit. It continues across the maxilla between the zygomatic bones and the roots of the maxillary teeth to the pterygomaxillary fissure.

3. A 19-year-old male presents following a fight, with left cheek swelling and complaining of double vision. On examination, there is left periorbital swelling and lateral sub-conjunctival haemorrhage. When viewed from above there is asymmetry of the left cheek.

Q2.40 Common condition of the face, mouth and jaws

A Acute ulcerative gingivitis
B Apical cysts
C Craniofacial clefts
D Craniosynostosis
E Hemifacial microsomia
F Lichen planus
G Mandibular-facial dysotosis
H Orthognathic deformities
I Solitary bone cyst

For each of the situations below, select the single most likely diagnosis from the list of options above. Each option may be used once, more than once or not at all.

1. A 4-year-old male presents with a congenital asymmetrical hypoplasia of the right face. The external ear, the vertical ramus of the mandible and temporomandibular joint are all hypoplastic.

2. A 38-year-old female presents with persistent white patches in her mouth. On examination, the patches cover the buccal mucosa of both cheeks and tongue. They are striated and form a lace-like pattern.

3. A 22-year-old man presents with toothache. A well-defined unilocular radiolucency is identified on the orthopantomograph in the mandible adjacent to the root of the first right molar.

Answer found on p. 161.

Q2.41 Common eye infections

A Blepharitis
B Chalazion
C Conjunctivitis
D Dacryocystitis
E Episcleritis
F Iritis
G Keratitis
H Scleritis

For each of the situations below, select the single most likely diagnosis from the list of options above. Each option may be used once, more than once or not at all.

1. A 32-year-old male presents with acute onset of right eye pain, photophobia, blurred vision and lacrimation. On examination, there is circumcorneal redness and a small pupil. Slit lamp examination reveals white precipitates on the back of the cornea and cells in the anterior chamber.

2. A 7-year-old female presents with bilateral red, sticky, watery eyes. The slit lamp reveals a normal intra-ocular examination and cornea.

3. A 16-year-old female presents with pain and swelling of the medial side of the left upper eyelid. On examination, there is tenderness over the medial lower eyelid extending on to the side of the nose. The eye is normal on slit lamp examination.

Answer found on pp. 161-162.

Paediatric surgery

Q2.42 Clinical problems in low birth weight babies

A Apnoeic attacks
B Hypocalcaemia
C Immature suckling and swallowing
D Impaired temperature control
E Intestinal ileus
F Necrotising enterocolitis
G Patent ductus arteriosus
H Periventricular haemorrhage
I Physiological jaundice
J Surfactant deficiency

For each of the situations below, select the single most likely diagnosis from the list of options above. Each option may be used once, more than once or not at all.

1. A male infant born at 33 weeks' gestation develops worsening tachypnoea in the hours after birth. On examination, there is an increased respiratory effort with grunting, flaring of the nasal alae, intercostal muscle recession and cyanosis. On the chest radiograph there is a diffuse granular appearance and air bronchograms (larger airways outlined).

2. A small for gestational age female infant is born at 35 weeks' gestation at 1.5 kg. Her oxygen consumption is higher than expected and she is found to have a core temperature of 36.2°C.

3. A full-term female infant with a birth weight of 3.2 kg develops visible jaundice on the third post-partum day. On examination, she is well and has a serum bilirubin level of 130 mmol/litre.

Answer found on p. 162-163. **99**

Q2.43 Correctable congenital abnormalities

A Anorectal atresia
B Diaphragmatic hernia
C Duodenal atresia
D Exomphalos
E Gastroschisis
F Hirschsprung's disease
G Malrotation volvulus neonatorum
H Oesophageal atresia
I Pyloric stenosis

For each of the situations below, select the single most likely diagnosis from the list of options above. Each option may be used once, more than once or not at all.

1. A full-term male presents at 4 weeks of age with projectile non-bilious vomiting. On examination, there is an 'olive-shaped' mass in the right hypochondrium. No other anomalies are noted on examination.

2. A full-term female infant is born by Caesarean section. Antenatally, she was found to have loops of bowel prolapsing from a cleft to the right of a normal umbilical cord. No other anomalies are noted on ultrasonography or by clinical examination.

3. A 39-week-gestation male is found to be difficult to resuscitate following an uneventful standard vaginal delivery. He is cyanosed with reduced breath sounds on the right.

Q2.44 Common paediatric surgical disorders
A Appendicitis
B Hydrocele
C Hypospadias
D Inguinal hernia
E Intussusception
F Patent urachal remnant
G Patent vitellointestinal duct
H Phimosis
I Umbilical hernia

For each of the situations below, select the single most likely disorder from the list of options above. Each option may be used once, more than once or not at all.

1. A 9-month-old male presents with vomiting, colicky abdominal pain and the passage of blood and mucus per rectum. The pain is intermittent lasting 1–2 minutes and recurs every 10–15 minutes.

2. A full-term female infant of Afro-Caribbean origin presents at 2 weeks of age with an umbilical lump which becomes prominent on crying. No lump is palpable when the infant is examined asleep.

3. A 5-year-old male presents with ballooning of the prepuce on micturition. With some assistance, he is able to pass urine. There are no signs of urinary retention.

Answer found on p. 164-165.

Q2.45 Orthopaedic disorders of infancy and childhood

A Developmental dysplasia of the hip
B Genu valgum
C Genu varum
D Perthes' disease
E Pes cavus
F Pes planus
G Talipes calcaneovalgus
H Talipes equinovarus
I Transient synovitis of the hip

For each of the situations below, select the single most likely diagnosis from the list of options above. Each option may be used once, more than once or not at all.

1. A full-term infant male is found to have a deformity of both feet in which the feet are inverted and supinated with the forefoot adducted. The heels are also inverted inwards and in plantar flexion with thinning of the calf muscles.

2. A full-term infant female is found to have a positive Barlow's manoeuvre (posterior dislocation out of the acetabulum) on neonatal screening.

3. A 7-year-old male presents with an insidious onset of left-sided hip pain and limp. There is marked sclerosis, irregularity and fragmentation of the left femoral head on the plain radiograph.

Plastic and reconstructive surgery

Q2.46 Cutaneous vascular anomalies

A Ataxia telangiectasia
B Familial glomangiomatosis
C Haemangioma
D Hereditary haemorrhagic telangiectasia (Osler–Weber–Rendu syndrome)
E Kaposiform haemangioendothelioma
F Klippel–Trenaunay syndrome
G Port-wine stain
H Pyogenic granuloma
I Sturge–Weber syndrome

For each of the situations below, select the single most likely diagnosis from the list of options above. Each option may be used once, more than once or not at all.

1. A 40-day-old female presents with a macular, dark red lesion over the right side of her forehead. The parents say that this lesion has been present since birth. It does not cross the midline. The baby is well otherwise and general examination is unremarkable.

2. A 2-year-old male is admitted to the Emergency unit with seizures, predominantly affecting the left side. On examination, there is a macular, reddish-brown stain along the left forehead extending up to his eyelids. The parents say that this discoloration has been present since birth. MR imaging of the brain reveals a left sided cortical atrophy.

3. A 13-year-old female presents with an increase in the length of her right leg. On examination, there are multiple, purplish, macular lesions over the anterolateral aspect of the right thigh. A few, clear-fluid filled vesicles are also seen.

Answer found on p. 167.

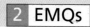

Q2.47 Disorders of the hand and wrist

A Bacterial flexor tenosynovitis
B Carpal tunnel syndrome
C De Quervain's tenosynovitis
D Dupuytren's contracture
E Flexor carpi radialis tenosynovitis
F Ganglion of the flexor sheath
G Mallet finger
H Stenosing tenosynovitis
I Volkmann's ischaemic contracture

For each of the situations below, select the single most likely diagnosis from the list of options above. Each option may be used once, more than once or not at all.

1. A 35-year-old female presents with aching pain over the radial side of her left wrist after strenuous domestic work. On examination, the pain is worsened by flexion and ulnar deviation of the wrist with the thumb adducted across the palm.

2. A 62-year-old diabetic male presents with a painless, hard lump beneath the skin in the palm along his left ring finger. On examination, there is a 10° fixed flexion deformity of the metacarpophalangeal joint of the ring finger.

3. A 38-year-old male gardener presents with a swollen and tender left ring finger. He sustained a thorn prick to this finger 3 days ago. On examination, the finger is partially flexed and there is severe pain on passive extension of the digit.

Q2.48 Non-malignant cutaneous lumps

A Dermatofibroma
B Dermoid cyst
C Lupus vulgaris
D Necrobiosis lipoidica
E Pilomatricoma
F Sebaceous cyst
G Seborrhoeic keratoses
H Stucco keratosis
I Xanthelasma

For each of the situations below, select the single most likely diagnosis from the list of options above. Each option may be used once, more than once or not at all.

1. A 3-year-old male presents with a painless swelling over the midline of the nose. The parents say that the swelling has been present since birth. On examination, the swelling is soft, non-tender and measures 5 cm in diameter. A small pit is visible.

2. A 34-year-old diabetic male presents with a painful, yellowish plaque over his right pre-tibial region. On examination, the plaque has an atrophic telangiectatic centre. There is also a small area of ulceration.

3. A 64-year-old male farmer presents with multiple, raised, pigmented lesions over his trunk and arms. On examination, the lesions are well circumscribed, oval in shape and have a greasy feel. The surface over some of the lesions shows a network of crypts.

Answer found on p. 169-170. **105**

Q2.49 Pre-malignant lesions/malignancies

A Actinic keratosis
B Basal cell carcinoma
C Basal cell naevus syndrome
D Bowen's disease
E Cutaneous malignant lymphoma
F Keratoacanthoma
G Marjolin's ulcer
H Squamous cell carcinoma
I Xeroderma pigmentosum

For each of the situations below, select the single most likely diagnosis from the list of options above. Each option may be used once, more than once or not at all.

1. A 75-year-old male gardener presents with a painless, well-defined ulcer over the lateral aspect of his left eye. On examination, it has a pearly rolled-out edge. He states that he noticed it 8 months ago as a small, pearly nodule which soon ulcerated.

2. A 64-year-old male builder presents with a 7-week history of a rapidly growing solitary, fleshy and dome shaped nodule over his right nasolabial region. On examination, it has a central hyperkeratotic core.

3. A 70-year-old male ex-sailor presents with an exophytic ulcer over his left cheek. On examination, the ulcer has an everted edge. A few enlarged lymph nodes are palpable in his neck.

Q2.50 Benign and malignant pigmented skin lesions

A Acral lentiginous melanoma
B Amelanotic melanoma
C Blue naevus
D Dysplastic naevi
E Ephelis
F Giant congenital naevus
G Lentigo maligna melanoma
H Nodular melanoma
I Solar lentigo

For each of the situations below, select the single most likely diagnosis from the list of options above. Each option may be used once, more than once or not at all.

1. A 32-year-old female presents with a raised, polypoidal and deeply pigmented lesion over her right knee. It is sharply delineated from the surrounding skin. She says that it feels itchy and it bleeds occasionally.

2. A 72-year-old male presents with an irregular, brown pigmented lesion over his right cheek. He says that he has had a brown patch over this area for nearly 10 years but this has recently got bigger. On examination, the patch feels thick and there is a discrete nodule within the lesion.

3. A 75-year-old female presents with an erythematous, irregular papule over the sole of her foot. It does not appear pigmented. On examination, lymph nodes are palpable in the inguinal region.

Answer found on p. 171.

Neurosurgery

Q2.51 Surgical disorders of the brain

A Astrocytoma
B Brain abscess
C Dural meningioma
D Hydrocephalus
E Medulloblastoma
F Neuroblastoma
G Pituitary adenoma
H Subdural empyema

For each of the situations below, select the single most likely diagnosis from the list of options above. Each option may be used once, more than once or not at all.

1. A 42-year-old male presents with generalised soft tissue swelling, headaches and excessive perspiration. On examination, he has bitemporal peripheral visual field defects. Basal concentrations of growth hormone are elevated.

2. A 55-year-old male presents with headaches and pyrexia; he has also suffered from chronic frontal sinusitis. On examination, he has drift of an out-stretched arm. There is papilloedema bilaterally on fundoscopy.

3. A 22-year-old female presents with recent onset of generalised seizures and gradual progressive cognitive changes. There is an ill-defined mass on T2-weighted MR scanning in the right cerebral hemisphere. Excision biopsy revealed increased staining for glial fibrillary acid protein.

Q2.52 Intracranial haemorrhage

A Cerebral arteriovenous malformation
B Extradural haematoma
C Intracranial aneurysm
D Intracranial arteriovenous malformation
E Intraparenchymal haemorrhage
F Intraventricular haemorrhage
G Subarachnoid haemorrhage
H Subdural haematoma

For each of the situations below, select the single most likely diagnosis from the list of options above. Each option may be used once, more than once or not at all.

1. A 69-year-old male presents with a sudden severe headache, dense right hemiparesis and loss of consciousness. There is a large haematoma within the substance of the left cerebral hemisphere on CT.

2. A 42-year-old female presents with a sudden severe headache which she describes 'as the worst of her life'. On examination, she is photophobic with neck stiffness. A lumbar puncture performed within 3 hours of the initial headache reveals uniformly bloodstained cerebrospinal fluid and xanthochromia in the supernatant.

3. A 19-year-old male presents following a single vehicle road traffic accident in which he had to be cut free. The driver of the vehicle was pronounced dead at the scene. On examination, he has a Glasgow Coma Scale of 6. A CT scan reveals major damage to the left hemisphere with a haematoma extending widely over the surface of the hemisphere.

Answer found on p. 172-173. **109**

Q2.53 Brain stem death

A Absent Babinski reflexes
B Absent vestibulo-ocular reflexes
C Anuria
D Asystole
E Brain stem function tests must be performed by the consultant in charge of the patients care
F Core temperature greater than 35°C
G Glasgow Coma Score of 0
H Patient is in a coma, receiving mechanical ventilation
I The immediate family must give their consent

For each of the situations below, select the single most likely option from the list of options above. Each option may be used once, more than once or not at all.

1. What precondition must be met before commencing tests of brain stem function?

2. What exclusion criteria must be met before commencing tests of brain stem function?

3. What brain stem function tests are included?

Q2.54 Surgical aspects of meningitis

A Bacterial
B Carcinomatous
C Chemical
D Cholesterol
E Head injury
F Communicating hydrocephalus
G Post-organ transplantation
H Tuberculosis
I Vertebral osteomyelitis
J Viral

For each of the situations below, select the single most likely diagnosis from the list of options above. Each option may be used once, more than once or not at all.

1. A 17-year-old female presenting with meningococcal meningitis develops ophthalmoplegia and increasing drowsiness. On fundoscopy, there is papilloedema.

2. A 62-year-old male developed a severe headache while undergoing a spinal anaesthetic for a right inguinal hernia repair. The anaesthetist realised later he had injected the prophylactic antibiotic instead of the local anaesthetic into the subarachnoid space.

3. A 23-year-old paraplegic male who previously sustained a gunshot wound to his lumbar spine has suffered with a discharging wound from the gunshot exit site. He has now developed pyrexia, headache, photophobia and neck stiffness.

Answer found on p. 174.   **111**

Q2.55 Rehabilitation
- **A** Axillary crutch
- **B** Elbow crutch
- **C** Graded activity exercises
- **D** Gutter crutch
- **E** Isometric exercises
- **F** Isotonic exercises
- **G** Rollator
- **H** Spinal support
- **I** Walking frame

For each of the situations below, select the single most likely option from the list of options above. Each option may be used once, more than once or not at all.

1. Activity aimed at widening the range of movement.
2. A functional aid that allows forearm weight bearing.
3. A brace used to provide spinal support in patients with cerebral palsy.

Trauma and orthopaedic surgery

Q2.56 Injuries to the upper arm and shoulder region

A Acromioclavicular joint subluxation
B Anterior dislocation of the shoulder
C Fracture of the acromion process
D Fracture of the coracoid process
E Fracture of the greater tuberosity
F Fracture of the head of the humerus
G Fracture of the neck of the humerus
H Fracture of the neck of the scapula
I Posterior dislocation of the shoulder
J Ruptured coraco-acromial ligament

For each of the situations below, select the single most likely diagnosis from the list of options above. Each option may be used once, more than once or not at all.

1. A 39-year-old male motorcyclist is admitted to the Emergency department after being involved in a high-speed road traffic collision. He sustained severe trauma to his right upper back when he fell onto the road. There is bruising and tenderness over this region. He has drooping of the right shoulder with lengthening of the arm. Movement of the shoulder is severely restricted and the arm is held in adduction.

2. An 18-year-old male is admitted to the Emergency department with a painful shoulder, after he fell awkwardly during a rugby tackle. On examination, there is a swelling in the deltopectoral groove with lowering of the anterior axillary fold and a prominent acromion process. The arm is slightly abducted and externally rotated.

3. An 80-year-old female presents to the Emergency department with extensive bruising and pain over her right upper/mid arm. She tripped while in the toilet and banged her right arm against the edge of the bath 2 days ago. She is unable to move her right shoulder. She suffers from osteoporosis.

Answer found on p. 175-176.

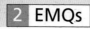

Q2.57 Injuries to the forearm and hand

A Colles' fracture
B Dislocated elbow
C Fracture of the coronoid process
D Fracture of the olecranon process
E Fracture of the radial head
F Galeazzi fracture
G Monteggia fracture
H Pulled elbow
I Scaphoid fracture
J Smith's fracture

For each of the situations below, select the single most likely diagnosis from the list of options above. Each option may be used once, more than once or not at all.

1. A 35-year-old male presents to the Accident and Emergency department with a painful upper forearm after being involved in a fight. There is pain and tenderness over the elbow region and upper forearm. Plain radiography reveals an angulated fracture at the junction of the proximal and middle third of ulna, and the head of the radius is dislocated anteriorly.

2. A 38-year-old female presents to the Emergency department with a painful right wrist after having fallen on her outstretched hand. On examination, there is mild swelling over the wrist and the movements are restricted. The pain is maximal over the distal end of radius in the snuffbox region, which is worsened on longitudinal compression of the thumb.

3. A 55-year-old female presents to the Emergency department with a painful swelling over her left distal forearm following a road traffic collision. On examination, there is tenderness, swelling and deformity over this region. Plain radiography reveals a fracture at the middle and distal thirds of the radius with the fragment of the radius tilted towards the ulna. There is disruption of the distal radio-ulnar joint.

Q2.58 Brachial plexus injuries

A Axillary nerve
B Lateral pectoral nerve
C Long thoracic nerve
D Medial pectoral nerve
E Median nerve
F Musculocutaneous nerve
G Nerve to rhomboid
H Radial nerve
I Suprascapular nerve
J Ulnar nerve

For each of the situations below, select the single most likely diagnosis from the list of options above. Each option may be used once, more than once or not at all.

1. A 55-year-old female presents with pain over her right upper arm after sustaining an injury to the region following a fall. On examination, there is bruising and tenderness over the mid-arm region. Neurological examination reveals sensory loss over the lateral side of the back of the hand and she is unable to extend her wrist.

2. A 32-year-old male presents with inability to raise his right arm. He had a deep intramuscular injection to his deltoid region 2 days ago. On examination, there is a small area of anaesthesia over the insertion of deltoid and loss of shoulder abduction beyond 10–15°.

3. A 68-year-old female presents to the orthopaedic clinic complaining of a 'prominent scapula'. She had recently undergone mastectomy for breast cancer. On examination, the scapula becomes prominent (standing out) over the vertebral border and the inferior angle when she is asked to push her arms against the wall.

Answer found on p. 178-179. **115**

Q2.59 Lower limb nerve injuries

A Common peroneal nerve
B Femoral nerve
C Lateral cutaneous nerve of thigh
D Lateral plantar nerve
E Medial plantar nerve
F Pudendal nerve
G Saphenous nerve
H Tibial nerve
I Sciatic nerve
J Sural nerve

For each of the situations below, select the single most likely nerve from the list of options above. Each option may be used once, more than once or not at all.

1. A 25-year-old male presents to the orthopaedic clinic with a painful right knee and difficulty walking. He was hit over the lateral side of his knee with a hockey stick 2 days ago. On examination, he is unable to dorsiflex and evert his left foot. He has reduced sensation over the lateral aspect of his lower leg and the dorsum of this foot and toes. Radiographs show a fracture of the fibular neck.

2. A 25-year-old male is admitted to the Emergency department following a deep stab wound injury to his upper left thigh. On examination, he has numbness over the anterior thigh and medial aspect of his leg. He is unable to extend his knee and the knee jerk is diminished.

3. A 37-year-old male is admitted to the Emergency department following a high-speed road traffic collision. He hit his flexed knee against the dashboard of his car. On examination, there is loss of sensation over the sole of the foot. He is unable to flex his toes and the ankle jerk is lost. Plain radiography reveals posterior dislocation of the knee.

 Answer found on pp. 179–180.

Urology

Q2.60 Urological trauma

A Anterior urethra
B Bladder
C Distal ureter
D Kidney
E Posterior urethral
F Proximal ureter

For each of the situations below, select the single most likely site of injury from the list of options above. Each option may be used once, more than once or not at all.

1. A 53-year-old female develops leakage of urine from the vagina 3 days following a hysterectomy for bulky fibroids.

2. A 34-year-old man presents following an assault. He reports being kicked once in the lower abdomen. He wants to void urine but is unable to do so. There is free intraperitoneal fluid on CT scanning.

3. A 10-year-old male presents unable to void urine following a straddle injury on a bicycle crossbar. On examination, there is blood at the external urethral meatus and ecchymosis of the shaft of the penis, scrotum and lower anterior abdominal wall.

Answer found on p. 180-181. **117**

Q2.61 Urinary tract infections and calculi

A Acute cystitis
B Acute prostatitis
C Acute pyelonephritis
D Calcium oxalate
E Calcium phosphate
F Cystine
G Struvite
H Uric acid
I Xanthogranulomatous pyelonephritis

For each of the situations below, select the single most likely diagnosis from the list of options above. Each option may be used once, more than once or not at all.

1. A 24-year-old female presents with rapid onset of loin to groin pain, fever and rigors. On examination, she has marked tenderness in the left loin.

2. A 52-year-old male presents with an acute onset of fever, dysuria, low back and perineal pain. Digital rectal examination is extremely painful.

3. A 34-year-old male present with an acute onset of intense right colicky loin pain. There is microscopic haematuria on urinalysis. There is a markedly radiodense spiculated calculus at the right vesicoureteric junction.

Answer found on pp. 181-182.

Q2.62 Haematuria

A Bladder outflow obstruction
B Glomerulonephritis
C Henoch–Schönlein disease
D Ureteric calculi
E Lower urinary tract infection
F Polycystic kidney
G Pyelonephritis
H Renal cell carcinoma
I Transitional cell carcinoma

For each of the situations below, select the single most likely diagnosis from the list of options above. Each option may be used once, more than once or not at all.

1. A 64-year-old male presents with fever, frank haematuria and left loin pain. On examination, there is a palpable mass in the left loin on balloting the kidney. He is also polycythaemic and hypercalcaemic.

2. A 71-year-old female presents with frank painless haematuria. The intravenous urogram reveals a filling defect within the bladder.

3. A 33-year-old female presents with fever and headache. On examination, she is hypertensive and has oedema of the face and legs. Urinalysis reveals protein and red blood cells.

Answer found on p. 182-183.   **119**

Q2.63 Urinary tract obstruction

A Aorto-iliac aneurysm
B Bladder outflow obstruction
C Calculi
D Crohn's disease
E Pelviureteric junction obstruction
F Primary megaureter
G Retrocaval ureter
H Retroperitoneal fibrosis
I Urothelial tumour

For each of the situations below, select the single most likely diagnosis from the list of options above. Each option may be used once, more than once or not at all.

1. An 18-year-old male presents with left loin pain following the ingestion of alcohol. On examination, there is a mass palpable on balloting the left kidney. There is microscopic haematuria on urinalysis.

2. A 68-year-old male presents with malaise, fever, weight loss, nausea and back-pain. On examination, he is found to be hypertensive and uraemic.

3. A 72-year-old male smoker presents with fever, weight loss and acute onset of anuria. On examination, he is hypertensive and has a pulsatile/expansile abdominal mass.

Answer found on pp. 183-184.

Q2.64 Pain and swelling in the scrotum

A Encysted hydrocele
B Epididymal cyst
C Epididymo-orchitis
D Haematocele
E Hydrocele
F Orchitis
G Sebaceous cyst of the scrotum
H Testicular torsion
I Testicular tumour
J Varicocele

For each of the situations below, select the single most likely diagnosis from the list of options above. Each option may be used once, more than once or not at all.

1. A 14-year-old male presents with a 4-hour history of lower abdominal pain and vomiting. On examination, there is oedema and erythema of the right hemiscrotum.

2. A 22-year-old male presents with a 1-day history of right testicular pain. On examination, the right testis is swollen and tender. White discharge is noted at the external urethral meatus.

3. A 47-year-old male presents with a painful right scrotal swelling. On examination, the swelling is fluctuant. The fluid aspirated is clear.

Answer found on p. 184-185.   **121**

Q2.65 Chronic renal failure

A Continuous ambulatory peritoneal dialysis (CAPD)
B Continuous arteriovenous haemofiltration (CAVH)
C Continuous cycling peritoneal dialysis (CCPD)
D Continuous veno-venous haemofiltration (CVVH)
E Continuous veno-venous haemofiltration and dialysis haemofiltration (CVVH-D)
F Standard machine driven haemodialysis (HD)
G Standard machine driven haemofiltration (HF)

For each of the situations below, select the single most likely option from the list of options above. Each option may be used once, more than once or not at all.

1. Plasma removed from the radial artery is passed under pressure through a semipermeable membrane with water and solute being added from a separate source to replace the essential components removed.

2. A method of dialysis, which does not require heparin.

3. Blood removed via a central vein is allowed to equilibrate across a semipermeable membrane by means of a concentration gradient.

Q2.66 Aspects of pelvic surgery

A Corpus cavernosum
B Distal urethral sphincter
C Dorsal nerve of the penis
D Parasympathetic pelvic splanchnic nerves
E Proximal urethral sphincter
F Pudendal nerve
G Seminal vesicle
H Superior hypogastric plexus

For each of the situations below, select the single most likely cause from the list of options above. Each option may be used once, more than once or not at all.

1. A 58-year-old male complains of erectile dysfunction following a low anterior resection.

2. A 62-year-old male complains of ejaculation dysfunction after abdominoperineal resection. He is able to achieve normal tumescence.

3. A 68-year-old male develops urinary stress incontinence after radical prostatectomy.

Answer found on p. 186.   **123**

ANSWERS

Cardiothoracic surgery

A2.1 Haemodynamic control

1. **F Sodium nitroprusside.** Sodium nitroprusside acts by relaxation of vascular smooth muscle resulting in dilatation of peripheral arteries and veins (more active on veins than on arteries). The resulting reduction in peripheral vascular resistance reduces workload on the heart by reducing preload and afterload. The hypotensive effect is seen within 1–2 minutes after the start of an adequate infusion, and it dissipates almost as rapidly after infusion is discontinued. Nitroprusside infusion is used to treat hypertensive crises (malignant hypertension, severe hypertension) or acute congestive heart failure.

2. **B Atropine.** In health, the sinoatrial node is under the tonic influence of the sympathetic and parasympathetic nervous systems. Atropine is a muscarinic receptor antagonist, which works by abolishing the parasympathetic influences (blocks acetylcholine released from the postganglionic vagus nerve endings in the cardiac tissue) resulting in an increased heart rate. Atropine is a naturally occurring alkaloid and is absorbed from the gastrointestinal tract, and is excreted in the urine. Atropine undergoes hepatic metabolism and has a plasma half-life of 2–3 hours. When used as pre-medication for anaesthesia, atropine decreases bronchial and salivary secretions, blocks the bradycardia associated with some drugs used in anaesthesia such as halothane, suxamethonium and neostigmine and also helps prevent bradycardia from excessive vagal stimulation.

3. **A Adenosine.** Adenosine is an endogenous purine nucleoside that slows atrioventricular nodal conduction and results in transient atrioventricular nodal block. It acts on a specific cell surface receptor and is used in the treatment of paroxysmal supraventricular tachycardia. Following administration, adenosine is rapidly cleared from the circulation by cellular uptake and metabolism (half-life of less than 5 seconds). Onset of action occurs within 30 seconds following intravenous infusion and has a duration of action of 1–2 minutes. Patients may experience transient dyspnoea or chest pain.

A2.2 Surgical disorders of the heart vessels and heart valves

1. **C Mitral regurgitation.** Papillary muscle rupture results in varying degrees of mitral regurgitation. Onset is rapid in ischaemic heart disease or more gradual in rheumatic heart disease or floppy valve disease (the most common cause of pure mitral valve disease characterised by the valve leaflets becoming soft and spongy and the chordae becoming elongated due to an underlying abnormality of the valve collagen).

Acute onset results in the heart being subjected to high pressures resulting in dyspnoea due to pulmonary oedema. On examination, the heart is enlarged and there are signs of left ventricular hypertrophy on electrocardiogram. Doppler-echocardiogram quantifies the regurgitation. Initial management is diuretic therapy, with mitral valve replacement usually being necessary in rapid onset cases. Mitral valve replacement is performed using cardiac bypass through a midline sternotomy, mechanical valves are predominately used in younger patients due to their excellent durability and to avoid the accelerated calcification and valve dysfunction seen in tissue valves. However, life-long anticoagulation is necessary.

2. **A** **Aortic regurgitation.** Aortic regurgitation is due to congenital causes (bicuspid or dome-shaped aortic valve) or acquired causes (rheumatic fever, dissecting aneurysm, bacterial endocarditis). The progress of aortic regurgitation may be insidious with the patient remaining apparently well until marked ventricular dilatation occurs. The natural history is variable and not all patients go on to develop cardiomegaly. Over a period of time, the increased pulse pressure results in massive arterial pulsation in the neck (Corrigan's sign) and collapsing (water hammer) pulse. The unpredictable course makes the timing of surgery difficult. Surgery is usually indicated when there are radiological signs of cardiomegaly or there is evidence of left ventricular deterioration. Aortic valve replacement is performed through a median sternotomy, cardioplegic (hypothermic total circulatory) arrest of the heart and direct coronary cannulation.

3. **B** **Aortic stenosis.** Aortic stenosis most frequently occurs on previously bicuspid valves, which become stiffened and calcified with age. Other causes include rheumatic heart disease (causing progressive commissural fusion and cup rigidity) and calcification in normal valves. Effort syncope is thought to arise from cardiac reflexes stimulated when the heart becomes overloaded. Most cases are discovered as an incidental finding or in the investigation of effort syncope or angina. Signs of left ventricular hypertrophy may be seen on the electrocardiogram with the echocardiogram confirming the diagnosis and the degree of thickening and calcification of the valve. The need for surgery is determined by the pressure gradient across the valve.

A2.3 Cardiopulmonary bypass and cardiac devices

1. **C** **Cardiopulmonary bypass.** Cardiopulmonary bypass allows whole body perfusion in which the pumping action of the heart and oxygenation of blood by the lungs are replaced by an extracorporeal circuit. The venous blood from the heart is diverted from the heart using a large bore cannula inserted in the right atrial appendage. When the right side of the heart has to be opened, separate cannulas are inserted into the superior and inferior vena cavae. Purse-string sutures are snared

around the incisions to produce a blood- and air-tight seal. The blood drained from the heart is passed through the oxygenator in which it is separated from a gas mixture by a system of membranes. The blood is then returned to the patient under pressure through a cannula, which is usually positioned in the ascending aorta.

2. **B** **Cardioplegia.** Cardiopulmonary bypass requires the ascending aorta to be cross-clamped to provide a bloodless field. This results in a cessation of the coronary circulation causing myocardial ischaemia. Paralysis of the heart (cardioplegia) reduces myocardial oxygen demand during the ischaemic period to such low levels that the myocardial energy stores are sufficient to maintain the heart. Various techniques, solutions and temperatures have been used. Cold potassium cardioplegia solutions raise the potassium level to 15–20 mmol/litre to arrest the heart in asystole and can be used for up to 2 hours without any irreversible affects. Administration of this solution aims to maintain a myocardial temperature below 20°C. Retrograde flow of the cardioplegic solution into the coronary sinus also lowers the risk of coronary occlusion. Reinfusion of the solution is often necessary at intervals of 30 minutes to maintain myocardial arrest and hypothermia.

3. **E** **Intra-aortic balloon pump.** The intra-aortic balloon pump is a method of circulatory support in patients awaiting surgery; in patients with left ventricular failure following coronary bypass grafting or in patients with cardiogenic support where there is a realistic prospect of the patient's condition improving. The balloon is delivered on a catheter to the descending aorta via the femoral artery. The balloon is inflated by a pump and is triggered by the patient's electrocardiogram or aortic pressure waveform. The balloon inflates in diastole producing counter-pulsation propelling blood into the coronary circulation. Use of this device increases the cardiac output by approximately 10%.

A2.4 Pathophysiology of thoracic trauma

1. **J** **Tension pneumothorax.** Tension pneumothorax develops when the wound in the parietal pleura seals but air continues to escape from the lung, then tension inside the pleura space rises. The increased volume of air in the pleural space causes the lung on the affected side to collapse and eventually causes the mediastinum to shift to the contralateral side. The shifted mediastinum impairs venous return and eventually compresses the contralateral lung impairing ventilation further. The diagnosis should be confirmed clinically by dyspnoea, unilateral absent breath sounds, tracheal deviation to the contralateral side and distended neck veins. Treatment is by immediate needle decompression followed soon after by insertion of a chest drain. Treatment should not be delayed by performing a chest radiograph (Fig. 2.4.1) to confirm the diagnosis.

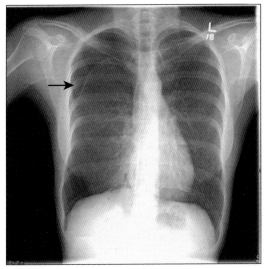

Fig. 2.4.1 A chest radiograph showing a right pneumothorax with lung collapse. There is slight displacement of the trachea and mediastinum medially.

2. **H** **Pulmonary contusion.** Pulmonary contusion usually results from severe blunt trauma to the chest. The contused lung is literally bruised although the process is usually self-limiting. Normal lung function does not usually return until the haematoma has resolved. The contused lung parenchyma is particularly susceptible to oedema which may extend to the adjacent lung tissue. Contusions may be exacerbated with vigorous crystalloid resuscitation or by infection. Left untreated, acute respiratory distress syndrome (ARDS) may develop. In the contused lung atelectasis, decreased lung compliance and increased airways resistance result in an increased workload of the injured chest to maintain adequate oxygenation. Patients are observed, preferably in a high dependency unit, with frequent chest physiotherapy and serial chest radiographs. Failure to maintain oxygenation requires tracheal intubation and mechanical ventilation.

3. **B** **Diaphragmatic rupture.** Blunt trauma to the abdomen resulting in a diaphragmatic perforation usually results in a large radial tear of the diaphragm. Left-sided herniation is more common, as the right hemidiaphragm is relatively protected by the liver. Herniation of stomach, spleen, omentum and small bowel may occur through the defect, with these structures being frequently traumatised by the force of injury. Chest radiograph findings may be mistaken for a loculated pneumothorax or a raised hemidiaphragm. The diagnosis is confirmed by a coiled NG tube in the left thorax or by CT. Presentation is either immediate with hypovolaemic shock (secondary to intraperitoneal or intrathoracic bleeding) or later with the effects of migration of the abdominal viscera

into the chest. Treatment is laparotomy ± thoracotomy, reduction of abdominal contents and repair of the hernia.

A2.5 Thoracotomy

1. **E Median sternotomy.** A midline sternotomy gives optimal access to the heart. However, median sternotomy affords a limited exposure of both pleural spaces and the anterior hilar structures. Median sternotomy causes the least compromise of pulmonary function in the early postoperative period of any thoracic approach. The procedure is performed with the patient in the supine position. A vertical incision is made in the midline from the suprasternal notch to just below the xiphoid process. The pectoralis fascia overlying the sternum is incised. The sternum is then cut and the two edges retracted. The sternum is closed with interosseous wire sutures.

2. **G Right posterolateral.** A posterolateral thoracotomy is the most common incision for pulmonary resection, bullectomy, chest wall re-section and oesophageal surgery. The patient is placed in the lateral decubitus position and the skin is incised in the fifth intercostal space (sixth or seventh in oesophageal surgery) in an S-shape from the ante-rior axillary line curved around the tip of the scapula to the posterior midline at the level of the spine of the scapula. The lower portions of latissimus dorsi and trapezius are divided and serratus anterior retracted. The incision is deepened to pleura on the upper border of the lower rib to avoid injury to the neurovascular bundle. The rib is divided at the costovertebral angle to avoid fracture. This technique provides optimal exposure of parenchymal and hilar structures but may be complicated by postoperative pain.

3. **H Transverse thoracosternotomy.** Transverse thoracosternotomy (clam shell) provides excellent exposure to both sides of the chest and mediastinum. The patient is placed in a supine position with the upper thoracic spine propped forward. Bilateral anterolateral incisions (mid-axillary line in the fifth intercostal space) are made in the inframammary fold and the sternum is transected. The thorax is then spread upwards with a rib-retractor. Complications of the procedure include severe postoperative pain and sternal instability.

A2.6 Surgical disorders of the lung

1. **H Pulmonary embolism.** Pulmonary embolism represents the worst outcome of thrombi originating from the pelvis or lower limbs. The effects of pulmonary embolism range from symptomless to fatal. Small emboli may be spontaneously and completely lysed with the patient experiencing no symptoms. Small emboli wedged in the peripheral lung may cause pleuritic chest pain with repeated small emboli causing pulmo-nary hypertension as progressively more of the pulmonary vascular tree is occluded. Larger emboli may obstruct a large part of the pulmonary

circulation resulting in central chest pain and circulatory collapse. Massive pulmonary emboli may prevent the right heart from emptying and is therefore rapidly fatal. The electrocardiogram may show sinus tachycardia, atrial fibrillation, T-wave inversion or right bundle branch block. The chest radiograph may be normal, or have a paucity of vascular markings or wedge opacity. The treatment of choice is intravenous or subcutaneous low-molecular weight heparin followed by warfarinisation for 3 months. Major emboli may be treated with thrombolysis or catheter embolectomy if cardiac output is severely affected.

2. **A** **Bronchiectasis.** Bronchiectasis is a chronic, necrotising infection resulting from destruction of the normal bronchial architecture. Clinically, the patient experiences a persistent cough, copious sputum production and recurrent bronchopulmonary infections. The damage is usually initiated in childhood when severe infections (whooping cough, measles or adenovirus infections) or chronic conditions (asthma, cystic fibrosis) are exacerbated by bronchial obstructions. With chronic infection, there is progressive bronchial dilatation and thickening (seen as tramlines on chest radiograph) and mucous gland hyperplasia. The dilated bronchi lack cilia, leading to pooling of secretions and chronic bronchial infections. Bronchopulmonary vascular anastomoses may rupture causing haemorrhage. Physiotherapy and postural drainage help to reduce the volume of retained sputum and resistant organisms. Infections are treated aggressively with antibiotics. Pulmonary resection is only indicated if bronchiectasis is localised and unilateral.

3. **B** **Carcinoma of the lung.** Bronchial carcinoma is the most common form of lung cancer and is the most frequent cause of deaths of men in the developed world. Most bronchial carcinomas develop in a main bronchus causing a partial or complete obstruction with distal collapse. Spread may be by direct invasion, via the lymphatics (hilar, mediastinal and supraclavicular lymph nodes) or blood-borne (liver, bones, brain). Symptoms are those of the primary tumour (cough, dyspnoea, pleuritic pain, haemoptysis), local spread (into the mediastinum causing left recurrent nerve paralysis resulting in a hoarse voice and bovine cough), metastases (bone pain, weight loss) or para-neoplastic syndrome. Pulmonary lobectomy or pneumonectomy are the treatment of choice as they provide the best chance of cure. Surgical resection is only possible in 10–15% of cases with a 5-year survival of approximately 30% in those operated on.

A2.7 Complications of thoracic operations

1. **E** **Haemothorax.** Complications of central venous catheterisation are related to the insertion of the line (air embolism, arrhythmia, catheter embolus, chylothorax, haemothorax, neurological injury, pneumothorax) or occur later (catheter-related infections and sepsis, central venous occlusion). Haemothorax presents with signs of hypovolaemic shock

with absent breath sounds and dullness to percussion on the affected side. Management of haemothorax requires aggressive resuscitation and simultaneous drainage of the chest via a large-bore chest drain. Thoracotomy is required if the initial output from the chest drain is greater than 1500 ml or if the subsequent output of the drain is greater than 200 ml/hour. A chest radiograph should be performed in patients treated conservatively to assess placement of the tube and a second chest drain inserted if necessary to achieve maximal drainage. Failure to drain a clotted haemothorax requires a thoracotomy as there is a high risk of a subsequent fibrothorax (progressive reduction in the size of the lung and compliance of the chest wall).

2. **F** **Mediastinitis.** Acute mediastinitis most frequently occurs following cardiac surgery or oesophageal resection, but may also result from penetrating trauma or rupture of the oesophagus. Left untreated the infection spreads to the pleural spaces and into the neck (potentially causing life threatening laryngeal obstruction) resulting in marked systemic disturbance and cardiovascular collapse. Patients present with tachycardia or other signs of sepsis. A pleural effusion is usually present in one or both sides. A mediastinal 'crunch' may be heard on auscultation if gas is present around the pericardium. Patients with mediastinitis require a thoracotomy, drainage of the mediastinum and broad-spectrum antibiotics. Mediastinitis following coronary artery bypass is more common in diabetic and obese patients and has a reported mortality rate of 20%. The mortality rate after oesophageal perforation is reported to be up to 50%.

3. **A** **Chylothorax.** Chylothorax presents congenitally (atresia, birth trauma) or as the result of damage to the thoracic duct by surgery (oesophagectomy, left pneumonectomy, thoracic aneurysm repair, radical neck resection), trauma or cancer. The thoracic duct originates from the cisterna chyli arising at the level of L2 and ascends behind the oesophagus, and between the aorta and azygous vein. At T5 the duct passes behind the aorta and aortic arch to join the venous system at the junction of the left jugular and subclavian veins. The thoracic duct is prone to injury throughout its course. Patients may present with insidious signs (dyspnoea) or with respiratory distress and shock if the injury to the thoracic duct is significant. Chest radiograph findings are suggestive of a pleural effusion or a haemothorax. Needle aspirate is the typical milky fluid of chyle. It must be differentiated from the chyliform appearance of a long-standing effusion or haemothorax. Chylomicrons and triglycerides are only found in true chylous effusions. Chylothorax following thoracotomy is unlikely to settle and re-exploration is usually necessary with ligation of the thoracic duct.

A2.8 Thoracic procedures

1. **A Chest drain.** Simple (spontaneous) pneumothorax results from a number of underlying lung conditions (asthma, chronic obstructive pulmonary disease, cystic fibrosis), mechanical ventilation or are idiopathic (probable due to a rupture of a congenital bulla). The majority of simple pneumothoraces are a result of an idiopathic cause. Air escaping into the pleural space allows the lung to contract in size due to elastic recoil. The pressure inside the pleural space rises because of the continuous leakage of air. A rise in pressure above atmospheric pressure causes occlusion of intrathoracic airways and trapping of air in expiration. Tension pneumothorax occurs when the pressure rises to a point which causes mediastinal shift, further reducing the cardiac output. Tension pneumothorax is a clinical diagnosis and is treated immediately with needle decompression followed by chest drain insertion. The decision to drain a simple pneumothorax depends on the radiological findings. A pneumothorax greater than 1.5 cm on chest radiograph (measured from the lung border to the inside of the thoracic wall at the level of the third rib) is considered significant and requires a chest drain.

2. **C Thoracotomy.** Pus in the pleural cavity (empyema thoracis) results from infection of the adjacent lung (pneumonia, tuberculosis, lung abscess), following thoracic surgery, penetrating trauma or oesophageal perforation. Empyema occurs more frequently in debilitated patients or in patients with bronchial obstruction. Empyema usually present as failure of pneumonia to resolve with antibiotic therapy with what appears to be a pleural effusion on chest radiograph. CT scan of the chest and culture of pleural aspirate confirm the diagnosis. Non-loculated empyema may be treated with chest drain insertion (ideally under radiological guidance) ± intrapleural fibrinolytics to aid breakdown of adhesions. Thoracotomy is indicated for chronic infection, where there is radiological evidence of gross pleural thickening and multiloculation, or when initial measures fail to achieve rapid resolution. Surgical treatment requires removal of the fibrous cortex (decortication) allowing re-expansion of the underlying lung.

3. **D Pleurodesis.** Pleural effusions are either transudates (cardiac failure, hypoalbuminaemia) or exudates (malignancy, secondary to inflammatory cause, e.g. pneumonia, subphrenic abscess). Transudates have a protein level less than 30 g/litre and exudates have a protein level greater than 30 g/litre. The fluid in the pleural space may be free or loculated. Clinically there is reduced chest movement, breath sounds and stony dullness to percussion on the affected side. The diagnosis is confirmed by chest radiograph and needle aspiration. Pleural effusions are initially managed with needle aspiration. Recurrent or malignant pleural effusions may require pleurodesis (obliteration of the pleural space) if symptom `tic. This procedure may also be used to prevent recurrence of pneumothorax, haemothorax or chylothorax. The procedure is performed by insertion of

a chest drain into the most dependent part of the effusion, instillation of a sclerosant and attachment of the chest drain to low-pressure suction for 4 days. A variety of sclerosants have been used including blood, tetracycline, bleomycin and talcum powder. Surgical pleurodesis may be achieved at thoracotomy by stripping the parietal pleura.

General surgery

A2.9 Causes of abdominal pain

1. **B Biliary disease.** Biliary disease presents with a range of clinical symptoms. Initially it is often difficult to differentiate between biliary colic and acute cholecystitis. Biliary colic arises from the impaction of a calculus (Fig. 2.9.1) in the cystic duct or gallbladder neck resulting in obstruction. Pain results from contraction of the gallbladder against the obstruction and usually lasts only a few hours. Cholecystitis results from acute inflammatory response within the gallbladder in the presence of continued obstruction. The pain is prolonged and may be exacerbated with systemic signs of raised temperature and white cell count. Bacterial colonisation may then develop in the obstructed gallbladder leading to ischaemic gangrene or perforation or resulting in empyema of the gallbladder.

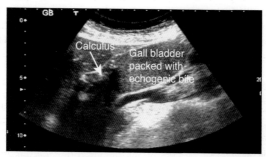

Fig. 2.9.1 An ultrasound scan showing the gallbladder to be distended with echogenic bile and post-acoustic shadowing from calculi in the neck of the gallbladder.

2. **H Perforated peptic ulcer.** Perforated peptic ulcers classically present with a severe onset of acute severe epigastric pain with rapid progression to signs of generalised peritonitis. Shoulder tip pain is common due to diaphragmatic irritation. Gas under the diaphragm may only be present in 50% of cases, however accuracy is increased by placing the patient in the erect position a few minutes prior to the investigation being performed. A radiological contrast study or CT may be performed if the diagnosis is in doubt. Signs of generalised peritonitis require an urgent laparotomy, lavage and omental patch repair of the ulcer. A sealed perforation may be treated conservatively with bowel rest, intravenous fluids and antibiotics. Clinical deterioration of a patient treated conservatively requires a laparotomy.

3. G Pancreatitis. The aetiology of acute pancreatitis includes gallstones (30–40%), alcohol (30–35%), or an idiopathic cause (20–30%); other causes are rare. Its presentation ranges from mild discomfort to overwhelming abdominal pain and systemic signs. Approximately 25% of patients presenting with acute pancreatitis have a severe attack with signs of cardiovascular and respiratory dysfunction. The diagnosis of acute pancreatitis is likely if the serum amylase is three times the upper limit of normal. The usual range may vary between laboratories. However, other conditions cause hyperamylasaemia and the serum amylase level drops rapidly following the initial attack of acute pancreatitis. The severity of the attack should be stratified using a validated prognostic scoring system, e.g. the Glasgow–Imrie scoring system for the initial prediction of severity in acute pancreatitis (age >55 years, white blood cell count $>15 \times 10^9$/litre, glucose >10 mmol/litre, urea >16 mmol/litre, PaO_2 <60 mmHg, calcium <2 mmol/litre, albumin <32 g/litre, lactate dehydrogenase >600 U/litre, aspartate/alanine aminotransferase >100 U/litre. Serum C-reactive protein concentration, although not part of the Glasgow criteria, has an independent prognostic value if the peak level is >210 mg/litre in the first 4 days of the attack). Other scoring systems exist, e.g. Ranson. Resuscitation and organ support is then dependent on severity classification. An ultrasound should be performed on all patients with acute pancreatitis to determine the presence of biliary calculi. A CT of the abdomen should be performed on all patients with severe acute pancreatitis between the third and tenth days following the onset of symptoms to ensure the pancreatitic blood supply (exclude a phlegmon or necrosis).

A2.10 Abdominal masses

1. D Colonic diverticular mass. Colonic diverticular masses result from the oedematous thickened inflamed segment of colon and adherent omentum. Suppuration may have occurred resulting in abscess formation. In the absence of peritonitis, patients are usually treated conservatively with bowel rest, intravenous fluids and intravenous broad-spectrum antibiotics. An ultrasound scan should be performed to exclude a gynaecological pathology in woman or to identify a collection. CT scan is highly sensitive in the acute phase. The patient is usually discharged within a few days when symptoms and signs have resolved. It is mandatory to perform a colonoscopy or barium enema and a sigmoidoscopy subsequently to exclude a colonic malignancy.

2. B Abdominal aortic aneurysm. Abdominal aortic aneurysm may cause symptoms due to pressure on surrounding structures, however approximately 75% may be asymptomatic at diagnosis. Abdominal aortic aneurysms primarily affect men over 65 years with a prevalence of 5%. Approximately 70% of presenting abdominal aortic aneurysms are detected before rupture and are treated electively, with 30% presenting as a rupture or with distal embolisation. Rupture is most often into the retroperitoneal space resulting in back pain, hypovolaemic shock and a pulsatile abdominal mass.

3. **E** **Colonic malignancy.** Colonic malignancy can present as an emergency or with chronic symptoms. Tumours of the caecum and the ascending colon typically present with anaemia and no change in bowel habit, due to the liquid nature of the faeces and the wide capacitance of the caecum. Tumours of the ileocaecal valve may present early with small bowel obstruction. Tumours of the descending or sigmoid colon tend to present with a change in bowel habit or colicky abdominal pain. Colonic malignancy is the second most common cause of death by cancer in the UK with an equal male to female ratio.

A2.11 The acute abdomen

1. **F** **Ruptured ectopic pregnancy.** Most ectopic pregnancies occur in the uterine tube due to defective transport of the fertilised ovum by scarring due to previous surgery or salpingitis. Eventually the increasing size of the embryo causes the tube to rupture. The symptoms of shock develop if bleeding is rapid with syncope resulting due to hypotension. Usually the woman reports vaginal bleeding which may be similar to a 'period', only rarely do patients experience a heavy vaginal bleed. Typically, the history is of one or two missed periods with other symptoms of early pregnancy. The pregnancy test is positive and must not be overlooked in women of childbearing age. This patient requires urgent resuscitation and surgical intervention.

2. **A** **Acute appendicitis.** Acute appendicitis can occur in any age group with the peak incidence occurring in young adults. The presentation varies widely with the 'classical history' being 12–24 hours of central abdominal pain localising to the right iliac fossa due to irritation of the parietal peritoneum. Abdominal tenderness is maximal over the inflamed appendix and may be atypical due to the variation in the position of the appendix. The diagnosis is based on clinical findings (i.e. facial flush, central pain moving to the right iliac fossa, rebound in the right iliac fossa), although urinalysis and inflammatory markers may be considered.

3. **C** **Crohn's disease.** Crohn's disease is frequently difficult to differentiate from acute appendicitis and is of course much rarer. However, the symptoms in Crohn's disease tend to be more insidious than in typical appendicitis. The non-specific inflammatory mediators (C-reactive protein) tend to be raised in Crohn's disease but may also be raised in appendicitis. Abdominal ultrasound, small bowel enemas and a CT scan may help to confirm the diagnosis. If doubt remains regarding the diagnosis and the patient is clinically unwell, a laparotomy should be performed.

A2.12 Intestinal obstruction

1. **B** **Adhesional small bowel obstruction.** Adhesional small bowel obstruction accounts for 90% of all small bowel obstructions, with small bowel obstructions making up 80–85% of all intestinal obstructions. Adhesions develop after all laparotomies to varying degrees, with those following appendicectomy and gynaecological procedures causing most trouble. The cardinal features of small bowel obstruction are early pain, vomiting, distension and later constipation with reduction in flatus, which then becomes absolute. The pain is usually colicky due to excessive peristalsis, but may become continuous if strangulation or perforation occurs. Vomiting is early in high small bowel obstruction, late in low bowel obstruction and delayed or absent in large bowel obstruction and may not occur at all in closed loop obstruction. Distension is usually absent in proximal small bowel obstruction, central and mild to moderate in distal small bowel obstruction, and generalised and moderate to gross in large bowel obstruction and is mostly related to gaseous distension.

2. **C** **Colonic carcinoma.** The symptoms experienced by patients with large bowel obstruction usually reflect the site of the tumour, with tumours of the ileocaecal valve presenting early with symptoms similar to those patients with lower small bowel obstruction. Obstructions due to tumours of the recto-sigmoid colon usually start with constipation-type symptoms leading to signs of obstruction. A 'closed loop obstruction' develops when large bowel obstruction develops in the presence of a competent ileocaecal valve, resulting in increasing distension of the large bowel with no back flow into the terminal ileum. Signs of right iliac fossa peritoneal irritation or a caecal diameter of >10 cm suggests that perforation is imminent or may have already occurred.

3. **E** **Gallstone ileus.** Gallstone ileus typically occurs in elderly females when a cholecystoduodenal fistula forms following an episode of cholecystitis. A large biliary calculus passes through the fistula escaping into the small bowel, usually lodging in the distal terminal ileum or at the ileocaecal valve. Occasionally the calculus can be seen on the plain abdominal radiograph, but more frequently, air is seen in the biliary tree. The obstruction is often incomplete thus making the condition more difficult to diagnose.

A2.13 Abdominal and pelvic abscess

1. **I** **Subphrenic abscess.** Subphrenic abscesses are often difficult to diagnose but are more common after upper abdominal procedures. The subphrenic space and the para-colic gutter are in direct contact, thereby allowing peritoneal contamination (e.g. bile, blood, bowel content) to spread. Direct contact causes diaphragmatic irritation resulting in a pleural effusion. An ultrasound scan is the investigation of choice as a percutaneous drainage catheter may be placed at the same time. Large cavities that fail to respond to percutaneous drainage and broad-spectrum antibiotics require open surgical drainage.

2. **A** **Anastomotic dehiscence.** Anastomotic leak presents with a spectrum of symptoms, with the clinical features being dependent on whether the leak is localised or is more extensive. Small localised leaks tend to have minor symptoms, while more extensive leaks may develop into frank peritonitis. Signs of a major leak include tachycardia, hypotension, pyrexia and abdominal pain. Contrast enemas usually confirm the diagnosis. Therefore, vigilance is required in any patient who is clinically deteriorating in the 2–3 weeks following an intestinal anastomosis. Unexplained sepsis should always raise the suspicion of an anastomotic leak. Localised leaks are treated with bowel rest and intravenous antibiotics; small abscess may be drained percutaneously. Major leaks require laparotomy and exteriorisation of the anastomosis following adequate resuscitation.

3. **D** **Pelvic abscess.** Pelvic abscesses following appendicectomy can present up to 10 days or more following the surgery. The diagnosis is confirmed with a pelvic ultrasound scan. Initially the patient may be treated with bowel rest and intravenous antibiotics. If not resolving, the abscess may be drained percutaneously. Some abscesses if left may spontaneously rupture through into the bowel or vagina in females. Patients deteriorating with conservative treatment require a formal laparotomy and drainage of the abscess.

A2.14 Gastrointestinal haemorrhage

1. **D** **Diverticular disease.** Diverticular disease accounts for approximately 50% of all lower intestinal bleeds. Diverticular bleeds result from erosion of the perforating blood vessels in the base of the diverticulum. Most patients presenting with lower intestinal bleeds are elderly, with most of these bleeds settling without any intervention. Lower intestinal bleeds are classified into mild (blood loss <20% of the circulating volume), moderate (20–40%) and massive (>40%). In mild bleeding, patients are usually observed in hospital until the bleeding stops, with a colonoscopy or barium enema and sigmoidoscopy performed as an outpatient procedure. Moderate and massive bleeds require resuscitation and may need localisation of the bleeding by gastroscopy in the case of upper gastrointestinal bleeding, colonoscopy, arteriography (Fig. 2.14.1) or radionuclide scanning.

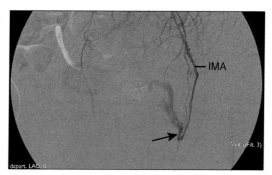

Fig. 2.14.1 A selective mesenteric angiogram showing a bleed from a branch of the inferior mesenteric artery (IMA).

2. **H** **Peptic ulcer.** Bleeding from peptic ulcers accounts for approximately 35% of upper gastrointestinal bleeds. Mucosal erosions develop commonly due to non-steroidal anti-inflammatory drugs, steroids or alcohol. Ulcers on the lesser curve of the stomach or posterior wall of the duodenum result from erosion into the left gastric and the gastroduodenal arteries respectively. Immediate management of the patient requires assessment of the airway, breathing, haemodynamic state and conscious level accompanied by rapid fluid and blood resuscitation. An urgent oesophago-gastro-duodenoscopy should be performed by a competent endoscopist. Failure to control the bleeding endoscopically requires an urgent laparotomy.

3. **F** **Oesophageal varices.** Approximately 30% of patients with liver cirrhosis die from oesophageal variceal haemorrhage. Approximately 50% of patients presenting with bleeding die on that admission. Oesophageal varices are dilated venous collaterals, which develop in the presence of portal venous hypertension in liver cirrhosis. Immediate management of the patient requires assessment of the airway, breathing, haemodynamic state and conscious level followed by rapid fluid and blood transfusion resuscitation. These patients, in addition to blood transfusion, require fresh frozen plasma, platelets and vitamin K. If bleeding is severe, a Sengtaken-Blakemore tube can be passed to achieve haemostatic tamponade in the lower oesophagus. An urgent oesophago-gastro-duodenoscopy should be performed by a competent endoscopist to attempt sclerotherapy or banding of the varices.

A2.15 Groin hernia repair

1. **G** **Tension-free prosthetic mesh repair.** Indirect inguinal hernias may be difficult to differentiate from direct inguinal hernias clinically. An indirect hernia travels along the spermatic cord, while a direct hernia comes directly forward from the posterior wall of the inguinal canal. The male to female ratio is 10:1 with 65% being indirect. Because of the risk of strangulation, it is sensible to advise repair of all inguinal hernias in

patients fit for the operation. Direct inguinal hernias with wide necks may be treated conservatively in elderly patients if relatively asymptomatic. Most surgeons in the UK now advocate the tension-free prosthetic mesh repair described by Lichtenstein. Initially a herniotomy of the indirect sac (if present) is performed then a synthetic mesh, cut to shape, is placed underneath the cord and sutured in place. The recurrence rate for this procedure has been reported to be as low as 0.77%. See 3.42 Inguinal hernia and 4.47 Inguinal hernia.

2. **C High approach.** Femoral hernias are the third most common hernia with a male to female ratio of 1:4, with the hernia occurring most frequently in elderly multiparous women. All femoral hernias should be repaired as 40% are strangulated on first presentation. Erythema of the overlying skin occurs in strangulation and is a sign of poor outcome. Several operative approaches have been described (low, inguinal and high approach) in the repair of femoral hernias. However, the low and inguinal approaches are only suited to elective repair. In the emergency situation, a small bowel resection may be required and therefore the high (McEvedy) approach is advocated. A vertical or transverse incision is made over the hernia with the rectus muscle being retracted medially, the preperitoneal space is entered by dividing the transversalis fascia. The femoral sac is reduced and the contents inspected. The defect is repaired with a non-absorbable suture or a synthetic mesh plug. See 3.43 Femoral hernia.

3. **B Herniotomy.** Congenital inguinal hernias have an incidence of 1–5% with the incidence being higher in infants born prematurely. The male to female ratio is up to 10:1 with the right side being more often involved. Herniotomy is performed as an early elective procedure because of the high risk of incarceration (12%). A groin crease incision is deepened until the inguinal ligament is identified and followed medially until the spermatic cord is seen at the external ring. The patent processus is separated from the rest of the cord and divided when the surgeon has insured that it is empty. The proximal end is then ligated close to the internal ring. Incarcerated hernias are reduced under sedation if there are no signs of gangrene followed by a herniotomy 24–48 hours later. Failure to reduce an incarcerated hernia is an indication for immediate surgery.

A2.16 Intestinal fistulas

1. **H Vesicocolic.** A vesicocolic fistula is an abnormal communication between the urinary bladder and the colon, which develops in association with diverticular disease, adenocarcinoma of the colon or inflammatory bowel disease. Diverticular disease is the most common cause of vesicocolic fistula due to an inflamed sigmoid diverticulum abutting the bladder, although fistulisation may occur with any adjacent hollow organ and an inflamed diverticulum. The typical symptoms are of urinary tract infection, pneumaturia and occasional debris in the urine.

Rhabdomyocytes on urinalysis is pathognomonic. A barium enema or CT is performed to exclude a malignant cause and to determine the site of communication. The treatment of choice is resection of the affected portion of the colon with anastomosis, with primary closure of the bladder and the placement of omentum between the bladder and colon (Fig. 2.16.1).

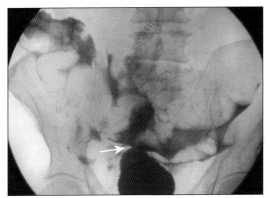

Fig. 2.16.1 Cystogram showing a leak of contrast from the bladder following repair of a vesicocolic fistula.

2. **C** **Enterocutaneous.** A postoperative enterocutaneous fistula is a communication between the bowel and the body wall. Predisposing factors include poor surgical technique, devascularisation, obstruction distal to the anastomosis or persistence of the original disease, e.g. Crohn's, carcinoma. Initially pus and often flatus discharge from the wound followed by intestinal contents. The quantity of discharge is related to the site of fistula with high output >500 ml/day (proximal small bowel) and low output <500 ml/day (distal small bowel). Postoperative fistulas often close spontaneously with conservative measures, provided there is no distal obstruction.

3. **D** **Enterocolic.** Enteric fistulas may affect patients with Crohn's disease, with approximately 40% being entero-enteric or enterocolic, occurring spontaneously or in the postoperative period. An enterocolic fistula usually presents with diarrhoea due to the large volume of small bowel contents passing directly into the colon. The degree of symptoms depends on the level of the small bowel and colon affected. The diagnosis is confirmed with a contrast study or CT scan. Enterocolic fistulas have an associated abscess in 60% of cases. The treatment of choice is en-bloc resection of the diseased or damaged bowel and the fistula tract with primary anastomosis.

A2.17 Gastrointestinal stomas

1. **D** **Mucous fistula.** In the emergency situation when the sigmoid colon has been resected (diverticular perforation, strangulated sigmoid volvulus) the proximal end colostomy is formed in the left iliac fossa, which

leaves enough distal bowel length to form a separate mucous fistula that can be sited in the lower end of the midline abdominal wound. It is rarely possible to form a mucous fistula after sigmoid colectomy performed for cancer as an adequate clearance distally usually renders the distal stump too short to be brought out through the wound.

2. **C Loop ileostomy.** The risk of leak from a low rectal anastomosis can be more than 20%, when assessed by clinical signs, colonoscopy or contrast enema. Therefore, most surgeons advocate a proximal stoma to divert the faecal stream until healing is confirmed. The choice lies between a loop transverse colostomy and a loop ileostomy. Loop transverse colostomies are sited in the right upper quadrant and therefore are unsightly and difficult to manage for the patient. They are also bulky and prone to prolapse. Loop ileostomies on the other hand are easier to construct in the right iliac fossa without tension and do not jeopardise the blood supply to the anastomosis. Loop ileostomies are usually reversed within 6 months depending on the health and wishes of the patient and the need for adjuvant therapy. More complications occur with the closure of ileostomies compared with colostomies.

3. **F Percutaneous endoscopic gastrostomy.** Percutaneous endoscopic gastrostomy (PEG) is the preferred method for long-term feeding in patients unable to swallow. In addition, it is also the optimal method for chronic gastric decompression. A number of commercially available PEG systems can be used. All combine a percutaneous cannula insertion under direct endoscopic vision. A wire loop connected to a thick suture is passed through the cannula, which is then grabbed by a polypectomy snare passed down the endoscope. The endoscope and snared wire are then removed, the suture is then pulled out of the patient's mouth and tied to the gastrostomy and is then pulled back through the patients abdominal wall by the assistant. The tube is then secured to the abdominal wall by an external bolster.

A2.18 Oesophageal disorders

1. **B Gastro-oesophageal reflux disease.** The physiological function of the lower oesophageal sphincter relates to its resting tone, the length of the intra-abdominal oesophagus, crural muscle of the diaphragm and the angle of insertion of the oesophagus into the stomach. Gastro-oesophageal reflux results from a transient or a persistently low resting tone of the lower oesophageal sphincter. The condition may or may not be associated with a hiatus hernia. Oesophagoscopy is required to assess the oesophageal mucosa while contrast studies may demonstrate reflux. Twenty-four hour pH studies and manometry are also required to allow for correlation with symptoms. Medical treatment consists of weight loss, cessation of smoking and avoidance of certain foods, followed by H_2 receptor antagonists or proton pump inhibitors. Surgical intervention is indicated when there has been a failure of medical therapy. Most anti-reflux surgery takes the form of a fundoplication undertaken

open or by minimally invasive approaches, where the proximal stomach is wrapped around the distal oesophagus.

2. **A** **Achalasia.** Achalasia results from defective peristalsis and failure of the lower oesophageal sphincter to relax. The condition is progressive, leading to gradual dilatation of the oesophagus above the sphincter. Achalasia can occur at any age but is most common in the third to fifth decade with an equal male to female ratio. Oesophagoscopy is necessary to exclude a carcinoma. A barium swallow may show a very dilated proximal oesophagus containing food matter, abnormal peristalsis and a functional obstruction at the lower oesophagus giving a 'birds beak' appearance. Manometry confirms failure of the lower oesophageal sphincter to relax. Treatment consists of medical therapy (nitrates, calcium channel blockers, anticholinergics), endoscopic balloon dilatation or surgical division of the lower oesophageal sphincter (Heller's cardiomyotomy).

3. **C** **Oesophageal carcinoma.** Oesophageal carcinoma occurs most frequently in the sixth to eighth decade with a male to female ratio of 5:1 in the UK. Risk factors include excessive alcohol, smoking and gastro-oesophageal reflux. A columnar-lining of the distal oesophagus (Barrett's oesophagus) is seen in 10% of patients with gastro-oesophageal reflux. The prevalence of adenocarcinoma in patients with Barrett's is 15%. Squamous carcinoma of the oesophagus is seen more frequently in southern Africa and China and is probably related to dietary factors. Oesophagoscopy and biopsy confirms the diagnosis, with a CT of the thorax and abdomen performed to stage the disease. Oesophagectomy is performed for cancers which have not invaded locally. The 5-year survival depends on the stage at presentation, location of the tumour (cervical, mid or lower oesophagus) and type of treatment (extent of surgery, use of radiotherapy or chemotherapy). The overall 5-year survival in most series is 22–32%.

A2.19 Carcinoma of the stomach

1. **E** **Total gastrectomy and lymphadenectomy.** Surgical resection with curative intent is the mainstay of gastric surgery: adequate surgical resection with an 8–10 cm clearance proximally and distally in the unstretched stomach. Therefore, centrally placed or large tumours usually require total gastrectomy to adequately clear the primary disease. The distal oesophagus is anastomosed to a loop or pouch of proximal jejunum. The extent of lymphadenectomy remains controversial. A lymphadenectomy of the perigastric nodes is performed routinely with a total gastrectomy. The role of a more extensive lymphadenectomy is not clear and it probably does not improve survival.

2. **D** **Oesophagogastrectomy.** Cancers at the region of the oesophagastric junction require a partial oesophageal resection plus resection of the proximal two-thirds of stomach. Oesophagogastrectomy requires

intrathoracic exposure of the oesophagus by a left-sided thoraco-abdominal incision or the preferred combination of an upper abdominal incision and a posterior right sided thoracotomy (Ivor–Lewis procedure). The distal oesophagus is anastomosed to the antrum of the stomach.

3. **C Gastro-enteric bypass.** A gastric outlet obstruction results from obstruction of the pylorus by scarring secondary to peptic ulceration or by an obstructing carcinoma. This patient is likely to have advanced malignant disease and is unlikely to withstand a major resection. The obstruction can be relieved by a gastrojejunostomy, which provides good palliation. Endoscopic stenting is an option if available. Palliative bypass procedures do not increase survival times.

A2.20 Jaundice

1. **D Increased bilirubin load.** Major incompatibility reactions are rare, even with emergency cross matching. Incompatibility reactions are most likely to occur when blood has been stored improperly or when the patient has had repeated transfusions. In this case, haemolysis results in an excess of unconjugated bilirubin, i.e. bilirubin which is not bound to serum albumin. Haemolytic jaundice tends to be mild with bilirubin levels <85 mmol/litre. In haemolytic jaundice, urinalysis shows no bilirubin in the urine although it contains excess urobilinogen because excess bilirubin reaches the intestine and is re-excreted as urobilinogen. A normal reticulocyte count virtually excludes haemolytic jaundice.

2. **B Disturbed bilirubin uptake.** Disturbed bilirubin uptake and reduced conjugation of bilirubin is seen in generalised liver cell disease (e.g. cirrhosis or viral hepatitis). The jaundice in generalised liver cell disease can be mild, moderate or severe. Urinalysis usually shows high levels of conjugated bilirubin, appearing secondary to the biliary stasis. The serum transaminases are elevated. Hepatitis serology should be performed. An abdominal ultrasound scan usually confirms a cirrhotic liver; if there is any doubt, a liver biopsy should be performed when the coagulopathy, if any has been corrected.

3. **A Disturbed bilirubin excretion.** Disturbed bilirubin excretion can result from intrahepatic (without mechanical obstruction) or extrahepatic cholestasis (mechanical obstruction). In this case, it is most likely that a biliary calculus has become lodged in the common bile duct. However, in this age group a cholangiocarcinoma or a carcinoma of the head of the pancreas needs to be excluded. Serum bilirubin tends to be higher in obstructive jaundice. Urinalysis reveals high levels of bilirubin and an absence of urobilinogen because no bilirubin reaches the gut due to the obstruction of the common bile duct and therefore cannot be re-absorbed and re-excreted. An ultrasound scan confirms an obstructed dilated common bile duct proximal to the obstruction ± intrahepatic duct dilatation. If there is any doubt, a CT scan should be performed to exclude malignancy.

A2.21 Acute pancreatitis

1. **A Glasgow–Imrie score = 0.** The original Glasgow score had age as one of the criteria but not the aminotransferases. The modified Glasgow criteria did not include age but included the aminotransferases. The following cut-off thresholds are used for the criteria, each given a score of one if present. Age >55 years, white blood cell count >15 × 10^9/litre, glucose >10 mmol/litre, urea >16 mmol/litre, PaO$_2$ <7.8 kPa, calcium <2 mmol/litre, albumin <32 g/litre, lactate dehydrogenase >600 U/litre, aspartate/alanine aminotransferase >100 U/litre. Following resuscitation, patients should be categorised into either mild or severe disease. A score of 0 or 1 is considered to be mild. These patients are treated with oxygen therapy, intravenous fluid, bowel rest and analgesia and are observed for signs of deterioration. Even patients with mild disease require rigorous intravenous fluid infusion to replace sequestration into the retroperitoneal space. In general, patients with mild acute pancreatitis improve spontaneously. Following resolution of symptoms therapy is aimed at identifying the aetiology and treatment, e.g. cholecystectomy for gallstone pancreatitis.

2. **C Glasgow–Imrie score = 2.** A Glasgow–Imrie score of 2 is stratified as acute pancreatitis. In addition to oxygen therapy, intravenous fluid, bowel rest and analgesia the patient needs to be moved to the high dependency unit as this patient is at high risk of deterioration. The patient should have a urinary catheter and central venous line placed for more accurate fluid replacement. Correction of biochemical abnormalities (hyperglycaemia, hypocalcaemia) is also usually required. Thromboprophylaxis and H$_2$ receptor antagonists should also be started as the patient is at risk of a thromboembolic episode and stress ulceration.

3. **D Glasgow–Imrie score = 3.** A Glasgow–Imrie score of 3 is stratified as severe acute pancreatitis. In addition to the measures listed above, the patient also needs to be transferred to the intensive care unit as she is developing three organ failure (cardiovascular, respiratory and renal) and requires organ support. Patients with severe acute pancreatitis have a mortality rate of approximately 30% with the rate increasing with the number of organs failing. Patients with severe acute pancreatitis are also at risk of developing pancreatic necrosis determined by triple phase contrast CT, therefore the use of prophylactic antibiotics in patients with severe acute pancreatitis is advocated.

A2.22 Chronic pancreatitis

1. **E Exocrine insufficiency.** Chronic pancreatitis is more common when the aetiology of the pancreatitis is alcohol. With repeated attacks of pancreatitis, the pancreas becomes atrophic and fibrotic which results in a reduction in the exocrine and endocrine function. Due to the large exocrine reserve of the pancreas, only 10% of patients with chronic pancreatitis develop steatorrhoea, i.e. offensive, pale, frothy stools,

which are difficult to flush away. Steatorrhoea may be exacerbated by a diet high in fat. Exocrine insufficiency is treated with pancreatic supplements which are supplied in enteric-coated capsules and which are swallowed when eating a meal. Patients with chronic pancreatitis are at risk of pancreatic failure, which presents clinically as gradual weight loss, anorexia, anaemia, exocrine and endocrine insufficiency and which in the most severe cases can lead to malnutrition and death.

2. **G Pancreatic pseudocyst.** Small peripancreatic effusions are common after an attack of acute pancreatitis, with most being reabsorbed spontaneously. Pseudocysts are so-called because they have a wall of granulation tissue which develops from a peripancreatic collection and not an epithelial lining as in a true cyst. Smaller cysts <6 cm usually resolve spontaneously while larger cysts form a thick wall, which can be drained percutaneously, or trans-gastrically using an endoscopic approach. Occasionally, a large cyst may require a cystogastrostomy or cystojejunostomy at open surgery. Open surgery should be delayed by 4–6 weeks to allow the cyst wall to mature.

3. **C Duodenal obstruction.** In chronic pancreatitis, obstruction of adjacent organs can occur due to fibrosis or due to peripancreatic collections. Compression of the second part of the duodenum can be so great as to cause a gastric outlet obstruction. If the obstruction is above the papilla, which it usually is jaundice will not be observed. The gastric outlet obstruction is treated by forming a gastrojejunostomy. The lower common bile duct running through the head of the pancreas is particularly vulnerable to compression. Common bile duct obstruction is treated with a stent placed at endoscopic retrograde cholangiopancreatography.

A2.23 Diseases of the biliary tract

1. **G Mirizzi syndrome.** Mirizzi syndrome is an obstruction of the common bile duct by a large gallbladder calculus in Hartmann's pouch pressing on (type I) or actually eroding (type II) into the common bile duct or as a result of adjacent inflammation of the gallbladder in cholecystitis. If the stone ulcerates into the common bile duct, it forms a cholecystocholedochal fistula. Treatment is by either open or laparoscopic cholecystectomy, common bile duct exploration and placement of a T-tube.

2. **F Iatrogenic.** Bile duct trauma may be recognised at the time of operation when one of the main ducts is damaged, accidentally ligated or completely transected. Frequently, the injury is not noted at the time of surgery and is identified in the early postoperative period when there is a persistent or increasing discharge in the drain or from the wound. Rapidly developing jaundice in the early postoperative period implies a ligated duct, usually the right hepatic. A bile duct injury may present in the late postoperative period with intermittent or progressive

jaundice, often associated with cholangitis. Iatrogenic bile duct injury is a potentially catastrophic complication. If identified at the time of the initial surgery the proximal common hepatic duct can be anastomosed onto a loop of jejunum (Roux-en Y loop).

3. **D** **Cholangiocarcinoma.** Cholangiocarcinoma is an uncommon tumour that can occur anywhere in the biliary tree. Most commonly, the bifurcation of the hepatic duct is involved (Klatskin tumour) with tumours of the distal common bile duct being the next most common. Surgical resection should be offered if appropriate as it produces the best long-term chance of survival. However, at presentation, more than 50% of patients have locally advanced disease or metastases. Palliative surgery in the form of cholecystectomy ± anastomosis of the hepatic duct to a loop of jejunum (hepaticojejunostomy) is offered to prevent acute cholecystitis. A biliary stent is placed to overcome the biliary obstruction and to prevent cholangitis.

A2.24 Portal hypertension and ascites

1. **E** **Intrahepatic portal hypertension.** Portal hypertension is defined as an increase in portal vein pressure of more than 10 mmHg (normal 5–10 mmHg). Portal hypertension has many different causes with liver cirrhosis accounting for 90% of cases in the UK. Classification is by site of obstruction, i.e. presinusoidal (absence of liver disease), sinusoidal (hepatocellular disease) and post-sinusoidal (may develop secondary hepatocellular disease). Portal hypertension is due to increased resistance to blood flow (classified into prehepatic, hepatic or posthepatic causes) or due to increased blood flow (e.g. increased splenic flow). Irrespective of the cause collateral channels develop between the portal and systemic circulation with oesophageal varices (oesophageal and gastric venous plexus to the splenic vein) being the most important clinically. Prognosis depends on the remaining hepatic reserves with 40% of patients dying from bleeding oesophageal varices.

2. **F** **Portal vein thrombosis.** Portal vein thrombosis is uncommon in adults but is the most common cause of portal hypertension in children. In adults portal vein thrombosis can result from abdominal sepsis, hypercoagulable states, chronic pancreatitis or cancer. In children, it can occur secondary to neonatal sepsis or umbilical vein catheterisation. The condition usually goes unnoticed for several years, where it presents with variceal bleeding, splenomegaly or pancytopenia. Liver function tests are usually normal and the diagnosis is confirmed by mesenteric angiography. A portosystemic shunt may be required when symptoms are severe.

3. **G** **Transudative ascites.** Traditionally, ascites has been classed as being either transudative or exudative, however some authors argue that a more precise classification is portal hypertensive and non-portal hypertensive. Ascites develops when there is flow of fluid from the

vascular space due to an excess of total body sodium (transudation) or when there is exudation of fluid through infection or peritoneal metastases. Liver cirrhosis accounts for 80% of the patients presenting in the UK with ascites. Alteration of renal function resulting in sodium retention occurs early in liver cirrhosis. In addition to sodium retention, portal venous hypertension in liver cirrhosis also causes transudation of fluid due to the increased filtration pressures linked to a decreased oncotic pressure due to hypoalbuminaemia. Needle paracentesis is performed to ascertain the level of protein: <25 g/litre (transudative), >25 g/litre (exudative). Management is aimed at treating the underlying cause. Salt restriction and diuretics (spironolactone) are also employed. In refractory cases, a transjugular intrahepatic portosystemic shunt (TIPS) or peritoneovenous shunt may be employed.

A2.25 Surgical disorders of the colon and rectum

1. **A** **Extended right hemicolectomy.** Radical surgical excision of a colonic tumour is the only advisable treatment in a patient who does not have advanced disseminated disease. The segment of colon containing the tumour is resected along with the appropriate vascular pedicle(s) and accompanying lymphatic drainage. Tumours of the caecum and ascending colon are treated by means of a right hemicolectomy and ligation of the ileocolic and right colic pedicles. Transverse colectomy is associated with a high rate of anastomotic leakage and therefore tumours of the proximal transverse colon are treated by means of extended right hemicolectomy, i.e. division of the ileocolic, right colic, middle colic ± ascending branch of the left colic. The bowel is divided proximally at the terminal ileum and distally across the descending/sigmoid colon, where the blood supply is plentiful, based on the inferior mesenteric and its branches. The bowel is then anastomosed using staples or a hand-sewn technique. See 3.50 Colectomy.

2. **B** **Left hemicolectomy.** Radical surgical excision of a sigmoid tumour requires ligation of the left colic pedicle, i.e. ligation of the inferior mesenteric artery at its origin from the aorta. This in turn devascularises the distal descending colon, necessitating resection of the descending and sigmoid colon. The operation is performed with the patient in the Lloyd–Davies position and requires mobilisation of the splenic flexure to allow for a tension-free colorectal anastomosis. Care should be taken when performing the dissection as the ureter and spleen is at risk. Most frequently, the anastomosis is performed using a circular anastomosing stapler to achieve a true end-to-end anastomosis.

3. **F** **Total mesorectal excision.** Patients with early rectal cancers may be treated by transanal local excision, although this is controversial. Tumours which have advanced to or through the bowel wall require a radical excision. Most surgeons now advocate a total mesorectal excision in conjunction with a low anterior or abdominoperineal resection as

the optimal treatment for mid- and low rectal tumours. This technique involves removal of the entire rectal mesentery to 5 cm below the tumour. The operation also requires mobilisation of the sigmoid and descending colon following identification of the ureters. In an anterior resection a low end-to-end anastomosis is performed, facilitated by a circular stapler passed transanally. Because of an anastomotic leak rate of up to 20%, most surgeons form a temporary proximal stoma (loop ileostomy) to allow the distal anastomosis to heal and minimises the effects of an anastomotic leak. In abdominoperineal resection, the colon is taken out in the left iliac fossa as an end colostomy, while the remaining anus is excised with the tumour-bearing specimen through the perineum. Rectal surgery should aim to remove all local disease, preserve continence, restore reasonable bowel frequency and to avoid permanent urinary and sexual dysfunction. See 3.52 Rectol surgery.

A2.26 Perianal disorders

1. **E** **Haemorrhoids.** Haemorrhoids relate to an abnormality of the vascular cushions of the anus. The three vascular cushions prevent incontinence of flatus and liquid. Degeneration of the supporting fibrous tissue and smooth muscle results in prolapse and the symptoms of haemorrhoids. Aetiological causes are unclear. Haemorrhoids may be complicated by thrombosis and acutely painful prolapse. Grading is clinical into bleeding alone (first degree), prolapse that spontaneously reduce (second degree), prolapse requiring reduction (third degree) and irreducible (fourth degree). Patients require proctoscopy to assess the anorectum and a minimum of a rigid sigmoidoscopy to assess the rectum. Assessment of the rest of the colon is necessary if there are any atypical features. Treatment may be conservative, injection sclerotherapy (bleeding haemorrhoids), rubber band ligation (prolapsing haemorrhoids) and operative (symptomatic external haemorrhoids). See 3.53 Haemorrhoids.

2. **B** **Anal fissure.** An anal fissure is a linear ulcer below the dentate line. They are divided into primary (not related to an underlying condition) or secondary to another condition, e.g. Crohn's disease. Anal fissures are related to a high resting tone of the internal anal sphincter. The high resting tone is thought to reduce perfusion of the anal mucosa. Fissures occur most frequently in the posterior midline ('6 o'clock position') in men and both the anterior and posterior midline in women. Proctoscopy and sigmoidoscopy ± biopsy are required to exclude other underlying pathologies. Usually these investigations are too painful and are performed under general anaesthetic. Treatment is initially with stool softeners. Topical smooth muscle dilators (nitrates, calcium channel blockers) reduce the resting tone of the sphincter and result in effective treatment in 50–70% of all fissures. Lateral internal sphincterotomy is reserved for patients refractory to medical treatment, but has a greater risk of incontinence.

3. **A** **Anal carcinoma.** Squamous carcinoma accounts for 80% of anal cancers. The incidence is particularly high in the male homosexual population. Human papilloma viruses 16, 18, 31 and 33 have been implicated. Anal tumours tend to spread proximally and therefore tend to be confused as a rectal cancer. Lymph node spread is common at presentation with spread initially to the peri-rectal nodes and thereafter to the inguinal, haemorrhoidal and lateral pelvic groups of lymph nodes. Local invasion into the sphincters can result in faecal incontinence. Patients are investigated by endoanal ultrasound and an examination under anaesthetic with biopsy. Treatment is chemo-radiotherapy with abdominoperineal resection reserved for refractory disease, recurrence or faecal incontinence.

A2.27 Common breast disorders

1. **E** **Fibrocystic disease.** Breast cysts are one of the most common causes of referral to the breast clinic. They are considered to be an aberration of normal development and involution (ANDI), with a prevalence of 7%. Cysts are classically seen in perimenopausal women. However, they may be seen in younger women, and older women on hormone replacement treatment. Cysts may be single or multiple. Patients report that cysts appear suddenly and are frequently uncomfortable. Cysts may be visible through the skin. They have a degree of mobility which is less than fibroadenomas. The diagnosis is confirmed by aspiration. Cystic fluid varies in colour from pale yellow to black. Cysts are divided into type according to the ratio of sodium and potassium within the cyst fluid. Sodium/potassium ratio >3 (have a low tendency to recur, no proven cancer link) <3 (apocrine origin, moderate tendency to recur, may have a loose association with breast cancer). Cystic fluid should be sent for cytology if blood stained to exclude ductal carcinoma. Mammogram/ultrasound should be performed with follow up if doubt remains over the diagnosis.

2. **D** **Fibroadenoma.** Fibroadenomas are benign tumours originating from the breast lobule and show proliferation of both epithelium and connective tissue and are another form of ANDI. They are considered to be an aberration of lobular development. Fibroadenomas are either classified into simple or giant. Simple fibroadenomas present in young women and, with the exception of those near the nipple, are very mobile; thus the term 'breast mouse' is often used. The diagnosis is confirmed by triple assessment (1) clinical, (2) radiological (ultrasound scan) and (3) cytological/histological (fine needle aspiration, core biopsy), although clinical diagnosis with adequate follow-up may be sufficient in women up to 25 years of age. The natural history is for the fibroadenoma to increase in size over 6–12 months, remain static in size with one-third regressing after 5 years. Surgical excision is no longer recommended unless requested by the patient. See 4.12 Fibroadenoma.

3. **A** **Carcinoma.** Breast cancer is the most common cause of malignancy in women in the UK. Risk factors include a previous breast cancer, nulliparity or first pregnancy after the age of 30 years, late menopause, early menarche, first degree level of breast cancer, prolonged exposure to oestrogen (oral contraceptive and hormone replacement therapy). Invasive ductal carcinoma accounts for 80% of breast cancers. Ductal carcinoma develops in a stepwise fashion from ductal hyperplasia to ductal atypia and on to ductal carcinoma *in situ* (DCIS). Grading of breast tumours is based on the resemblance to normal breast tissue (differentiation). The breast screening programme has resulted in more breast cancers being picked up at the non-invasive stage. The diagnosis and stage is confirmed by triple assessments. Staging can be classified using the TNM system. Prognosis may be predicted by the Nottingham prognostic index (G + N + 0.2 S – tumour grade 'G' is scored as 1, 2 or 3 and lymph node status 'N' scored 1, 2 or 3 and the tumour size is measured in centimetres). Surgical excision of early breast cancer takes the form of tumour excision with a 1 cm margin of surrounding normal breast tissue (wide local excision), simple mastectomy (removal of breast tissue and nipple-areolar complex). Axillary surgery is necessary to accurately stage the disease, this traditionally took the form of axillary node clearance but is being superseded by selective node sampling (sentinel node biopsy). See 3.31 Breast disorders and surgical anatomy; 3.54 Malignant breast lumps.

A2.28 Surgery of the thyroid gland

1. **E** **Thyroid lobectomy.** Papillary carcinoma accounts for 50–60% of all thyroid tumours. Approximately 85% of papillary carcinomas are considered low risk, as they are usually small primary lesions occurring in young adults, well-differentiated with no metastases. The remaining 15% are considered high risk, as they are usually large primary tumours occurring in older patients, poorly-differentiated, locally invasive with distant metastases. Patients at low risk are therefore treated with total lobectomy and isthmusectomy. Postoperatively, the patient undergoes life-long thyroxine suppression, i.e. the TSH is maintained below 0.1 mU/ litre. Total thyroidectomy is reserved for high-risk patients.

2. **A** **Isthmusectomy.** Anaplastic carcinoma accounts for 10–15% of all thyroid tumours. They frequently affect the elderly with females affected more frequently than males. The tumour grows rapidly with early invasion into local structures. Histology shows few or no differentiated structures. Death occurs within 1 year in 90% of patients. Surgery has usually little to offer these patients, as the tumour rapidly fungates through the wound. However, pressure on the trachea can be relieved by isthmusectomy.

3. **D** **Total thyroidectomy.** Hyperthyroidism results from diffuse toxic goitre (Graves' disease), hyperfunctioning adenomas or multinodular goitres (Plummer's disease). Graves' disease is an autoimmune condition in which immunoglobulins activate thyroid-stimulating hormone receptors on the thyroid cell membrane. Graves' disease has a male to female ratio of 1:10 and is most common in the second to fourth decades. Clinical features include weight loss despite a good appetite, preference for cool environments, sweating and tremors. Signs occur in the eyes (lid lag, proptosis, paresis of the extraocular muscles), cardiovascular system (sinus tachycardia, atrial fibrillation) and skin (increased pigmentation, thyroid acropathy, palmar erythema, pretibial myxoedema). Cardiovascular symptoms are more common in Plummer's disease whereas central nervous system symptoms are more common in Graves' disease. Treatment is medical or surgical. Carbimazole is administered with thyroxine until the patient has been rendered euthyroid and is reduced and stopped slowly. Relapse occurs in 50–60% of patients, with 15% suffering drug related reactions. Radioactive iodine is slow to act and leaves 40% of patients hypothyroid at 10 years. Surgery has the advantage of working immediately with a low recurrence rate. Disadvantages include recurrent and external laryngeal nerve injury. Prior to surgery, the patient is required to be euthyroid (2 weeks of carbimazole or propylthiouracil) with β-adrenergic blockade (propranolol). A total thyroidectomy is performed and the patient commenced on thyroxine postoperatively. See 4.14 Multinodular goitre.

A2.29 Parathyroid disorders

1. **E** **Primary hyperparathyroidism.** Hyperparathyroidism results from the excess production of PTH and is primary (adenoma of a single parathyroid 80%; hyperplasia of two or more parathyroids 10–15%; parathyroid carcinoma 1%), secondary (prolonged hypocalcaemia, e.g. chronic renal failure) or tertiary (seen in patients with long standing secondary hyperparathyroidism who undergo dialysis/renal transplantation, parathyroids act autonomously resulting in raised calcium and PTH). Primary hyperparathyroidism has a male to female ratio of 1:2 with an incidence of 0.01–0.02% increasing with age. The clinical features of 'painful bones, stones, abdominal groans and psychic moans' result from hypercalcaemia. Hypercalcaemia can also result from metastatic bone disease and myeloma and needs to be excluded by measuring PTH. Surgery is indicated even in asymptomatic patients as hypercalcaemia predisposes to atherosclerotic heart disease and stroke.

2. **A** **Multiple Endocrine Neoplasia I.** The multiple endocrine neoplasia syndromes are characterised by tumours involving two or more endocrine glands. Their inheritance is autosomal-dominant or sporadic. MEN I is characterised by anterior pituitary adenoma, pancreatic tumours (gastrinomas, insulinomas) and parathyroid hyperplasia.

3. **B** **Multiple Endocrine Neoplasia IIa.** Multiple Endocrine Neoplasia II describes the association of medullary thyroid carcinoma, phaeochromocytomas and parathyroid tumours. MEN II is subdivided into IIa,

IIb and medullary thyroid carcinoma only. MEN IIa is the most common variant with parathyroid disease commonly following the development of medullary thyroid cancer, 50% of patients develop phaeochromocytomas (i.e. MEN IIa: 100% medullary thyroid carcinoma, 50% phaeochromocytomas and less than 10% have mild hyperparathyroidism). MEN IIb is characterised by MEN IIa plus Marfanoid features and mucosal neuromas. In MEN IIb, the medullary cancer is very aggressive with most patients dying before developing either a phaeochromocytoma or hyperparathyroidism. The genetic mutation should be identified and all family members tested (following counselling).

A2.30 Adrenal disorders and secondary hypertension

1. **B** **Adrenocortical hyperfunction.** Adrenocortical hyperfunction (Cushing's syndrome) results from an increased circulating level of glucocorticoids. The most common cause is iatrogenic (therapeutic steroids), with the second most common cause being microadenomas of the anterior pituitary gland. Other causes include ectopic ACTH secretion (small cell carcinoma of the lung) and adrenal causes (adenoma, hyperplasia, carcinoma). Complications include fractures secondary to osteoporosis. Initially, a 24-hour urinary free cortisol measurement is performed, if elevated a low-dose dexamethasone suppression test is performed with the diagnosis confirmed by failure to suppress the free cortisol. ACTH assay and a CT scan is performed to confirm the origin. Treatment is aimed at the source, e.g. adrenalectomy, trans-sphenoidal microsurgical adenoma excision.

2. **H** **Primary aldosteronism.** Primary aldosteronism (Conn's syndrome) results from excessive autonomous secretion of aldosterone by an adrenal cortex adenoma (85%) or by bilateral hyperplasia (15%) of the zona glomerulosa. Aldosterone causes the retention of sodium in exchange for potassium and hydrogen ions in the distal nephron. Therefore, raised levels of aldosterone results in hypokalaemia and hypertension due to intravascular fluid retention secondary to sodium retention. Primary aldosteronism needs to be distinguished from hypertension treated with loop or thiazide diuretics, and renin-induced secondary hypertension secondary to renovascular disease. The diagnosis is confirmed by elevated plasma aldosterone level, which is not suppressed by a saline infusion. Treatment is with spironolactone (a specific antagonist to aldosterone). Unilateral adrenalectomy is performed for adenomas.

3. **F** **Phaeochromocytoma.** Phaeochromocytomas are uncommon tumours of the chromaffin cells of the sympathetic nervous system, which secrete excessive quantities of catecholamines into the circulation. They are an important cause of treatable hypertension. They occur most frequently between the third and sixth decades with an equal male to female ratio. They can arise anywhere along the distribution of neural crest-derived sympathetic/adrenal system with 90% in the adrenal

medulla. Approximately 10% are bilateral, malignant or extra-adrenal. Symptoms can be episodic or paroxysmal. Metanephrines and vanillyl-mandelic acid are the major breakdown products of catecholamines and are therefore screened for in the urine passed in 24 hours. The diagnosis is confirmed by elevated plasma catecholamines. CT, MR and MIBG scans are used to localise the tumour. Preoperatively, the patient requires an α-adrenergic blockade with phenoxybenzamine for at least 2 weeks followed by a β-adrenergic blockade for those who develop a reflex tachycardia.

A2.31 Endocrine disorders of the pancreas

1. **E** **Insulinoma.** Insulinomas are the most common pancreatic islet cell tumours. Pancreatic islet cell tumours are considered to be functioning (symptomatic) or non-functioning (asymptomatic). With the exception of insulinomas, islet cell tumours are usually malignant. Insulinomas have symptoms related to hypoglycaemia. They are generally small, solitary, benign tumours located within the pancreas. Some 5–10% may occur as part of the MEN I syndrome. The diagnosis should be considered if there is a raised serum insulin or raised C-peptide and a reduced serum glucose. The diagnosis is confirmed by fasting the patient for 72 hours, with the serum glucose and insulin measured every 6 hours. Patients with insulinomas usually become symptomatic within 12–24 hours. CT is performed to exclude metastases. Due to the malignant potential, all insulinomas should be resected by enucleation or partial pancreatectomy.

2. **C** **Gastrinoma.** Of patients with gastrinomas, 90% develop peptic ulceration. They may occur as part of Zollinger–Ellison syndrome (peptic ulceration, gastric acid hypersecretion and an islet cell tumour of the pancreas). Approximately 20% of patients with Zollinger–Ellison have MEN I. Sporadic Zollinger–Ellison occurs most frequently in the fifth decade of life. Patients with Zollinger–Ellison and MEN I tend to present in the third decade. There is a male to female ratio of 2:1. An elevated basal gastric acid output >15 mEq/hour and a serum gastrin >1000 pg/ml are diagnostic of a gastrinoma. For equivocal results, a secretin stimulation test is required. Gastrinomas are frequently malignant and may be extrahepatic. Lesions are localised by somatostatin-receptor scintography with a CT being performed to exclude metastases. Gastrinomas are treated with high dose proton pump inhibitors to alleviate symptoms. Surgical resection is performed aided by intraoperative ultrasound and intraoperative endoscopy.

3. **D** **Glucagonoma.** Glucagonoma is usually a malignant islet cell tumour, which occurs most frequently in the fifth and sixth decades of life. Patients present with the characteristic rash as described, which is termed necrolytic migratory erythema. The rash can progress to bullous lesions which can slough. Weight loss is due to hypoaminoacidaemia.

The diagnosis is confirmed if the serum glucagon is >500 pg/ml. Glucagonomas are usually located within the pancreas, metastatic and unresectable. Prior to surgery, most patients are severely cachectic and may require parenteral nutrition.

A2.32 Arterial surgery

1. **J Femoro-popliteal bypass.** Intermittent claudication is an aching pain usually experienced in the calf on exercise but may also occur in the buttock and thigh. The pain is relieved within 2–3 minutes of standing still. It is important to determine how long the patient has suffered with claudication, whether it is getting worse and the impact on the patient's quality of life and particularly work. The ankle–brachial pressure index provides a quantitative assessment of global arterial disease with a ratio >1 being normal; 0.5–0.9 representing moderate arterial disease; <0.5 severe arterial disease. Duplex Doppler scanning provides an accurate non-invasive method of quantifying arterial disease. However, angiography still remains the gold standard. Initial management should involve risk factor modification (smoking cessation, weight loss, control of hypertension and diabetes mellitus) and best medical treatment (e.g. antiplatelet agent, ACE inhibitor, statins). Angioplasty may be performed for isolated superficial femoral artery stenosis/occlusions <10 cm in length. Above knee femoro-popliteal bypass grafting is indicated if the stenosis/occlusion is >10 cm in length, with *in situ* vein grafts giving the best long-term patency of 60% at 3 years.

2. **E Embolectomy.** Acute limb ischaemia is defined as deterioration in the blood supply of a previously stable limb of less than 2 weeks duration. Frequently, onset can be sudden, i.e. complete occlusion of a proximal artery in the absence of collaterals resulting in the classic presentation of: pain, paralysis, paraesthesia, pallor, pulselessness and a perishingly cold limb. Initially, the limb is white with venous dilatation giving a mottled appearance. Sensorimotor deficit results from muscle and nerve ischaemia. At this stage, the limb is still salvageable. If flow is not restored, thrombus propagation and capillary rupture result in fixed mottling and tense muscle compartments. Acute limb ischaemia results from embolisation (left atrium in atrial fibrillation, proximal aneurysm, myocardial infarction) or more commonly, thrombosis (usually at the site of atherosclerotic stenosis). Initial management is balloon catheter embolectomy (local or general anaesthetic) or intra-arterial thrombolysis. Limb salvage is reported to be 70%, with a 22% mortality. Fasciotomy may need to be considered.

3. **I Femoro-femoral bypass.** Bilateral aorto-iliac disease in a fit patient is best treated by an aortobifemoral bypass as the 5-year patency rate is approximately 90%. However, the mortality rate for this procedure is 3–5% and there is also a risk of graft infection and impotence. Unilateral iliac disease is best treated with an extra-anatomic femoro-femoral

crossover graft. Inflow disease of the donor site can be treated by angioplasty ± stenting. The 1-year patency rate is approximately 90%. At surgery, both femoral arteries are approached through longitudinal incisions. The graft used is an 8 or 10 mm externally-supported synthetic graft and is tunnelled subcutaneously.

A guide to the ankle-brachial pressure index (ABPI) in arterial disease

	ABPI	Signs and symptoms	Severity of disease	Action
A	≥0.7	Mild intermittent claudication. Some patients may be symptom-free	Mild arterial disease	Reduce risk factors and change in lifestyle: smoking cessation, weight reduction, regular exercise. Prescribe an anti-platelet agent
B	0.7–0.5	Varying degrees of intermittent claudication	Mild to moderate arterial disease	As in 'A' + referral to out-patient vascular specialist ± appropriate arterial imaging (Duplex scan and/or angiogram)
C	0.5–0.3	Severe intermittent claudication. Rest pain	Severe arterial disease	As in 'A' + urgent referral to the vascular specialist ± appropriate arterial imaging (Duplex scan and/or angiogram)
D	≤0.3 or ankle systolic pressure <50 mmHg	Critical ischemia, as defined as rest pain >2 weeks ± tissue loss (ulcer, gangrene)	Severe arterial disease; patients at risk of limb loss	Urgent referral to the vascular emergency on-call ± surgical or radiological intervention as appropriate

Notes:
1. An ABPI of 1–1.1 is considered to be normal.
2. The above figures should be used as an adjunct to the clinical findings. Erroneous readings may arise due to incompressible arteries due to presence of calcification (e.g. diabetes) or presence of tissue oedema. Patients may present with an arterial ulcer even with a normal ABPI.
3. Patients with arterial disease may present with an acutely ischemic limb (6Ps: pale, pulseless, pain, paresthesia, perishing with cold, paralysis – loss of function) either due to an embolus or a thrombus (acute-on-chronic ischaemia). These patients should be referred as an emergency to a vascular specialist for urgent intervention to prevent imminent limb loss.

A2.33 Venous disorders of the lower limb

1. **C** **Long saphenous vein reflux.** Primary varicose veins are due to valvular failure and are derived from the long or short saphenous veins or their major tributaries. Secondary varicose veins develop in the presence of damaged or occluded deep leg veins. Presentations of primary varicose veins are either uncomplicated (disease confined to superficial system) or complicated (combined superficial and deep venous disease and at risk of developing chronic venous insufficiency). Patients presenting with varicose veins are assessed by history and general examination with the patient standing (presence, nature and distribution of varicose veins and skin changes). Common sites of deep to superficial reflux give rise to typical distributions of varices. Hand-held Doppler examination is performed with the patient standing. The probe is placed over the saphenofemoral junction; incompetence is confirmed by squeezing the calf and releasing which results in prograde and retrograde signal if incompetence is present. Compression of the long saphenous vein results in abolition of the signal. Hand-held Doppler testing is inferior to duplex Doppler and is particularly inaccurate in assessing recurrent varicose veins.

2. **B** **Deep venous occlusion.** Deep venous occlusion can present with a spectrum of severity ranging from minimal symptoms through to venous gangrene. Thrombosis extending up to the iliofemoral segment may present with a swollen painful leg, which is typically pale (phlegmasia alba dolens). Extension of thrombosis to the venular and capillary level ± secondary development of acute arterial ischaemia produces a cyanosis and an extremely painful leg (phlegmasia caerulea dolens); left untreated venous gangrene occurs in 50% of patients. Phlegmasia caerulea dolens results in fluid sequestration due to obstruction at the capillary level, this may be severe with the patient presenting with shock. Management is directed at improving tissue perfusion by aggressive fluid resuscitation, limb elevation to reduce oedema and intravenous heparin. The role of thrombectomy and thrombolysis in deep venous occlusion remains controversial.

3. **E** **Post-thrombotic syndrome.** Chronic venous insufficiency results from impaired venous return over a prolonged period of time. The resulting venous hypertension results in varicosities mainly confined to the calf around associated perforators, oedema, varicose eczema, pigmentation due to local deposition of haemosiderin, subcutaneous atrophy (lipodermatosclerosis), atrophie blanche and ultimately ulceration, usually in the gaiter region. Chronic venous insufficiency secondary to previous deep vein thrombosis is referred to as post-thrombotic syndrome (or post-phlebitic limb). The risk of developing this condition increases the more proximal the DVT. Venous reflux and residual venous obstruction are largely responsible for the development of this syndrome. Therefore, DVT treatment should be aimed at preventing thrombus propagation, pulmonary embolism, preventing further venous damage and restoring venous function.

A2.34 Swollen limb

1. **H** **Pedal oedema.** Pedal oedema is the most likely cause as the condition is bilateral and of short duration. It develops in the presence of heart failure, i.e. inadequacy of the heart muscle secondary to intrinsic disease or overloading. Failure of the right heart pump causes an increased pre-load resulting in an increased blood volume and sequestration of fluid into the dependent tissues. It is usual for the left ventricle to fail before the right (e.g. ischaemic heart disease, systemic arterial hypertension), with left ventricular failure being the most common cause of right ventricular heart failure. Congestive heart failure refers to a combination of right and left heart failure, with symptoms and signs of systemic and pulmonary venous hypertension.

2. **E** **Lymphoedema praecox.** Lymphoedema is an excessive accumulation of interstitial fluid as a result of defective lymphatic drainage. The causes are divided into primary or secondary. Primary lymphoedema has a male to female ratio of 1:3 and has no known cause, but one-third of patients have a family history of the condition. Secondary lymphoedema is more common than primary and occurs when the lymphatic channels become blocked due to an acquired cause. Primary lymphoedema is classified into congenital when it occurs soon after birth (Milroy's disease is the inherited form), lymphoedema praecox when it presents before the age of 35 years and lymphoedema tarda when it presents over the age of 35 years. Primary lymphoedema is thought to be due to aplasia, hypoplasia or hyperplasia of the lymphatic vessels during development. Isotope lymphography is performed to confirm the diagnosis and to assess the prognosis for both limbs. Treatment is aimed at reducing swelling and weight, reducing the risk of infection and improving function. Surgery (debulking or bypass procedures) is occasionally required in severe cases but is of limited value.

3. **I** **Post radiotherapy.** Secondary lymphoedema results when the lymphatic channels distal to the obstruction become dilated and the valves secondarily incompetent. Worldwide the most common cause is infection with the filariasis parasite; in developed countries, obstruction is most commonly due to malignant disease, lymph node dissection or radiotherapy. Radiotherapy results in nodal fibrosis, which in turn causes obstruction of the lymphatic vessels, although recurrence should always be suspected if the swelling develops a number of years following the radiotherapy. Soft tissue sarcomas are treated with aggressive surgical resection (i.e. whole muscle) and adjuvant radiotherapy. Secondary lymphoedema of the upper limb is also common in patients who have undergone axillary node clearance and irradiation for breast cancer.

A2.35 Renal transplantation complications

1. **C Acute tubular necrosis.** A diuresis is expected following revascularisation in all living donor kidneys and in approximately 70% of cadaveric transplants. When urine is not produced, a technical complication is sought, e.g. vascular, urological. When the surgeon is confident that the anuria is not due to a technical cause, the wound is closed and the patient undergoes haemodialysis in the postoperative period. If hyperacute rejection is suspected, a biopsy is taken at the time of surgery and repeated at 24 hours. Delayed graft function is invariably due to acute tubular necrosis secondary to pre-transplant renal ischaemia and commonly seen in kidneys that have been stored on ice for prolonged periods. Postoperatively, the renal function is assessed with serial serum creatinine measurements and accurate fluid balance.

2. **G Renal vein thrombosis.** The complications of transplant surgery are either due to technical complications or related to immunosuppressive therapy (infection, cancer). Renal vein thrombosis has increased in incidence since the introduction of cyclosporin. It usually occurs in the first few days following transplantation and is associated with an abrupt cessation of renal function with a tender swollen graft. Re-exploration and thrombectomy is usually unsuccessful with graft loss being the usual outcome. The prophylactic use of low dose aspirin significantly reduces this complication. Renal artery stenosis is a late complication in approximately 10% of patients undergoing transplantation. Urological complications are usually due to devascularisation of the distal ureter at the time of organ retrieval. This may present early with a urine leak or late with a ureteric stenosis or obstruction.

3. **E Hyperacute rejection.** Four types of rejection are seen after transplantation: hyperacute, accelerated, acute and chronic. Hyperacute rejection occurs within 24 hours of transplantation and results from an immediate antibody rejection. The classic hyperacute rejection is no longer seen, which occurred within 1 hour due to HLA class I antibody or an ABO incompatible kidney. However, these florid hyperacute reactions still occur in sensitised patients or in patients receiving a re-graft. Accelerated rejection is cell-mediated and is seen in sensitised patients 2–4 days following transplantation. A biopsy reveals a florid cellular infiltrate (macrophages and T-lymphocytes). A Duplex ultrasound scan is also necessary to exclude a vascular complication. Cyclosporin levels should also be performed to exclude cyclosporin toxicity. Acute rejection is the outcome of the immune response of the allograft in a non-sensitised patient and most commonly occurs between 7 and 21 days post transplantation. Ultrasonography should be performed to exclude ureteric obstruction, but cyclosporin toxicity should also be excluded. Chronic rejection is the most common cause of late graft loss and is characterised by an insidious, irreversible deterioration of function in the months following transplantation.

Otorhinolaryngology, head and neck surgery

A2.36 Ear, nose and throat disorders

1. **A** **Acute otitis media.** Acute middle ear infections are common following upper respiratory viral infections. They affect all ages but are particularly common in children. The patient usually complains of ear pain, a sensation of pressure in the ear and hearing loss. In young children, the features are more generalised and often mask the ear symptoms. There is initially hyperaemia of the tympanic membrane, followed by an accumulation of serous fluid, which becomes purulent if bacterial infection (*Streptococcus pneumonia* and *Haemophilus influenzae* being the most common infecting organism) is present. The drum looks dull and bulges on otoscopy. The drum eventually perforates with relief of symptoms. Children are treated with oral amoxicillin and adults with phenoxymethylpenicillin. Left untreated, rare complications include: mastoiditis, labyrinthitis, meningitis and intracerebral abscesses.

2. **G** **Pharyngeal pouch.** Pharyngeal pouch (pharyngo-oesophageal diverticulum) is an out-pouching of mucosa through an area of weakness (Killian's dehiscence) between the inferior constrictor of the pharynx (thyropharyngeus) and the cricopharyngeus posteriorly. This results from an incoordination of the pharyngeal muscles during swallowing. The patients are usually elderly and present with progressive dysphagia or regurgitation of undigested food. They may also present with recurrent chest infections due to "silent" aspirations. Patients are offered surgery as symptoms usually progress. Surgery is performed through a two-beaked endoscope or fibreoptic pharyngoscope under general anaesthetic. The contents of the pouch are aspirated. A stapling gun is passed down the endoscope. The beaks of the gun are passed over the cricopharyngeal bar, locked in position and fired, cutting through the cricopharyngeal bar and sealing the defect with three layers of staples.

3. **F** **Peritonsillar abscess.** Peritonsillar abscess (quinsy) follows an acute tonsillar infection, which results in pus collecting in the peritonsillar space. The abscess usually points in the soft palate. The abscess requires drainage under local anaesthetic.

A2.37 Common neck swellings

1. **D** **Cystic hygroma.** Cystic hygroma (cavernous lymphangioma) is a congenital, cystic lymphatic malformation. This results in lymphatic fluid collecting in thin-walled, single or multiple interconnecting cysts situated at the base of the neck. Presentation is usually at birth (50–65%) and occasionally it is of such a size to require emergency decompression to free the airway. Otherwise it is seen in childhood or adolescence. They are often treated with aspiration and injection of sclerosant, but many recur. If they recur, surgical excision is indicated. CT scanning is required preoperatively to assess caudal extent and involvement of

important neurovascular structures. Dissection should be performed cautiously as important structures lie in or adjacent to the cystic hygroma.

2. **A Branchial cyst.** Branchial (lateral cervical) cysts are thought to develop from persistence of the embryonic branchial clefts (lateral clefts). Incomplete obliteration of the medial clefts results in a deep connection to the nasal or oral pharynx. However, most branchial cysts do not have a deep connection and result from epithelial inclusions within upper deep cervical lymph nodes, which subsequently undergo cystic degeneration. Most present as an enlarging lump ± signs of infection at the junction of the upper- and middle-thirds of the sternocleidomastoid in the third decade of life. The diagnosis is confirmed by fine needle aspiration, which reveals pus-like fluid with a characteristic cytology of cell debris and cholesterol crystals. A branchial fistula may also be present with a discharging point on the anterior border of the sterno-cleidomastoid low in the neck. Surgical excision is advised. This is performed through an oblique skin crease incision. A careful dissection is required as the cyst lies deep to the fascia and is closely related to the deep structures.

3. **B Carotid body tumour.** Carotid body tumours (chemodectomas) arise from the chemoreceptor cells found at the carotid bifurcation. Patients usually present in the fifth or sixth decade of life. Most of these tumours are benign (80%) and do not secrete adrenaline or nor-adrenaline and therefore do not affect the blood pressure. The diagnosis is confirmed with Duplex, a carotid angiogram and fine needle aspiration cytology. Surgical excision is advised even in benign cases as enlarge-ment results in compression of the local structures. Preoperatively, the tumour is selectively embolised radiologically. The carotid is approached as for a carotid endarterectomy. It is usually possible to develop a plane of dissection between the adventitia and the tumour (enucleation). Local invasion requires arterial excision and long saphenous vein grafting.

A2.38 Salivary gland disorders

1. **G Sialolithiasis.** Sialolithiasis (salivary calculi) affects 1% of the popu-lation usually in the fifth decade of life and most frequently occurs in the submandibular gland. Predisposing factors include reduced salivary flow rates, duct obstruction, dehydration and salivary pH. Submandibular gland saliva has a higher pH and is more viscid than saliva produced from the other glands. Sialolithiasis may be complicated by acute bacterial sialadenitis. The diagnosis is confirmed by sialography or CT scanning. Submandibular calculi are removed trans-orally by incising the duct directly over the stone and then the duct marsupialised, i.e. the opened duct is sutured to the adjacent mucosa. A recurrent calculus requires excision of the whole submandibular gland.

2. **A** **Acute sialadenitis.** Acute parotid sialadenitis is usually due to paramyxovirus (mumps) in children, and due to infection by echo virus or coxsackie virus in adolescents. The acute inflammatory response within the parotid glands leads to oedema of the gland parenchyma with obstruction of the intraglandular ducts. Eating results in an exacerbation of pain and swelling. Tuberculosis or HIV/AIDS-associated lymphoma must be considered as possible aetiological causes in high-risk groups which present in a similar fashion.

3. **B** **Salivary gland tumour.** A total of 80% of salivary gland tumours are in the parotid, 80% of these are pleomorphic adenomas and 80% of these are in the superficial lobe; 15% of salivary gland tumours arise in the submandibular gland and of these 50% are benign. Salivary gland neoplasms are derived from the ductal and acinar tissue and are classified as: benign (pleomorphic salivary adenoma, monomorphic adenoma, adenolymphoma) and malignant (well-differentiated, e.g. muco-epidermoid carcinoma, adenoid cystic carcinoma and poorly-differentiated, e.g. malignant change within a pleomorphic adenoma). Parotid masses are assessed and treated with ultrasound, fine needle aspiration cytology and superficial/total parotidectomy. See 3.55 Parotidectomy, 4.9 Parotid odenome.

Oral and maxillo-facial surgery

A2.39 Maxillo-facial trauma

1. **H** **Mandibular ramus.** Mandibular rami fractures can occur through the neck, body, symphysis or ramus. The fracture can be recognised by the deranged dental occlusion and palpating or squeezing over the fracture site. Soft tissue swellings around a fracture may enlarge and obstruct the airway. The diagnosis is confirmed with orthopantomograph; lateral oblique and anterior views of the mandible. Treatment is conservative (if the fracture is undisplaced and stable), intermaxillary fixation (interdental wiring between the respective teeth of the lower and upper jaws) or open reduction and internal fixation ± plate fixation (for displaced or unstable fractures).

2. **B** **Le Fort II.** Fractures of the maxilla occur at three levels: Le Fort I, II and III, and may be unilateral or bilateral. Le Fort fractures are classified as follows: I, through the maxilla, leaving the nose and orbits intact; II, through the maxilla into the orbits and across the nose, leaving the middle-third of the face mobile; and III, through the lateral walls of the orbit and across the nose. All maxillary fractures require urgent treatment as the middle-third of the face may fall backwards and obstruct the airway. They are managed by securing the airway and assessed with CT. Fractures are approached through various incisions, anatomically reduced and fixed with plates and screws, placed along the axes of the major facial buttresses.

3. **K** **Zygomatic.** Zygomatic fractures usually result from direct blows to the face and may be missed due to soft tissue swelling. A depressed zygoma results in asymmetry when viewed from above. The zygoma also forms the inferolateral part of the orbit, where it tends to fracture (zygomatic-frontal suture). Diplopia results particularly on upward gaze due to injury to the extraocular muscles. Zygomatic fractures are best seen on oblique postero-anterior (Waters') view with CT scanning required for orbital involvement. Stable undisplaced fractures are treated conservatively; closed reduction may also be possible for some displaced fractures, while open reduction and internal fixation is required when closed reduction fails or when there is orbital involvement.

A2.40 Common condition of the face, mouth and jaws

1. **E** **Hemifacial microsomia.** Hemifacial microsomia is centred on the structures derived from the first and second branchial arches. When fusion of the fingers or toes (syndactyly) is present, the condition is termed Goldenhar's syndrome. The treatment varies according to severity. Surgery may be carried out in childhood to improve the appearance but needs to be repeated in adolescents when growth has ceased. Usually an inverted "L" osteotomy of the ramus of the mandible is employed. When there is marked hypoplasia, a costochondral graft is employed to lengthen the mandible. Hypoplasia of the soft tissues are treated with a free tissue transfer.

2. **F** **Lichen planus.** White patches arising in the oral cavity are common. Causes include: lichen planus, frictional keratosis (e.g. sharp teeth), smoker's keratosis (usually found on the palate and is not pre-malignant), leucoplakia (diagnosis of exclusion, 2% proceed to malignancy) and candidiasis. Lichen planus is an autoimmune disorder and is the most common cause of persistent white patches in the oral cavity. They are usually flat but may become papular and confluent. The condition is associated with anxiety and stress. Erosive lesions are treated with topical corticosteroids.

3. **B** **Apical cysts.** Apical cysts are the most common inflammatory odontogenic cysts. They result from the spread of dental infection into the bone, stimulating epithelial remnants to coalesce. They are usually painless but may present with secondary infection which may be painful. Most small cysts (<1 cm) resolve spontaneously. Larger cysts require excision ± marsupialisation.

A2.41 Common eye infections

1. **F** **Iritis.** Acute iritis (anterior uveitis) affects the uveal tract, which is the vascular-pigmented part of the eye including the iris, ciliary body and choroid. The inflammation is sterile and is associated with immunological-based disorders, e.g. ankylosing spondylitis. White blood cells deposit on the posterior surface of the cornea (keratic precipitates) and when

inflammation is severe, a layer of white cells may deposit in the inferior part of the anterior chamber (hypopyon). The pupil is initially small due to iris spasm but may become irregular due to adhesions. Treatment (0.5% prednisolone eye-drops) is aimed at preventing prolonged inflammation in the eye. Cataracts may develop as a long-term complication if not treated adequately.

2. **C** **Conjunctivitis.** Infectious conjunctivitis is most often caused by viruses (adenovirus) or less commonly by bacteria (*streptococci, pneumococci*). On examination, there is a diffuse reddening of the conjunctival sac with the greatest inflammation being furthest from the corneal margins. Viral infections are associated with small lymphoid aggregates appearing as follicles on the tarsal conjunctiva. Viral conjunctivitis is best treated symptomatically with bland antibiotic ointments as they provide soothing comfort. Antibiotic treatment of bacterial conjunctivitis is based on culture sensitivities.

3. **D** **Dacryocystitis.** Dacryocystitis is an acute inflammation of the lacrimal sac (located medial to the medial canthus) resulting in pain and epiphora (overflow of tears onto the cheek). Treatment is with broad-spectrum systemic antibiotics. Most infections resolve without requiring drainage. This condition may result in blockage of the tear duct requiring dacryocystorhinostomy. Dacryocystorhinostomy is performed through a nasofacial crease to expose the medial side of the lacrimal sac. The sac is incised and the flaps anastomosed to the nasal mucosa through a surgically formed defect in the bone.

Paediatric surgery

A2.42 Clinical problems in low birth weight babies

1. **J** **Surfactant deficiency.** Respiratory distress syndrome (RDS) results from a deficiency of surfactant, the mixture of lipoproteins excreted by the alveolar epithelium which lowers the surface tension. This results in alveolar collapse (unable to stay inflated between breaths) resulting in inadequate gas exchange. Re-inflation between breaths exhausts the baby and respiratory failure follows. The more preterm the infant, the higher the incidence of RDS. If there is a sufficient interval (>48 hours) antenatal glucocorticoids can stimulate fetal surfactant production. Synthetic surfactant preparations may be given in addition to supplementary oxygen delivered with continuous positive airway pressure. These babies must be managed on the special care baby unit.

2. **D** **Impaired temperature control.** Newborn infants have a larger surface area relative to their body weight than older children. The skin of the preterm is thin and poorly keratinised. Therefore, babies lose body heat very quickly unless nursed in an environment with an optimal temperature (the core temperature should be maintained

at 36.7–37.3°C). Preterm infants are unable to shiver, cannot curl up and are usually nursed naked. Oxygen consumption is increased if the environment is too cold or too hot. Closed incubators provide a constant temperature and ambient humidity.

3. ◘ **Physiological jaundice.** Overall, a majority of newborn infants become visibly jaundiced due to haemolysis of fetal red cells in the first few days of life coupled to a less efficient bilirubin metabolism. Jaundice within the first 24 hours is always pathological (Rhesus or ABO incompatibility, G6PD deficiency, congenital infections). If left untreated, elevated hyperbilirubinaemia results in deposition in the brain causing bilirubin neurotoxicity (kernicterus). Mild cases (full-term infant: serum bilirubin <300 mmol/litre) are treated with phototherapy which breaks down unconjugated bilirubin in the skin. More severe cases require exchange transfusions.

A2.43 Correctable congenital abnormalities

1. ◘ **Pyloric stenosis.** Infantile hypertrophic pyloric stenosis usually presents between 4 and 6 weeks of age with a male to female ratio of 4:1 and is more common in the first-born. The aetiology is unknown. Microscopically, there is marked hypertrophy of the circular muscle and some hypertrophy of the longitudinal muscle. An ultrasound scan confirms the diagnosis. Initial management is rehydration and correction of the electrolyte disturbance (hypochloraemic metabolic alkalosis) using 0.45% sodium chloride with added potassium. A Ramstedt pylorotomy is performed through a right upper quadrant, periumbilical incision or laparoscopically.

2. ◨ **Gastroschisis.** The developing embryonic mid-gut passes into the umbilical cord as a physiological hernia between the 4-5th weeks of gestation. An abnormality in the development of the anterior abdominal wall or alteration of the usual forces involved in the normal retraction of the herniated intestine at 12 weeks' gestation results in exomphalos. The bowel is covered in a sac within the umbilical cord which may also contain the liver, spleen, stomach or gonads. Almost 50% of the infants have other major congenital anomalies (chromosomal; trisomy 13 and 18, or congenital heart disease). In gastroschisis the herniated bowel is not covered by a sac, the defect is usually to the right of the midline and other congenital anomalies are rare. The cause is obscure but a failure of mesodermal migration, a defect in involution of the right umbilical vein or a prenatal rupture of the amniotic sac have been suggested. Both conditions are nearly always diagnosed antenatally. At birth, the eviscerated bowel should be wrapped in cling-film to minimise fluid and heat loss, a large bore nasogastric tube passed, intravenous maintenance and fluid boluses provided together with prophylactic antibiotics. Most gastroschisis defects are small and closed primarily. Larger defects may require graded daily reductions within a Silastic bowel bag prior to formal closure at 7–10 days of age.

3. **B Diaphragmatic hernia.** Congenital diaphragmatic hernias are usually diagnosed on antenatal ultrasonography. Most are left-sided hernias (the liver prevents herniation on the right) through the postero-lateral foramen. The diagnosis is confirmed by noting intestinal loops ± nasogastric tube on chest radiograph. Following a number of days of stabilisation, the infant has the intestines reduced and the diaphragm repaired primarily through a subcostal incision. Pulmonary hypoplasia due to compression by the herniated viscera is a major problem in these infants and carries a mortality rate of 30–60%.

A2.44 Common paediatric surgical disorders

1. **E Intussusception.** Intussusception is the invagination of one segment of bowel into an adjacent lower segment. It is the most common abdominal emergency in infants aged between 3 months and 2 years. The cause is usually idiopathic with the leading point being an enlarged Peyer's patch that develops secondary to a viral infection. The ileocaecal region is most frequently involved, although any part of the intestine may be involved. The diagnosis may be made clinically if a sausage-shaped mass is palpable. Ultrasound scanning confirms the diagnosis with accuracy approaching 100% in skilled hands. Treatment consists of fluid resuscitation, electrolyte correction and nasogastric decompression. Most cases are treated successfully by air insufflation under radiological guidance with laparotomy reserved for unsuccessful insufflation or signs of peritonitis. If clinical suspicion remains despite a normal ultrasound scan then air enema is undertaken. Two or three attempts at air reduction are attempted with 1–2 hours between attempts. Peritonitis is the only indication to proceed straight to laparotomy.

2. **I Umbilical hernia.** An infantile umbilical hernia is present in 10% of Caucasian infants (male to female ratio of 2:1) and 90% of children of African descent. The incidence is higher in children of low birth weight. The hernia sac penetrates through the linea alba umbilical cicatrix (ring) to lie in the subcutaneous tissue. The hernia results from failure of the umbilical stump scar to fuse with the cicatrix. The hernia is usually symptomless and presents as an easily reducible lump. Incarceration or strangulation is extremely rare with most hernias resolving spontaneously by the age of 2 years.

3. **H Phimosis.** Phimosis is a term which encompasses a normal non-retractile prepuce, a non-retractile prepuce due to scarring (usually due to ill-advised attempts at retraction), or lichen sclerosis (balanitis xerotica obliterans) when the tip of the prepuce becomes thickened, white and fixed to the glans. The natural history of the prepuce is to separate well before 3 years old (90% foreskins fully retractable by 3 years; 92% by age 6 and 99% by age 17). Expansion of the prepuce on micturition (ballooning) rarely leads to urinary retention. The parents are advised on gentle retraction to allow the passage of urine.

Circumcision is not indicated. However, ballooning of the prepuce occurs with both physiological and pathological phimosis and the latter can lead to outflow obstruction. Circumcision is therefore indicated for balanitis xerotica obliterans.

A2.45 Orthopaedic disorders of infancy and childhood

1. **H Talipes equinovarus.** Congenital talipes equinovarus (club foot) results from a pathological dislocation of the talonavicular joint and is of an unknown aetiology. The condition is often bilateral, affecting approximately 1.5 per 1000 births with a male to female ratio of 2:1. On examination, the position of the foot is fixed and cannot be completely corrected. Treatment is started soon after birth with serial plaster casts or strapping and splinting. Corrective surgery is required if conservative therapies fail. Surgery is usually performed at 6–9 months of age and takes the form of releasing the tight medial soft tissues and lengthening the Achilles and medial tendons.

2. **A Developmental dysplasia of the hip.** Developmental dysplasia of the hip (congenital dislocation of the hip) is a spectrum of disease from dysplasia through to frank dislocation due to an abnormality of the capsule, proximal femur or acetabulum. The aetiology is thought to be due to the maternal hormone relaxin. Screening detects six cases per 1000 births with a female to male ratio of 6:1. If suspected, the diagnosis and degree of dysplasia/dislocation is assessed by ultrasonography. The infant is initially managed in abduction using a restraining device (Pavlik harness) for several months. Open reduction and derotation femoral osteotomy is required if conservative measures fail.

3. **D Perthes' disease.** Perthes' disease (Fig. 2.45.1a) is due to idiopathic ischaemia of the femoral epiphysis, resulting in avascular necrosis, followed by revascularisation and reossification. The condition is bilateral in 20% of cases with a male to female ratio of 3:1. The diagnosis is usually made on the plain radiograph. A bone scan or MR scan may be performed if the diagnosis remains in doubt. The prognosis is good in most children with most being treated conservatively (regular review). Surgery is only required if there is a dislocation of the femoral head from the acetabulum. Slipped capital femoral epiphysis (SCFE) (Fig. 2.45.1b) is a condition of adolescents in which the capital epiphysis slips posteriorly and inferiorly. Classically, the condition occurs in overweight boys following minor trauma. Moderate and severe displacement is treated with AO or cannulated screws.

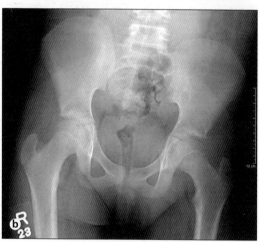

Fig. 2.45.1 **(a)** Perthes' disease of the left hip characterised by sclerosis and irregularity of the capital epiphysis. **(b)** Bilateral slipped capital femoral epiphysis (SCFE).

Plastic and reconstructive surgery

A2.46 Cutaneous vascular anomalies

1. **G** **Port-wine stain.** Port-wine stain is a form of capillary malformation that is present at birth and persists throughout life. It usually presents as a macular, dark red vascular stain over the face, trunk or limbs. It can be either well localised or could have an extensive spread. These lesions do not cross the midline. Port-wine stain must be differentiated from the common fading macular stain (naevus flammeus neonatorum) that occurs in up to 50% of neonates, commonly over the glabella, eyelids, nose, upper lip (angel kiss) and nuchal area (stork bite). It should also be differentiated from haemangiomas which are not usually present at birth but rapidly increase in size before involuting. Most port-wine stains are harmless cutaneous birthmarks, and no general or systemic abnormalities are present.

2. **I** **Sturge–Weber syndrome.** Sturge–Weber syndrome is a congenital vascular malformation affecting the head, face and brain associated with ipsilateral pial and ocular vascular anomalies. The leptomeningeal vascular abnormalities can cause seizures, contralateral hemiplegia and variable developmental delay of motor and cognitive skills. Seizures usually present within the first 2 years of life. Development of the brain usually proceeds to a normal size, but after birth, there is progressive atrophy of the affected hemisphere. The disease is usually unilateral, but bilateral cases can occur. The capillary stain involves the ophthalmic trigeminal dermatome. Children who have evidence of ipsilateral increased choroidal vascularity are at an increased risk for retinal detachment, glaucoma and blindness, which is even more likely if the capillary malformation involves both ophthalmic and maxillary neurosensory area.

3. **F** **Klippel–Trenaunay syndrome.** Klippel–Trenaunay syndrome is a combination of combined slow-flow anomaly and patchy port-wine stain associated with limb hypertrophy. The limb hypertrophy is usually not present at birth, but may appear within the first few months or years of life; the problem worsening with puberty. There may be periods of rapid enlargement and then cessation of growth. The anomaly may involve one or more limbs as well as the face or trunk. The capillary malformations are multiple, usually studded with haemolymphatic vesicles, and typically located in a geographic pattern on the anterolateral aspect of the thigh, buttock or trunk. Anomalous lateral veins are prominent because of insufficient or absent valves; deep vein anomalies can occur. Lymphatic hypoplasia is another primary defect.

A2.47 Disorders of the hand and wrist

1. **C** **De Quervain's tenosynovitis.** De Quervain's stenosing tenosynovitis is caused due to swelling and inflammation of the abductor pollicis longus and/or the extensor pollicis brevis tendons at the radial styloid

process. There is myxomatous degeneration to the wall of the first extensor compartment surrounding these tendons. This is the most common tenosynovitis of the wrist. Symptoms may occur spontaneously, or following unaccustomed or repetitive use of the wrist. The main symptom is aching pain along the ulnar side of the wrist and at the base of the thumb; the symptoms are exacerbated by flexion and ulnar deviation of the wrist with the thumb adducted across the palm (the Finkelstein test). Direct tenderness and swelling may be found over the first dorsal compartment at the radial styloid process. Rest, NSAIDs and wrist splintage may relieve the condition in many patients. If unsuccessful, local steroid injection into the first dorsal extensor compartment provides relief in about 80–90% of patients. Surgical treatment comprises decompression of both the abductor pollicis longus and the extensor pollicis brevis tendons.

2. **D** **Dupuytren's contracture.** Dupuytren's contracture is a disease of the palmar fascia. It is characterised by progressive thickening and contracture of the palmar fascia leading to the development of fibrous bands along the palmar surface of the hand and fingers. This disease is more common in Celtic races, has a possible genetic link and the majority of the patients have a positive family history. It has a male to female ratio of 7:1. The ring finger is the most commonly affected finger, followed by the little finger; any digit may, however, be affected. The disease is associated with epilepsy, diabetes mellitus, alcoholism (with or without cirrhosis of the liver) and trauma. In the early stages, the patient usually notices a painless, small, hard lump below the skin in the mid-palm region along the line of the ring or little fingers. As the disease progresses, the overlying skin becomes increasingly puckered and rough bands of thickened tissue can be felt along the affected area. Nodules and bands (cords) develop with progressive contracture of the metacarpophalangeal, proximal interphalangeal joints, or, rarely, the distal interphalangeal joints. The other clinical features include: palmar nodule, skin pits, knuckle pads and eventually contracting cords.

3. **A** **Bacterial flexor tenosynovitis.** Flexor tenosynovitis is caused due to bacterial infections, commonly from penetrating injuries to the digit. Penetrating trauma introduces bacteria into the deep structures and tendon sheaths, allowing the spread of infection along the tendon and its sheath. The majority are due to Staphylococcus aureus infection. Any digit can be affected depending on the site of injury. Bacterial flexor tenosynovitis should be distinguished from stenosing tenosynovitis ('trigger' finger) of the digital flexor tendons which commonly affects the thumb or the ring finger. Finger movements are severely restricted and the four cardinal signs of tendon sheath infection are: partially flexed finger, fusiform swelling of the finger, tenderness along the entire flexor tendon sheath and severe pain on passive extension of the finger. These four signs, however, may not be present together. The tenosynovitis can rapidly destroy the synovial gliding surfaces and

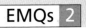

result in healing with restrictive adhesions. Bacterial flexor tenosynovitis is a medical emergency requiring, intravenous antibiotics, elevation and splinting. If no definite signs of improvement are seen after 24–36 hours, surgical exploration and drainage of the affected digit (area) must be considered.

A2.48 Non-malignant cutaneous lumps

1. **B** **Dermoid cyst.** Dermoid cysts are congenital hamartomas (also known as congenital subcutaneous cysts) and result from anomalous developmental inclusion of embryonic epidermis along embryonic cleft closure lines (along the lines of fusion). The cyst is lined by stratified squamous epithelium but, unlike an epidermal cyst, the wall may contain functioning epidermal appendages such as hair follicles, sweat and sebaceous glands. At times, even cartilage and bone are present. They are of variable size, at times as large as 10 cm. Common sites are the medial and the lateral ends of the eyebrows (where they are called external and internal angular dermoid cysts), the midline of the nose (called nasal dermoid cysts), sublingual, sternum, scrotum and the midline of the neck, perineum and the sacrum. They are subcutaneous in location and could resemble epidermoid cysts. Treatment consists of complete excision of the lesion.

2. **D** **Necrobiosis lipoidica.** Necrobiosis lipoidica is commonly, although not exclusively, associated with diabetes mellitus. It may precede the clinical onset of diabetes mellitus and has a predilection for the pretibial region. The lesion begins as a dusky red plaque that slowly progresses to atrophy of the skin; it may ulcerate in the centre secondary to minimal trauma. A distinctive yellowish cast in the atrophic telangiectatic centre of the lesion is characteristic. Typically, ulceration due to necrobiosis lipoidica is slow to heal, painful and frequently complicated by infection. Tight diabetic control, good wound care and topical corticosteroids are the recommended form of management. Topical PUVA therapy may also have a role. Although surgical resection of the involved area and resurfacing with split-thickness skin grafts has been advocated, it is seldom undertaken.

3. **G** **Seborrhoeic keratoses.** Seborrhoeic keratoses (basal cell papilloma, seborrhoeic wart) are benign tumours caused by the overgrowth of epidermal keratinocytes. They are seen in large numbers, especially on the trunk, face and arms of middle-aged and older individuals. They are sharply circumscribed, and often develop as single or multiple, round or oval shaped, slightly greasy lesions with a 'stuck on' appearance. It has also been described as cauliflower-like, waxy papillomatous lesion, with a friable hyperkeratotic surface. Pigmentation of seborrhoeic keratosis is variable, ranging from mild to deep black. They are often characterised by a network of crypts. Multiple seborrhoeic keratoses may be associated with an internal malignancy (Leser–Trelat sign). Appropriate treatment

consists of shave-excision curettage, superficial electrodesiccation, or cryotherapy using liquid nitrogen.

A2.49 Pre-malignant lesions/malignancies

1. **B** **Basal cell carcinoma.** Basal cell carcinoma (BCC) is the most common cutaneous malignancy. It may be single or multiple, and commonly occurs in the sun-exposed areas of the elderly. There is an increased incidence in smokers. Nodular or the nodulo-ulcerative type is the most common form of BCC. In this type, the tumour is usually single, and commences as a small, waxy or pearly nodule with clearly defined margins. The pearly appearance is more apparent on lightly stretched skin and it may be covered with surface telangiectasia. As the tumour enlarges, central ulceration occurs, resulting in the characteristic rolled-up edge. BCC is frequently painless in the early stages; pain signifies deeper extension with underlying tissue involvement. The common modalities of treatment for BCC includes surgical excision, fractionated radiotherapy, Mohs micrographic surgery, cryosurgery, electrodesiccation and curettage and topical chemotherapy (with 5-fluorouracil).

2. **F** **Keratoacanthoma.** Keratoacanthoma (*molluscum sebaceum*) is a cutaneous lesion commonly seen in sun-exposed sites. Although it is commonly thought to be benign, some authorities maintain that they are, in fact, well-differentiated SCCs rather than a distinct clinical entity; hence it is also known as the 'self-healing' SCC. These tumours may be solitary or multiple, and are more common in males. It presents as a fleshy, elevated and nodular lesion with an irregular crater shape and a characteristic central hyperkeratotic core. The most significant histological feature is its rapid growth (6–8 weeks). The short history and a rapid increase in size suggest keratoacanthoma rather than a squamous cell carcinoma. In some cases, it undergoes spontaneous resolution within 6 months of onset, leaving a depressed scar behind. If it fails to resolve, complete surgical excision is the treatment of choice. Topical chemotherapy with intra-lesional 5-fluorouracil is also useful in its management. See 4.6 Keratoacanthoma.

3. **H** **Squamous cell carcinoma.** Squamous cell carcinoma (SCC) is seen primarily in older patients, mostly men. They originate from the keratinising or Malpighian (spindle) cell layer of the epithelium. Like BCC, the prime aetiologic factor is excessive exposure to solar radiation. Farmers, sailors and all those whose occupation require excessive sun exposure are predisposed to SCC. In addition to radiation, chemicals, cytotoxic drugs, immunosuppressant drug treatment, chronic lesions and a wide variety of dermatoses also play a role in its development. There are two main types of SCC: (1) a slow growing variety that is verrucous in nature and exophytic in appearance. This is locally invasive, penetrating deeper structures, and is more likely to metastasise, and (2) a nodular and indurated type, with rapid growth and early ulceration

combined with local invasiveness. Metastasis is late compared with the verrucous type. Small isolated skin ulceration suspicious of carcinoma can be observed for 2–3 weeks before definitive treatment is undertaken. Any lesion that has not healed after this period must be considered as a skin cancer until proven otherwise. Treatment of SCC depends on the age of the patient, the site, size and type of lesion and the presence or absence of metastases.

A2.50 Benign and malignant pigmented skin lesions

1. **H Nodular melanoma.** Nodular melanoma is the second most common subtype of all melanomas. These may occur over any part of the body although they are more common over the legs and trunk. These are frequently raised, palpable, deeply pigmented and usually convex in shape; they may bleed or ulcerate. It is well demarcated from the surrounding skin. Histologically, there is no recognisable intra-epidermal component at the margin of the tumour mass, all the cells being in vertical growth phase; there is no identifiable radial growth phase. Lymphatic involvement occurs early. This type of melanoma has the worst prognosis among all forms of melanomas. See 4.5 Malignant melanoma.

2. **G Lentigo maligna melanoma.** Lentigo maligna melanoma (Hutchinson's melanotic freckle) almost always arises over the sun-damaged skin of the face, neck, arms and legs of elderly individuals. It is the least malignant variety and it presents as an irregular brown patch. The precursor *in situ* lesion, lentigo maligna, is usually present for more than 10–15 years and attains a large size (4–8 cm diameter) before progressing to malignancy. Malignant degeneration is characterised by thickening and the development of discrete tumour nodule within the lesion. Histologically, there are features of lentigo maligna with gross sun damage to the dermal collagen. There are islands of malignant melanocytic cells within the dermis.

3. **B Amelanotic melanoma.** Amelanotic melanoma is a variant of melanoma in which the cells do not make melanin. It does not hence appear darkly pigmented. It may, however, occasionally appear light brown or tan with grey edges. Classically, the lesions are pink or red appearing as erythematous papules or nodules. They have irregular edges/margins. Amelanotic melanoma may occur in any one of the four clinico-pathological variants (lentigo maligna melanoma, superficial spreading melanoma, nodular melanoma and acral-lentiginous melanoma). Patients with amelanotic melanoma frequently present with advanced disease and lymph node involvement. Their prognosis is poor, probably because of their delayed presentation and/or diagnosis. It is often confused with other cutaneous malignancies including basal cell carcinoma and squamous cell carcinoma.

Neurosurgery

A2.51 Surgical disorders of the brain

1. **G Pituitary adenoma.** Pituitary adenomas arise from the anterior lobe and are classified by size (when >2 cm in diameter they expand into the suprasellar space causing optic chiasmal compression) or endocrine activity. The most common pituitary tumours secrete prolactin, growth hormone (causing acromegaly as in this case) or ACTH. Non-secreting tumours are less common and usually present with tumour compression of the optic chiasma. Pituitary adenomas may be treated medically, surgically or with radiotherapy with the aim of decompressing neural structures and to restore and maintain normal hormone secretion. Pituitary adenomas are best imaged with MR scanning. Preoperatively the patient is commenced on intravenous hydrocortisone. The pituitary is approached trans-sphenoidally with the aim of decompression, correction of endocrine dysfunction and to obtain a histological diagnosis. Cure is only possible with surgery. Complications include diabetes insipidus which is usually transient.

2. **B Brain abscess.** Brain abscesses most frequently result from spread of infection from a nearby site, usually from the frontal sinuses or middle ear. The remainder result from direct blood-borne infection from a distant source (e.g. dental abscesses). The clinical features consist of pyrexia, headache and focal neurological signs. Headache is the most frequent, with other signs of raised intracranial pressure ranging from papilloedema through to coma. Diagnosis is confirmed by CT (cystic lesion with a fine regular capsule and surrounding oedema). Treatment is drainage via a burr-hole centred over the abscess, repeated daily until no further pus is drained. Craniotomy may be necessary if the capsule is too thick. The offending sinus or middle ear should be drained at the same time.

3. **A Astrocytoma.** Primary intracranial tumours are intrinsic (arising from the brain parenchyma and make up 50% of all primary brain tumours) or extrinsic (arise from the meninges and make up 30% of all primary brain tumours). Glial cells are the connective tissue of the brain and are of three main types: astrocytes, ependymal cells and oligodendrocytes. Astrocytomas occur most frequently and are grade I–IV, with grade IV carrying the worst prognosis. Treatment is aimed at complete resection. However, complete resection may not be possible in lesions involving functionally important areas. Radiation therapy may be used when a significant amount of tumour is left behind. The 3-year survival for grade I astrocytomas is approximately 50%.

A2.52 Intracranial haemorrhage

1. **E Intraparenchymal haemorrhage.** Spontaneous intracranial haemorrhages are classified as: intraparenchymal, intraventricular or subarachnoid. They are most frequently due to hypertension but are also

due to cerebral saccular (berry) aneurysms, arteriovenous malformations and blood coagulopathies. The most common site of haemorrhage is in the basal ganglia and external capsule (supplied by a perforating branch of the middle cerebral artery). Craniotomy and evacuation of haematoma is performed if the patient is considered to be salvageable.

2. **G Subarachnoid haemorrhage.** Spontaneous subarachnoid haemorrhages are most frequently due to intracranial saccular aneurysms (85%) but are also due to arteriovenous malformations, vasculitis and coagulopathies. Bleeding results in chemically-induced meningitis, vasospasm of the cerebral arteries and obstructive hydrocephalus. Management is aimed at maintaining the patient's airway and blood pressure. CT scanning ± angiography is the investigation of choice in establishing the diagnosis if performed in the first 24 hours following the onset of symptoms. Lumbar puncture is required if radiological investigation is normal or equivocal. The timing of craniotomy and clipping of an aneurysm is controversial. Early surgery (<3 days) reduces the risk of re-bleeding but is technically more difficult.

3. **H Subdural haematoma.** Acute subdural haematomas are seen more commonly than extradural haematomas following high-velocity injuries. They are associated with more severe brain injuries and other systemic injuries. Affected patients are usually found unconscious and do not have a period of consciousness (lucid interval) following the injury as seen in extradural haematomas. Acute subdural haematomas require prompt surgical evacuation usually through several, linear, unconnected incisions in the dura. The overall outcome is worse than with extradural haematomas, with mortality being as high as 45%.

A2.53 Brain stem death

1. **H Patient is in a coma, receiving mechanical ventilation.** Death can be defined as an irreversible loss of capacity for consciousness combined with an irreversible loss of the capacity to breathe. Both of these functions are controlled by the brain stem. Before undertaking brain stem death testing in a comatose patient, several preconditions must be satisfied and include: (1) the patient is in a coma, receiving mechanical ventilation; (2) the definitive cause for the coma has been diagnosed; (3) enough time has elapsed to ensure irreversibility; and (4) two doctors of sufficiently senior rank perform the tests independently.

2. **F Core temperature greater than 35°C.** The patient must have a core temperature greater than 35°C. Exclusions to performing the tests include: (1) complicated medical conditions confounding clinical assessment; (2) the patient must not be hypothermic (core temperature <35°C) and have no residual affects of drugs (e.g. sedatives or anaesthetics).

3. **B Absent vestibulo-ocular reflexes.** The diagnosis of brain stem death is performed by demonstrating the absence of the following brain

stem reflexes: papillary, corneal and vestibulo-ocular reflexes, response to painful stimulus in the trigeminal nerve territory and gag reflex. The results should be carefully recorded in the patient's case notes preferably on a standard form (declaration of brain stem death).

A2.54 Surgical aspects of meningitis

1. **F Communicating hydrocephalus.** Cerebrospinal fluid (CSF) is normally produced at 20 ml/hour by the choroid plexus, flows through the ventricles and is eventually reabsorbed by the arachnoid villi at 20 ml/hour. Hydrocephalus is classified as: non-communicating (obstruction in the circulation pathway of CSF) or communicating (impairment of circulation in the subarachnoid space or abnormal absorption). Hydrocephalus in infancy is commonly due to a congenital structural abnormality of the brain. It may also result from severe bacterial meningitis, brain trauma, subarachnoid haemorrhage or tumour. The investigation of choice is CT. Lumbar puncture should not be performed if the intracranial pressure is raised. Placement of a shunt (ventriculoperitoneal shunts are most frequently used) offers the only effective treatment of hydrocephalus in adults. However, temporary benefits may be obtained with acetazolamide or furosemide.

2. **C Chemical.** Chemical meningitis usually results from the iatrogenic introduction of substances into the subarachnoid space during lumbar puncture or spinal anaesthetic. Injecting the wrong drug can be catastrophic for both patient and subsequently the doctor. Most drugs excluding local anaesthetics are neurotoxic either directly or as a result of their pH. Local anaesthetic should only be drawn up immediately before use and should be clearly labelled. Occasionally chemical meningitis results from rupture of a dermoid or epidermoid cyst present in the subarachnoid space.

3. **I Vertebral osteomyelitis.** Vertebral osteomyelitis most frequently results from entrapment of septic emboli (e.g. from cutaneous abscesses, urinary tract infection) in the arteriolar networks of the vertebral bodies. Infection then advances into the spinal canal in approximately 10% of patients. The diagnosis is confirmed by MR imaging or isotope bone scanning. Ideally, a bone biopsy should be performed to obtain cultures and sensitivities. Most cases of osteomyelitis and associated meningitis settle with systemic antibiotics. A surgical debridement may also be necessary.

A2.55 Rehabilitation

1. **F Isotonic exercises.** As early as possible following any intervention, the patient should be encouraged to exercise. Effective analgesia is necessary to facilitate passive movement and to allow the patient to cooperate in graded activity exercises to improve breathing and limb mobility. Isometric exercises (tension in the muscle increases without

muscle shortening) are performed to increase muscle strength; while isotonic exercises (muscle contraction results in muscle shortening) are performed to increase the range of movement.

2. **D** **Gutter crutch.** Functional (walking) aids take the form of walking sticks, crutches or walking frames. Crutches produce greater load reductions than walking sticks but are more unstable than walking frames. Crutches consist of three types: axillary, elbow and gutter. Axillary crutches that are not used properly (i.e. elbows locked straight) may result in radial nerve palsy. Elbow crutches overcome this problem but have the disadvantage of being easily broken. Gutter crutches provide weight bearing through the forearms and are ideal for elderly patients with hand deformities.

3. **H** **Spinal support.** Neuromuscular conditions (i.e. cerebral palsy, Duchenne's muscular dystrophy) may result in progressive spinal deformity, which compromises cardiorespiratory function and quality of life. Semi-rigid or total contact external spinal orthoses are used in neuromuscular scoliosis to facilitate seating and function. Orthoses act on the spine via pressure applied to the skin, soft tissues, ribs and abdomen. The corrective force transmitted to the spine is limited by the tolerance of the soft tissues.

Trauma and orthopaedic surgery

A2.56 Injuries to the upper arm and shoulder region

1. **H** **Fracture of the neck of scapula.** Scapular neck fractures are usually caused by direct trauma to the upper back, as in a fall from height, or by high-speed road traffic collisions. It can also result from an anterior or posterior force applied to the shoulder region. Patients present with bruising and tenderness over the scapular region on the affected side; maximal tenderness is over the lateral humeral head. There is also drooping of the affected shoulder with apparent lengthening of the arm, particularly with a fractured neck of the scapula. Patients with scapular neck fractures resist all shoulder movements and hold the limb in adduction. Fractures of the scapula, first or second ribs, or the sternum, suggest a magnitude of injury so severe that associated injuries to the head, neck, spinal cord, lungs and the great vessels should be ruled out. Most scapular neck fractures can be treated conservatively. Internal fixation is indicated for some articular fractures of the glenoid cavity.

2. **B** **Anterior dislocation of the shoulder.** Anterior (subcoracoid) dislocation is the most common type of dislocation of the shoulder. The usual mechanism of injury is a fall onto the outstretched arm with the arm abducted and externally rotated. It can also result from various sporting injuries, commonly basketball and rugby. Pain is severe, and the

patient is unwilling to attempt movements of the shoulder. A swelling may be noticed in the deltopectoral groove (displaced head) with an undue prominence of the acromion process. The arm is held in slight abduction and external rotation. There may be flattening and loss of contour of the shoulder just below the acromion process, and lowering of the anterior axillary fold. If the axillary nerve is damaged, patients may present with loss of sensation over the upper, outer aspect of the arm (Regimental Badge area).

3. **G Fracture of the neck of the humerus.** Fractured neck of the humerus is common in the middle aged and the elderly. The fracture can result from direct trauma to the upper arm. In elderly patients, particularly women, the bone is frequently osteoporotic; the possibility of a pathological fracture secondary to malignancy should also be borne in mind. The patient may present with extensive bruising and pain over the upper- and mid-parts of the arm. Sometimes the presentation is delayed because the patient may be able to use the arm to some extent without much pain. This is particularly true for impacted fractures. The modern Neer classification for fractures of the proximal end of humerus is based on the involvement of the four parts: (1) articular segment of the head, (2) the greater tuberosity, (3) the lesser tuberosity and (4) the surgical neck. Depending on the number of parts displaced, they are classified as two-part, three-part, or four-part fractures. See 4.24 Heal of humerus fracture.

A2.57 Injuries to the forearm and hand

1. **G Monteggia fracture.** Monteggia fractures, comprising less than 5% of forearm fractures, are primarily associated with falls on an out-stretched hand with forced pronation. The mechanism of injury is that of transmission of force through the hand and forearm with the elbow partially flexed. It can also result from direct trauma to the forearm. A Monteggia fracture is characterised by angulation at the junction of the proximal and middle-third of the ulna, accompanied by anterior dislocation of the radial head. Following injury, patients may present with elbow pain. Depending on the type of fracture and severity, they may also have elbow swelling, deformity, crepitus and paraesthesia. Elbow flexion and forearm rotation are limited and painful. Radial head dislocation may lead to radial nerve injury. The posterior interosseous branch of the radial nerve, which courses around the neck of the radius, is especially at risk, especially in Bado type II injuries. See 4.25 Forearm fracture.

2. **I Scaphoid fracture.** The scaphoid is the most commonly fractured carpal bone (Fig. 2.57.1). The mechanism of injury is usually a fall on the outstretched hand with the wrist extended and radially deviated. This causes extreme dorsiflexion at the wrist and compression to the radial side of the hand, leading to fracture of the scaphoid. The patient usually

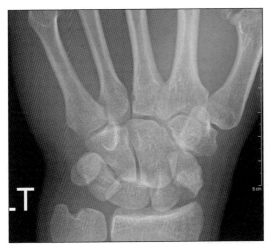

Fig. 2.57.1 The antero-posterior view shows a fracture of the waist of the scaphoid. The lunate also appears more triangular than normal and is suggestive of a perilunate dislocation.

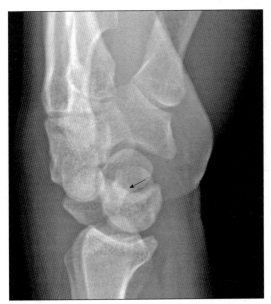

Fig. 2.57.2 The lateral view confirms the perilunate dislocation (arrow).

complains of a deep, dull pain on the radial side of the wrist, which is worsened by gripping or squeezing. It is also exacerbated by active extension and adduction of the thumb. Tenderness in the anatomical snuffbox and pain on longitudinal compression of the thumb (scaphoid compression test) are the most accurate signs of scaphoid fracture, although the former is more commonly performed. There may be mild wrist swelling or bruising and, possibly, fullness in the anatomical snuffbox, suggesting a wrist effusion. Early accurate diagnosis and management of scaphoid fractures is vital. A delay can lead to a variety of adverse outcomes including persistent pain, non-union, delayed union, decreased grip strength, decreased range of wrist motion and osteoarthritis of the radiocarpal joint. The differential diagnosis for suspected scaphoid injuries includes distal radial fracture, fractures of other metacarpal bones, scapholunate dissociation (Fig. 2.57.2), tenosynovitis or strains. See Case 3.4.

3. **F** **Galeazzi fracture.** A Galeazzi fracture is a fracture of the junction of the distal-third and middle-third of the radius with associated sub-luxation or dislocation of the distal radio-ulnar joint. They usually occur after a fall on the hand with a rotational force superimposed on it (axial load placed on a hyperpronated forearm). It can also occur following a direct blow to the middle/distal forearm as in road traffic collisions. Patients present with pain and soft-tissue swelling at the distal-third radius fracture site and at the wrist joint. On examination, there is bruising, swelling and tenderness over the lower end of the forearm. Deformity may be present. Plain radiography reveals the displaced fracture of the radius and the fragments of the radius are usually tilted medially towards the ulna. The ulnar head is prominent due to dislocation of the inferior radio-ulnar joint. Galeazzi fractures in adults should be treated by open reduction and internal fixation. Surgical reduction of both the radius and distal radio-ulnar joint provides the best opportunity for healing. See 4.25 Forearm fracture.

A2.58 Brachial plexus injuries

1. **H** **Radial nerve.** Radial nerve compression or injury may occur at any point along the anatomical course of the nerve. It may be associated with fracture of the humerus, especially in the middle-third or at the junction of the middle- and distal-thirds; the radial nerve lies in the spiral groove in this region. The presentation may be at the time of the injury or secondary to fracture manipulation; delayed presentation may be seen related to a healing callus. The other important site of compression of the radial nerve is in the proximal forearm in the area of the supinator muscle and involves the posterior interosseous branch. Such injuries cause wrist drop (paralysis of the extensor muscles of the wrist, finger and thumb) and also paralysis of the brachioradialis and the supinator muscles. Very proximal lesions may affect the triceps muscle. There is sensory loss over the dorsoradial aspect of the hand and the dorsal aspect of the radial $3^1/_2$ digits.

2. **A** **Axillary nerve.** The axillary (circumflex) nerve can be injured or damaged after fracture dislocation of the upper humerus, shoulder dislocation, pressure from casts or splints, improper use of crutches,

or deep intramuscular injections. There may be wasting and weakness of the deltoid resulting in the loss of shoulder abduction. The patient is unable to initiate abduction of the shoulder because the supraspinatus and the deltoid help the early phase of abduction; supraspinatus causes the first 10–15° of abduction followed by deltoid, which helps in further 90–100° of abduction. There may be a small area of sensory loss over the insertion of deltoid (upper outer aspect of the deltoid region; also called the 'Regimental Badge area'). Relevant investigations in patients with suspected axillary nerve injuries secondary to intramuscular injection include electromyography, nerve biopsy and MR imaging.

3. **C Long thoracic nerve.** The long thoracic nerve (nerve of Bell), comprising the C5, 6, 7 nerve roots, supplies the serratus anterior muscle which helps to stabilise the scapula. This nerve may be damaged following brachial plexus injury or during surgery to the chest wall, breast (including mastectomy and breast augmentation) or the axillary region. Other causes include radiotherapy, trauma, anaesthetic nerve block and transaxillary incision. Paralysis of the serratus anterior muscle causes winging of the scapula particularly when the patient is asked to push his/her arms against resistance.

A2.59 Lower limb nerve injuries

1. **A Common peroneal nerve.** The common peroneal nerve (lateral popliteal nerve; L4-S2) injury is common following fibular neck fractures because the nerve winds down the neck and is relatively superficial at this point. Isolated fractures of the proximal fibula or fibular shaft are however uncommon and are usually due to a direct blow producing transverse or comminuted fractures. The fibula can also be injured by indirect forces, with the proximal fibula most commonly fractured by external rotation forces and the distal fibula by internal rotation forces. The common peroneal nerve can also be injured following a trauma or injury to the knee, use of tight plaster casts and pressure to the fibular neck region from positions during deep sleep or coma. The common peroneal nerve gives motor supply to the dorsiflexor and evertor muscles of the ankle and toes. Its sensory branches supply the anterior and lateral aspect of the leg and whole of the dorsum of the foot and toes except the lateral aspect of the foot (supplied by the sural nerve). Injury to this nerve results in foot drop and the patient is unable to dorsiflex and evert the foot. The sensory loss is over the anterior and lateral aspect of the leg, and dorsum of the foot and the toes.

2. **B Femoral nerve.** The femoral nerve (L2-4) reaches the front of the leg by penetrating the psoas muscle before it exits the pelvis by passing beneath the medial inguinal ligament to enter the femoral triangle. In the femoral triangle, it lies immediately lateral to the femoral artery and vein. It may be injured by direct penetrating wounds, gunshot wounds, traction during surgery, injuries to the femoral triangle, by massive

haematoma within the thigh, psoas abscess, fractured pelvis, or by hip dislocation. It innervates the iliopsoas (a hip flexor) and the quadriceps (a knee extensor). The motor branch to the iliopsoas originates in the pelvis proximal to the inguinal ligament, and injury at or above this level leads to loss of hip flexion. The sensory branch of the femoral nerve, the saphenous nerve, innervates skin of the medial thigh and the anterior and medial aspects of the calf. Damage to the femoral nerve causes weakness of the quadriceps muscle and decreased patellar reflex. The patient finds that the knee gives way on walking and has difficulty climbing stairs. There is numbness over the anterior thigh and medial aspect of the leg.

3. **H** **Tibial nerve.** The tibial nerve (S1-S2) may be damaged by posterior dislocation of the knee, posteriorly displaced fractures of the tibia, sports injuries, and severe fractures around the knee joint. It may also be compressed behind the medial malleolus by the posterior tarsal tunnel. The tibial nerve supplies the flexor compartment giving muscular branches to the deep surface of soleus, flexor digitorum longus and hallucis longus, and tibialis posterior. It divides into medial and lateral plantar branches to supply the intrinsic muscles of the foot and provides sensation to the plantar surface of the foot. It also provides cutaneous and articular branches to the medial side of the ankle and foot. Injury to the tibial nerve results in loss of toe flexion and inability to invert the ankle and the ankle jerk is lost. There is complete sensory loss over the plantar surface of the foot.

Urology

A2.60 Urological trauma

1. **C** **Distal ureter.** The ureter descends through the retroperitoneum on the psoas major muscle, it crosses the pelvic brim at the bifurcation of the common iliac artery and lies on the levator ani muscle before swinging forward and medially into the base of the bladder at the level of the ischial spine. Iatrogenic ureteric injuries, in particular, occur during resection of the large bowel, aortic aneurysm surgery and hysterectomy. The ureter is most prone to injury below the pelvic brim (distal ureter). An unrecognised division of a ureter results in a urinary fistula which may drain through the vagina or wound. If a ureteric injury is recognised at the time of surgery, immediate repair is performed over a JJ ureteric stent. Delayed recognition usually requires re-implantation of the ureter into the bladder. A tube of bladder needs to be fashioned (Boari flap) if the ureter is short.

2. **B** **Bladder.** Bladder injuries most commonly result from blunt trauma. The most common mode of injury is a direct blow over a full bladder. Full thickness tears anteriorly or posteriorly result in extraperitoneal extravasation of urine causing suprapubic pain, tenderness and swelling.

A full thickness tear in the dome results in an intraperitoneal rupture resulting in pain initially, with later signs of uraemia as the peritoneum reabsorbs urea from the urine. The diagnosis is confirmed by CT cystography. Extraperitoneal ruptures are usually managed conservatively while intraperitoneal ruptures require laparotomy and two-layered closure of the bladder.

3. **A** **Anterior urethra.** Anterior (bulbous) urethral trauma usually results from iatrogenic manipulation or straddle injuries, whereas most posterior urethral injuries result from pelvic fractures sustained in motorcycle injuries. The diagnosis of urethral trauma is confirmed by a retrograde urethrogram. Most anterior urethral injuries are treated conservatively with urethral catheterisation and systemic antibiotics. A completely transected urethra requires debridement, mobilisation and urethral anastomosis over a urethral catheter.

A2.61 Urinary tract infections and calculi

1. **C** **Acute pyelonephritis.** Acute pyelonephritis results from a bacterial infection (usually Gram-negative organisms, predominantly *Escherichia coli*) of the upper urinary tract and is an important manifestation of lower urinary tract infections. Predisposing factors include urinary tract obstruction, e.g. benign prostatic hypertrophy, pregnancy or incompetence of the vesicoureteral orifice. Acute pyelonephritis is frequently mistaken for appendicitis when present on the right. However, high fever is uncommon in appendicitis but commonly a feature in acute pyelonephritis. The patient may also report nausea, vomiting, increased urinary frequency or dysuria prior to the onset of fever. Urinalysis reveals bacteria and white cells. Ultrasonography is performed to identify any obstruction. Systemic antibiotics are required because of the risk of septicaemia.

2. **B** **Acute prostatitis.** Acute prostatitis is seen in men of all ages and is typically associated with lower urinary tract symptoms, suprapubic and perineal pain. The mid-stream urine sample frequently shows no growth. The causative organisms are usually Gram-negative (e.g. *Escherichia coli* or *Klebsiella*). Patients require a prolonged course of antibiotics (approximately 6 weeks). Chronic bacterial prostatitis may follow acute infection and is diagnosed by culture of the mid-stream urine following prostatic massage.

3. **D** **Calcium oxalate.** Urinary tract calculi result from inadequate drainage of the renal tract (e.g. abnormal renal tract anatomy), urinary tract infection (e.g. those caused by *Proteus* spp.), metabolic causes (e.g. raised calcium in hyperparathyroidism, raised uric acid (e.g. patients with ileostomies or chronic diarrhoea), hyperoxaluria, dehydration or idiopathic causes. The composition of calculi varies, with calcium oxalate lithiasis being most frequently found in Western societies. Calcium oxalate calculi are hard, irregular (jackstones) and brittle and are the most radiodense

of all renal calculi. These calculi usually result from hypercalciuria and hyperoxaluria of dietary origin. The treatment of urinary tract calculi includes open surgery, percutaneous techniques and fragmentation of calculi (extracorporeal or endoscopic). Patients should also be given dietary advice to prevent recurrence. See 4.53 Renal tract calculi.

A2.62 Haematuria

1. **H** **Renal cell carcinoma.** Renal cell carcinoma is an adenocarcinoma arising from the proximal convoluted tubule. The tumour spreads locally through the renal capsule and along the renal vein to the inferior vena cava. Presentation is usually due to direct, lymphatic (approximately 25% to para-aortic, paracaval or mediastinal lymph nodes) or haematogenous spread (approximately 25%, e.g. lung 'cannonball metastases' or bone) or due to paraneoplastic syndrome (e.g. increased renin production results in hypertension, elevated erythropoietin results in polycythaemia, increased parathyroid hormone results in hypercalcaemia). Left renal vein involvement may cause a rapid onset varicocele (Fig. 2.62.1). Staging is by CT: I, confined to kidney; II, through capsule; III, to renal vein; IV, local invasion or distant metastases. Treatment is by radical nephrectomy with removal of any venous thrombus. See 3.58 Nephrectomy.

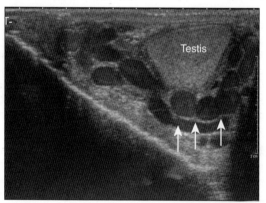

Fig. 2.62.1 Ultrasound of a left varicocele. Varicoceles are more common on the left due to their drainage to the left renal vein. Drainage is to the inferior vena cava on the right.

2. **I** **Transitional cell carcinoma.** Transitional cell carcinoma accounts for 97% of all bladder urothelial cancers. Squamous cell and adeno-carcinomas are extremely rare. Cigarette smoking is the most common aetiological cause. Most patients present with painless haematuria although increasingly, patients are being identified earlier with micro-scopic haematuria on routine urinalysis. Patients with haematuria are screened with mid-stream urinalysis, intravenous urogram and flexible cystourethroscopy. Superficial tumours (T0 and T1) are resected with a rigid cystoscope (transurethral resection of bladder tumour), treated with

intravesical immunotherapy (attenuated *Mycobacterium bovis*) and followed up at regular intervals with cystoscopy. Invasive tumours (T2 and T3) require radical radiotherapy or radical cystectomy and formation of an ileal conduit.

3. **B** **Glomerulonephritis.** Acute glomerulonephritis usually follows 2–3 weeks after an upper respiratory infection (β haemolytic, Lancefield group *A Streptococcus*). The bacterial antigen becomes attached in the glomerulus and leads to an acute diffuse proliferative glomerulonephritis. The congestion of the glomeruli results in hypervolaemia due to sodium retention and impaired renal function. The anti-Streptolysin O titre is usually raised. Treatment is usually supportive (control of fluid retention and hypertension). Most patients recover fully with only a small number progressing to develop renal failure.

A2.63 Urinary tract obstruction

1. **E** **Pelviureteric junction obstruction.** Pelviureteric junction obstruction most frequently presents in infancy or childhood. It results from intrinsic (disorder of the smooth muscle of the ureter), extrinsic (pressure from an aberrant vessel) or secondary causes (severe vesicoureteric reflux) and has a male to female ratio of 2:1. Most cases are now detected on antenatal ultrasonography (hydronephrotic kidney). Presentation in adulthood is usually with urinary infection, abdominal pain, loin mass and haematuria. Stasis of urine may also lead to stone formation (ingestion of large volumes of fluid leads to a build-up of urine proximal to the obstruction, resulting in pain). The diagnosis is confirmed by ultrasonography. A voiding cystogram should also be performed to exclude vesicoureteral reflux. Treatment is by refashioning of the pelviureteric junction (pyeloplasty). Non-functioning kidneys are treated with nephrectomy.

2. **H** **Retroperitoneal fibrosis.** Retroperitoneal fibrosis is a benign or malignant fibro-inflammatory process which spreads proximally to encase the ureter and renal pelvis from the sacroiliac joints. The condition may involve the inferior vena cava and aorta. Approximately 60% of cases result from idiopathic retroperitoneal fibrosis (which is benign). The most common cause of malignant retroperitoneal fibrosis is lymphoma although metastasis from breast, colon, stomach or pancreas may also be the cause. The diagnosis is confirmed by CT and a raised erythrocyte sedimentation rate. Initial management involves treatment of renal failure and the placement of JJ ureteric stents to relieve the obstruction. Definitive treatment is with laparotomy and ureterolysis.

3. **A** **Aorto-iliac aneurysm.** Aorto-iliac aneurysms may produce obstruction of one or both ureters by extrinsic compression or by inflammation. Inflammatory abdominal aortic aneurysms account for 10% of all aortic aneurysms below the level of the renal arteries. The reason for the inflammation remains unclear. At operation, there is a dense white peri-aortic

fibrosis which obscures anatomical tissue planes and frequently involves the ureters, duodenum and left renal vein. A characteristic rind of fibrosis outside the calcified wall of the aneurysm is commonly seen on CT. JJ ureteric stents should be placed prior to aneurysm repair. Ureterolysis is rarely required as the condition usually resolves following aneurysm repair.

A2.64 Pain and swelling in the scrotum

1. **H Testicular torsion.** Testicular torsion (more correctly torsion of the spermatic cord) is of two types: extravaginal, occurring in the neonatal period, or intravaginal which can occur at any age (peak incidence 14–20 years). Intravaginal torsion results from a high investment of the tunica vaginalis producing a horizontally lying ('bell-clapper') testis; this position allows the testes and spermatic cord to rotate within the tunica. Patients present with scrotal pain, which is often referred to the groin or iliac fossa in the early stages. Nausea and vomiting are also common. Oedema and erythema are common in testicular torsion while uncommon in epididymo-orchitis. Testicular torsion requires an emergency surgical exploration, the testes detorted and assessment of viability made. Viable testes are fixed at three points to the tunica with the contralateral testis fixed in a similar fashion (as horizontally lying testes are frequently bilateral). A necrotic testis requires immediate orchidectomy. Torsion of a testicular appendage, orchitis and idiopathic scrotal oedema are also common in adolescent males. If there is doubt over the diagnosis the scrotum should be explored surgically. See 3.57 Orchidopexy.

2. **C Epididymo-orchitis.** Epididymo-orchitis is most frequently transmitted sexually in men younger than 35 years (*Chlamydia trachomatis*, *Neisseria gonorrhoeae*). In older men it is usually caused by non-sexually transmitted Gram-negative enteric organisms following urethral catheterisation or due to an anatomical abnormality of the urinary tract. Patients present with unilateral testicular pain. This pain needs to be differentiated from the pain of testicular torsion (in which pain is usually sudden and severe). The patient may report a history of urethritis or a urethral discharge if the epididymo-orchitis is sexually transmitted. On examination, the testis is swollen and tender on the affected side with a swollen epididymis. The patient is usually pyrexial and a hydrocele may be present. Urethral swabs or first-void urine should be sent for culture and sensitivity. Management consists of bed rest, analgesia, scrotal elevation and support. Patients are also advised to abstain from sexual intercourse and screened for other sexually transmitted infections. Prior to sensitivities becoming available, the patient should be treated empirically with ceftriaxone or ciprofloxacin and doxycycline (if thought to be sexually transmitted). If testicular torsion cannot be excluded an immediate scrotal exploration should be performed.

3. **B Epididymal cyst.** Epididymal cysts most frequently arise in the head of the epididymis from one of the tubules of the epididymis. The fluid

aspirate is clear. Occasionally the fluid is white and opaque due to the presence of spermatozoa and in this case, the cyst is called a spermatocele. The cyst is thin-walled, smooth to palpation and occasionally loculated. When large, they may be difficult to differentiate from a hydrocele. However, the fluid aspirated from a hydrocele is usually clear and straw coloured. These cysts are usually treated conservatively, but enucleation may be performed if persistently painful. Surgery should be avoided in young men as postoperative fibrosis may impair sperm transfer. Recurrent, symptomatic cysts may be treated with epididymectomy.

A2.65 Chronic renal failure

1. **B** **Continuous arteriovenous haemofiltration (CAVH).** Renal replacement therapy is required when acute renal insufficiency is not adequately corrected by general measures. Renal replacement therapy may be dialysis, haemofiltration or a combination of both. Haemofiltration is either continuous arteriovenous or veno-venous. The removed plasma is driven under pressure through a semipermeable membrane in large volumes. The filtrate is discarded and replaced by water and solute. The clearance of intermolecular weight solutes is higher than in haemodialysis, while the clearance of small molecular solutes is greater in haemodialysis. Continuous haemofiltration can be used in patients with low systolic blood pressures to provide continuous metabolic control and fluid balance. CAVH requires heparinisation and should only be used in immobilised patients and where there is continuous nursing supervision.

2. **A** **Continuous ambulatory peritoneal (CAPD).** Continuous ambulatory peritoneal dialysis is performed via a rigid or soft (Tenckhoff) catheter inserted percutaneously into an intact peritoneum. CAPD has the advantage of being relatively cheap and simple to set up. In continuous ambulatory peritoneal dialysis, fluid is passed into the peritoneum via the peritoneal catheter and the dialysate changed four times daily. In this technique, the uraemic toxins diffuse from the blood of the mesentery across the peritoneum (semipermeable membrane) into the dialysate. Disadvantages are relatively high re-admission rates with complications (leakage of fluid, infection/peritonitis, catheter displacement) and a tendency to obesity following glucose absorption.

3. **F** **Standard machine driven haemodialysis (HD).** Haemodialysis produces ultrafiltration of blood across a semipermeable membrane to allow the removal of water and solutes. Filtration occurs across the membrane which separates the blood from water mixed with concentrated electrolytes (dialysate). Blood is transported to the membrane via an arteriovenous (usually between the radial artery and the cephalic vein) fistula into which two needles are inserted. Continuous ambulatory peritoneal dialysis is an alternative to haemodialysis. See 4.39 Haemodialysis access.

A2.66 Aspects of pelvic surgery

1. **D Parasympathetic pelvic splanchnic nerves.** The neural control of erection comes from the genital branches of the parasympathetic pelvic splanchnic nerves S2-S4 (still often referred to as the nervi erigentes), resulting in vasodilatation of the arteries of the erectile tissue of the corpora and a degree of venous occlusion. These nerves lie anterolaterally in the angle between the seminal vesicles and the prostate and are prone to injury during pelvic surgery. In rectal surgery early division and retraction of Denonvilliers' fascia protects the nerves. Erectile dysfunction following radical prostatectomy has been reported to be approximately 30% and has been reported to be as high as 50% following abdominoperineal excision. Patients should therefore be warned of the risks of sexual and urinary dysfunction if pelvic surgery is anticipated.

2. **H Superior hypogastric plexus.** The first part of ejaculation process (emission) is under control of the superior hypogastric plexus (sympathetic nerves T11-L2) and consists of transmission of seminal fluid from the vasa, prostate and seminal vesicles by contraction of the smooth muscle within these structures into the prostatic urethra. The second part (ejaculation) is under both autonomic and somatic control and consists of constriction of the internal urethral opening (to prevent retrograde flow into the bladder) and compression of the penile urethra by the contractions of the bulbospongiosus (perineal branch of the pudendal nerve S2, S3), which results in expulsion of the semen. Ejaculatory dysfunction can occur following bladder neck surgery, resection of the rectum or open prostatectomy. The superior hypogastric plexus (still occasionally referred to as the pre-sacral nerves) divides on the anterior surface of the sacral promontory into the right and left hypogastric nerves which run on each pelvic side-wall. These nerves should be identified at the start of a posterior dissection to prevent injury. Disruption of any of the above may result in an ejaculation or retrograde ejaculation (semen passes into the bladder). The patient should be assessed to exclude a psychogenic cause.

3. **B Distal urethral sphincter.** Male stress incontinence is rare and usually results from prostate surgery. The rates of stress incontinence following transurethral prostatectomy are approximately 4% with rates up to 80% reported after radical prostatectomy. The male functional sphincter unit is divided into proximal urethral sphincter (bladder neck) and distal urethral sphincter (urethral muscularis and periurethral striated muscle). The proximal sphincter is removed at open and transurethral prostatectomy, therefore relying on the distal sphincter for continence. Damage to the distal sphincter unit renders the patient incontinent.

SAQs

CHAPTER 3

The viva

QUESTION AND ANSWER

Applied surgical anatomy

Case 3.1 Thorax

Q A 35-year-old motorcyclist involved in a road traffic accident (RTA) presents with severe bruising over his left chest wall. On examination, the lower four ribs on the left side are fractured and bowel sounds are heard in the chest. What is the most likely diagnosis?

A The most likely diagnosis is rupture of the left hemi-diaphragm. There is injury (and rupture) of the hemi-diaphragm in approximately 5% of all abdomino-thoracic injuries.

Q What are the causes for diaphragmatic rupture?

A A common cause for diaphragmatic rupture is direct penetrating injuries to the thoraco-abdominal region. The injury could be at any level between the 4th or 5th to the 10th intercostal space (ICS), depending on the state of the patient's respiratory pattern (see below). Trauma causing fracture of the ribs is another important cause. The final, albeit uncommon, cause of diaphragmatic rupture is a sudden, severe increase in thoraco-abdominal pressure. This occurs when there is blunt abdominal trauma with the individual having a closed glottis.

Q What do you know about the levels of the two domes of the diaphragm and what is its clinical significance?

A The diaphragm is the thin sheet of muscle caudal to the lungs, consisting of two domes with the central tendon lying at the level of the xiphisternal junction (level of T8 vertebrae). Since the liver lies underneath the right dome and pushes it upwards, the right dome lies anatomically higher than the left. In full expiration, the right dome ascends up to the 4th ICS (level of the nipple) while the left reaches the 5th rib. In stab injuries to the thoraco-abdominal region, it should be borne in mind that even in high chest injuries the diaphragm can be injured if the patient was in full expiration and, likewise, intra-abdominal organs such as the liver may be injured even if the wound appears to be in the thoracic cavity.

Q What structures traverse the diaphragm?

A The diaphragm has three large openings for the passage of structures between the thorax and abdomen. The aortic opening lies opposite the T12 vertebra. It transmits the aorta along with the azygos vein and thoracic duct. The oesophageal opening lies opposite the T10 vertebra. It transmits the oesophagus. The vena caval opening lies opposite the T8 vertebra and transmits the inferior vena cava along with the right phrenic nerve.

Q **Which nerve supplies the diaphragm and what is its clinical significance?**

A The diaphragm is supplied by the phrenic nerve (C3, C4, C5) on each side. Complete transaction of the cervical cord at or above this level leads to total paralysis of the diaphragm and thus fatal respiratory compromise. In such instances, the patient will become fully dependent on an external ventilatory support. In cases of unilateral phrenic nerve damage, the affected hemi-dome is paralysed. The unaffected side can sustain respiratory function but the patient is likely to develop frequent lung infections in the affected side.

Q **How will you manage injuries to the diaphragm?**

A Diaphragmatic injury, especially in blunt trauma has a high proportion of associated injuries such as pelvic injuries and visceral injuries (e.g. spleen, liver) which need to be identified and treated. Diaphragmatic rupture is difficult to detect clinically and this leads to significant morbidity and even mortality. Rupture may be suggested on a plain chest radiograph, especially with an abnormal location of the naso-gastric tube but the accuracy of this method is only modest. Helical CT scanning identifies most injuries and the investigation of choice in the trauma setting. MR scanning while very sensitive and specific, is not feasible in most trauma situations, but remains a useful tool to explore abnormalities or uncertainties from a prior CT scan, in stable patients. An exploratory laparotomy or laparoscopy may be necessary to confirm or rule out the diagnosis.

At laparotomy or thoracotomy, associated injuries which often take precedence, should be sought and treated. The diaphragm may be sutured using non-absorbable sutures without tension. An intercostal chest drain is placed and connected to an underwater seal drain system.

Case 3.2 Mediastinum

Q **A 40-year-old motorcyclist involved in a RTA presents with bruises and lacerations over his left chest wall. On examination, breath sounds are normal bilaterally but the heart sounds are muffled. His blood pressure is 90/68 mmHg; the jugular venous pressure is elevated. A chest radiograph shows fractured 4th, 5th and 6th ribs on the left. What is your most likely diagnosis?**

A The most likely diagnosis is cardiac tamponade.

Q   **What is the aetiology of cardiac tamponade?**

A   Direct penetrating injury to the heart is the mostly likely aetiology for a cardiac tamponade. However, blunt injuries to the heart may also cause cardiac tamponade by injuring the pericardial vessels. Likewise, high velocity injuries to the great vessels could result in pooling of blood in the pericardium leading to tamponade. Apart from trauma, it can occur following lung or breast carcinomas, pericarditis and myocardial infarction.

Q   **How would you make a diagnosis of cardiac tamponade?**

A   Cardiac tamponade can be difficult to detect clinically, especially in a trauma setting. The classic (and diagnostic) signs include: a fall in blood pressure; rising jugular venous pulse and muffled heart sounds (Beck's triad). Pulsus paradoxus may also be an associated finding (normally, there is a physiological decrease in systolic blood pressure during spontaneous inspiration. When this change exceeds 10 mmHg, it is termed pulsus paradoxus). In addition, the jugular venous pulse may paradoxically rise with inspiration (Kussmaul's sign). Chest radiograph may reveal a globular heart, a convex or straight left heart border and a right cardiophrenic angle of <90°.

Q   **Describe the surface anatomy of the heart.**

A   The heart has three borders: the right, the inferior and the left. The right heart border is made up entirely of the right atrium with the superior and the inferior vena cava. This extends from the 3rd to the 6th right costal cartilage, approximately 3 cm away from the midline. The inferior border consists of the right ventricle and the apex of the left ventricle. It extends from approximately 3 cm to the right of the midline at the level of the 6th costal cartilage to the apex which lies in the 5th inter-costal space in the mid-clavicular line (approximately 6 cm away from the midline). The left border extends from the apex up to the 2nd inter-space, approximately 3 cm away from the midline.

Q   **How would you perform a pericardiocentesis?**

A   The procedure should be performed under ECG monitoring. The patient should be (preferably) sat up with a 30–45° head elevation. This increases pooling of blood (or fluid) toward the inferior and anterior surface, thus maximising fluid drainage. The selected site for needle insertion is infiltrated with local anaesthesia. Under sterile conditions, after cleaning and draping the area, a needle, connected to a 3-way tap, is directed from the left xiphichondral junction at an angle of 45° pointing to the left shoulder (care should be taken to prevent injury to vital structures such as the internal mammary artery, lungs, liver, neurovascular bundle at the inferior margin of each rib and the great vessels). The needle and the syringe are advanced until the needle tip is posterior to the rib cage. The syringe should be aspirated while advancing the needle toward the pericardial space. The needle is advanced until blood (or fluid) is aspirated in the syringe or the ECG monitor shows ST elevation. The needle is withdrawn slowly with negative pressure on the syringe if the ECG shows ST elevation (current of injury). The needle is reinserted in a different direction very slowly until blood (or fluid) is aspirated in the syringe. In cardiac tamponade, aspiration of as little as 20 ml of blood relieves the complication. If continuous drainage is required, using the Seldinger technique, a pericardial catheter should be inserted. The catheter can be left in place for 24 hours. Gravity or negative suction can be used to increase the drainage. The catheter should be removed after 24 hours, if possible, because of the risk of infection in the pericardial space. However, keeping the catheter in the pericardial space often is necessary to maintain drainage for longer periods. If exploration of the pericardial wound is required (preferably in the operating theatre), a small pericardial window can be created by using a short sub-xiphoid incision in the skin and the underlying linea alba (under local or general anaesthesia). The underlying subcutaneous tissue is separated using blunt dissection. The wound can then be explored down to the pericardial sac.

Q   **What are the risks associated with this procedure and how would you monitor it?**

A   Injuries to the cardiac muscle, chamber(s) of the heart and, rarely, to the great vessels are the most common and serious risks associated with this procedure. If the needle enters the cardiac muscle, commonly into the ventricular muscle, an injury pattern known as the 'current of injury' appears on the ECG monitor. This is characterised by extreme ST-T wave changes or a widening and enlarged QRS complex. This pattern dictates that the pericardiocentesis needle should be withdrawn until the previous baseline ECG tracing reappears. If the needle is advanced too far, it enters the chamber(s) of the heart with the appearance of fresh blood into the syringe at relatively high pressure (the blood in the pericardial sac causing the tamponade is usually altered and unclotted). If the needle enters the left ventricle or ascending aorta then there is bright red, arterial blood.

Case 3.3 Abdominal wall

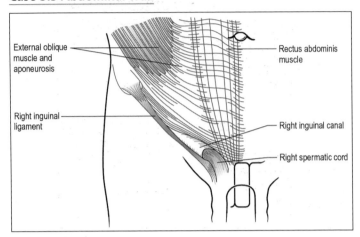

External oblique muscle and aponeurosis

Right inguinal ligament

Rectus abdominis muscle

Right inguinal canal

Right spermatic cord

Fig. 3.3.1 Interior abdominal wall.

Q   **What muscles make up the anterior abdominal wall?**

A   The anterior abdominal wall comprises of four muscles (Fig. 3.3.1) on each side of the midline: three of these are arranged in layers in the lateral part of the abdominal wall – external oblique, internal oblique and transversus abdominis. As these muscles traverse medially, the fleshy part gives way to an aponeurosis which forms a sheath (rectus sheath) around the fourth muscle – the rectus abdominis.

Q   **What are the other contents within the rectus sheath?**

A   The rectus sheath also contains the superior and inferior epigastric vessels, the lower six intercostal (thoracic) nerves and the small pyramidalis muscles.

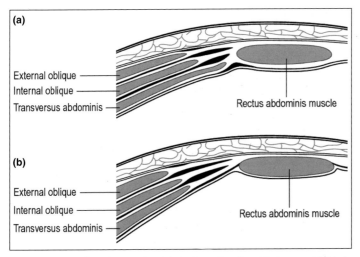

(a)

External oblique

Internal oblique

Transversus abdominis

Rectus abdominis muscle

(b)

External oblique

Internal oblique

Transversus abdominis

Rectus abdominis muscle

Fig. 3.3.2 Formation of rectus sheath in horizontal section, **(a)** above and **(b)** below the arcuate line.

Q   **Does the rectus sheath enclose the rectus muscle uniformly throughout the anterior abdominal wall?**

A   No, the composition of the rectus sheath varies at different levels. The posterior wall of the rectus sheath thins out abruptly a short distance below the umbilicus to form the arcuate line (Fig. 3.3.2). Above this line, the posterior wall of the sheath comprises the transversus abdominis aponeurosis and the posterior layer of the internal oblique aponeurosis. Below the arcuate line, all three aponeuroses pass anterior to the rectus and thus at this level the posterior surface of the rectus muscle is in direct contact with the transversalis fascia, which is a complete fascial sheet lying deep to the abdominal wall muscles surrounding the peritoneal cavity.

Q   **What do you understand by the term 'linea alba' and what is its significance?**

A   Between the two recti, all the aponeuroses fuse to form the linea alba, a strong midline fibrous structure. Median incisions through the linea alba are relatively bloodless and also allow quick access to all four quadrants of the abdomen.

Q   **Can you describe the lymphatic drainage of the anterior abdominal wall?**

A   Above the umbilicus, the superficial tissues of the anterolateral abdominal wall drain to the pectoral group of axillary nodes and below the umbilicus, to the superficial inguinal nodes. The deeper parts of the wall, above the umbilicus, pierce the diaphragm to reach the mediastinal nodes and below it, they run to the external iliac and para-aortic nodes. Umbilical tumours (squamous carcinoma) metastasise to the inguinal nodes.

Case 3.4 Upper limb

Q   What do you know about scaphoid fractures?

A   The scaphoid is the most frequently fractured carpal bone, accounting for approximately 80% of all carpal bone fractures. It is more common in young adults although elderly patients can also be affected. The mechanism of injury is usually a fall on to the outstretched hand, with the wrist extended to about 95°. The common causes of such injuries are a simple fall, sports accidents or road traffic accidents.

Q   What are the signs and symptoms of scaphoid fractures?

A   The classical signs of scaphoid fractures are: pain on wrist movements; swelling (fullness) over the anatomical snuffbox region and tenderness on direct pressure over the anatomical snuffbox region with worsening of the pain when the wrist is ulnar deviated.

Q   How would you manage a scaphoid fracture?

A   If the fracture is proven radiologically (and clinically), immobilisation of the fracture using a scaphoid plaster cast for 6 weeks is the recommended line of management. The patient should be referred for physiotherapy during this period. If a scaphoid fracture is a strong possibility but the initial radiographs are negative (as happens in a majority of cases), then the fracture should be immobilised in a scaphoid plaster cast for 2 weeks. A repeat radiograph should be done after this period by which time the fracture may be visible. If the radiograph is still inconclusive, a bone scan, CT or MR scan may be required to confirm the diagnosis, while the fracture is continued to be immobilised in plaster. Surgical intervention, including open reduction and internal fixation, is indicated in grossly comminuted or unstable fractures. In cases of non-union, internal fixation (with or without a bone graft) using a Herbert screw may be required.

Q   What one major complication is associated with scaphoid fractures and why?

A   Avascular necrosis is one of the major complications associated with fractures of the scaphoid bone. The blood supply to the scaphoid is from the radial and anterior interosseous arteries, with 70% of the blood supply entering through the distal ridge. Normally no vessels enter through the proximal pole and there is no intraosseous anastomosis between the vessels entering the tuberosity and dorsal ridge. The proximal pole receives its blood supply via retrograde flow from vessels that enter the cortex at or distal to the scaphoid waist; therefore, fracture through the waist causes devascularisation of the proximal pole resulting in avascular necrosis (this also explains the high healing rate in distal scaphoid fractures).

Q What is the prognosis of scaphoid fractures?

A The majority of stable, non-displaced, acute scaphoid fractures heal with conservative treatment. As a general rule, well-managed fractures involving the distal pole have a nearly 100% healing rate, while fractures of the waist have an 80–90% healing rate and proximal pole fractures treated by immobilisation have only a 60–70% rate of union. Degeneration of the wrist and early osteoarthritis are recognised late complications of scaphoid fractures.

Case 3.5 Joints and bones

Q How do you classify the various joints in the body?

A All joints in the body could be broadly divided into three types: (1) fibrous; (2) cartilaginous of which there are primary and secondary cartilaginous types and (3) synovial, which could be divided into typical and atypical types.

Q What is the difference between a fibrous and primary cartilaginous joint?

A The bone ends in a fibrous joint are united by fibrous tissue. The bones of the vault of the skull at the sutures are united by fibrous joints; the movement in such type of joints is negligible. Primary cartilaginous joints are formed when bone joins cartilage. They are immobile and strong. The adjacent bone may fracture but the bone-cartilage interface seldom separates. All epiphyses and the ribs attaching to their costal cartilages are examples of primary cartilaginous joints.

Q Can you explain a secondary cartilaginous joint with some examples?

A A secondary cartilaginous joint is a union between bones whose articular surfaces are covered with a thin lamina of hyaline cartilage, which in turn is frequently united by a fibrocartilage. All midline joints – symphysis pubis, sternal angle, xiphisternum and intervertebral discs – are examples of secondary cartilaginous joints.

Q What is a synovial joint and explain the types you know of with examples?

A A synovial joint is one in which the articular surfaces of the bone are covered by hyaline cartilage and surrounded by a capsule enclosing a joint cavity. The capsule is lined internally by synovial membrane (containing synovial fluid) and the capsule is reinforced internally or externally, or both, by ligaments. The joint is capable of varying degrees of movement. All limb joints fall in this category. In atypical synovial joints, such as the sternoclavicular joint and the acromioclavicular joint, there is no hyaline cartilage in the joint. The cartilaginous epiphysis, like all hyaline cartilage, has no blood supply. The synovial membrane, joint mesenchyme and its derivatives are supplied from a vascular plexus that surrounds the epiphysis and sends branches to the joint structures. As ossification of the cartilaginous epiphysis begins, branches from this vascular circle penetrate the ossification centre.

Q **What are the important differences between the bones of children and adults?**

A The most obvious difference between the bones of children and adults is the presence of cartilaginous growth plates at bone ends in children. In major long bones, they are present at either ends but usually at only one end of the 'short' long bones such as the metacarpals and the metatarsals. In childhood, the long bones also differ from the adult state in that they are more resilient and springy, withstanding greater deflection without fracture. This accounts for the incomplete fractures of the 'green-stick' type frequently seen in children. Another striking feature of children's bones is that the periosteum is only loosely attached to the diaphysis. The consequence of this feature is that when blood collects beneath the periosteum due to fractures, it might be easily stripped (denuded) from the bone over a considerable length. The subperiosteal haematoma is soon replaced by callus; this therefore extends a long way up and down the shaft, even when there has been little displacement of the bony fragments.

Case 3.6 Spinal cord

Q **Can spinal cord injuries occur without fractures of the vertebra?**

A Yes, it is possible to have spinal cord injuries without bony injury. This is particularly common in children. Due to the high mobility of the bony spine, fractures are less common in children than in adults. Spinal cord injury occurs in more than 50% of children without an associated fracture or radiological abnormality. This is called spinal cord injury without associated radiological abnormality (SCIWORA). The cervical region, particularly in children <8 years old, is the most common site for such pattern of injury. Although common in children, this can also occur in adults and there should be a high index of suspicion if the history and mechanism suggests a possible spinal cord injury.

Q **What are the types of spinal cord injury you know of?**

A Complete transaction of the spinal cord is the frequently observed pattern of injury. In addition, other types of injury can occur if the damage is only partial or incomplete. This is more common in direct stab or penetrating wounds to the spinal cord.

Brown-Sequard syndrome is due to hemisection of the cord. There is ipsilateral paralysis and loss of vibration and joint sense on the affected side; there is contralateral loss of pain and temperature sensation.

Central cord syndrome causes more selective damage to the central grey matter leading to paralysis of the affected group of muscles. The upper limbs are more affected due to the position of the fibre position within the cord; the sensory loss is variable. Patients may also have urinary retention.

Anterior cord syndrome is caused due to damage to the anterior spinal artery which leads to cord ischaemia. This can occur from aortic trauma or cross-clamping of the aorta during repair of abdominal aortic aneurysm. This condition results in paralysis of the affected group of muscles (cortico-spinal) with loss of light touch, pain and temperature sensations (spino-thalamic tracts). Posterior column function is preserved and normal vibration and joint position sensation are maintained.

Cauda Equina syndrome is associated with fractures of the lumbar vertebrae. The patients have dysfunction of the gastrointestinal and genito-urinary tracts. In addition, there are lower motor neuron signs in the lower limbs. Sensory changes are variable.

Q   **Describe the physiological and autonomic changes seen in early spinal cord injury.**

A   The pattern of injury depends upon the level and nature of the injury but all injuries have some common characteristics. Spinal cord trauma causes massive sympathetic discharge, leading to a sudden profound rise in blood pressure and systemic vascular resistance. Direct sequelae of this include myocardial infarction, strokes and severe arrhythmias. If there is associated airway loss, due to impaired reflexes and gastric stasis, there is the risk of vomiting and subsequent aspiration. Fractures at or above the level of C5 damage the phrenic nerve resulting in loss of diaphragmatic movement causing respiratory embarrassment. Fractures affecting T2–12 vertebrae affect the inter-costal muscles. Interference with breathing results in reduced tidal volumes, sputum retention and subsequent lower respiratory tract infection. Other effects include development of neurogenic pulmonary oedema and ARDS. Loss of sympathetic tone causes vaso-dilatation resulting in neurogenic shock. If the damage is high (cervical level), cardiac innervation is affected; unopposed vagal tone may result in severe bradycardia and even asystolic cardiac arrest. Muscle flaccidity and areflexia may be present which may last for many weeks. Over 50% of T7 or higher lesions are associated with autonomic dysreflexia. Other features include hypothermia from peripheral vasodilatation, paralytic ileus, urinary retention, water retention and hyponatraemia due to a syndrome of inappropriate ADH secretion, glucose intolerance, thrombo-embolism, stress ulceration in the stomach and pressure ulcers over bony prominences.

Physiology

Case 3.7 Wound healing

Q   **What are the various stages involved in acute wound healing?**

A   There are four different stages in acute wound healing. They are: (1) haemostasis; (2) inflammation; (3) proliferation and (4) remodelling and scar formation.

Q   **Briefly describe each of these phases.**

A   Extravasation of blood into a wound causes constriction of nearby vessel walls and initiates the coagulation cascade leading to clot formation and platelet aggregation. The platelets also secrete several growth factors such as PDGF, IGF-1, EGF and TGF-β which initiate the wound healing cascade by attracting and activating fibroblasts, endothelial cells and macrophages.

Haemostasis is followed by the inflammatory phase. Within 24–48 hours of injury, the wound is infiltrated with neutrophils. They phagocytose bacteria and other foreign particles by releasing degrading enzymes. The neutrophil activity usually ceases within a few days of wounding after any contaminating bacteria have been cleared. Macrophages (phenotypic variation of blood monocytes) arrive at the wound site between 48–72 hours. They also function as phagocytic cells as well as producing growth factors responsible for the production and proliferation of extracellular matrix, proliferation of fibroblasts and stimulating angiogenesis. They release proteolytic enzymes, such as collagenase, which help to debride the wound.

The proliferative phase starts at approximately day three and lasts after wounding for 2–4 weeks. This phase is characterised by migration of fibroblasts, extracellular matrix deposition, angiogenesis and formation of granulation tissue. With progression of the proliferative phase, the provisional fibrin/fibronectin matrix is replaced by newly formed granulation tissue. Epithelialisation (regeneration) of the wound represents the final stage of the proliferative phase.

The final phase is the remodelling phase and maturation of the resulting scar. The remodelling phase is initiated concurrently with the development of granulation tissue and continues over prolonged periods of time up to 2 years after injury. There is continuous collagen synthesis and breakdown as the extracellular matrix is constantly remodelled, equilibrating to a steady state approximately 21 days after wounding. Ultimately, the granulation tissue scaffolding evolves into an avascular scar which is composed of largely inactive, spindle-shaped fibroblasts, dense collagen, fragments of elastic tissue and other ECM components.

Q   What do you understand by the term growth factor?

A   Growth factors represent a variety of proteins involved in the coordination of the regulated and interrelated processes which occur during wound healing. They may exert their effects in an endocrine, paracrine or autocrine fashion.

Q   Briefly describe the actions of growth factors in wound healing.

A   The combined action of the various naturally occurring growth factors such as platelet derived growth factor, transforming growth factors-α and β, platelet derived growth factors, epidermal growth factor, fibroblast growth factor, hepatocyte growth factor and vascular endothelial growth factor are: control of cell proliferation; cell migration; angiogenesis; granulation tissue formation and formation, accumulation and degradation of extracellular matrix components. All these actions contribute to the wound healing process. In addition, the balance between the various isoforms of transforming growth factor-β play an important role during the remodelling phase of wound healing and thus in the mechanism of scarring or scarless healing (as seen in the fetus).

Case 3.8 Stress response to surgery

Q   What is meant by 'stress response' to surgery?

A   The 'stress response' is a phenomenon seen not just after surgery but also after other causes of trauma including burns or haemorrhagic shock. This is a series of metabolic and hormonal changes that occur in the body due to polypeptides released from damaged tissues. Whatever causes the stress response, the neuroendocrine pathway is initiated.

Q   Can you briefly describe the reason for this stress response and what clinical effect this might have?

A   The body responds to any form of injury with local and systemic responses that attempt to contain and heal the tissue damage; it thus helps to protect the body while it is injured. The systemic response, produced by many different mediators (sympathetic nervous system, acute phase response, endocrine response and vascular endothelial cell system response), increases the metabolic rate, mobilises carbohydrate, protein and fat stores, conserves salt and water, stimulates immunological and coagulation systems and diverts blood preferentially to vital organs. Blood is redistributed from the viscera and skin to the heart, brain and skeletal muscles and there is an increase in heart rate and contractility. The overall result is an increase in cardiac output, an increase in respiratory rate (leading to alkalosis), hypoalbuminaemia and an activation of the clotting cascade (which may result in Disseminated Intravascular Coagulation, DIC).

Q   **What do you understand by the terms 'ebb' and 'flow' phases and what happens during these phases?**

A   'Ebb' is the initial phase which occurs within first 24 hours of injury. During this phase, there is a decrease in the metabolic rate and a fall in the plasma insulin concentration (with resultant hyperglycaemia). The fall in plasma insulin concentration is due to the action of catecholamines and cortisol which make the β-islet cells of the pancreas less sensitive to glucose. Glucagon also inhibits insulin release and cortisol reduces the peripheral action of insulin; less carbohydrate is transported into cells and blood sugar rises. The next phase is the 'flow' phase which is associated with an increase in metabolic rate. This may be associated with glucose intolerance and a catabolic state.

Q   **Can you briefly describe the other neuroendocrine responses and their effects?**

A   ACTH stimulates aldosterone secretion (in addition to glucocorticoids) through the renin-angiotensin axis, leading to increased reabsorption of sodium and secretion of potassium (and hydrogen ions) in the distal convoluted tubules and collecting ducts. This leads to metabolic alkalosis as well as a reduction in the urine volume. In more severe injuries, however, a metabolic acidosis is common due to poor tissue perfusion and anaerobic metabolism. Arginine vasopressin (from the posterior pituitary) acts on the distal tubules and collecting ducts in the kidney and leads to increased reabsorption of solute-free water; it causes peripheral vasoconstriction especially in the splanchnic bed and it also stimulates hepatic glycogenolysis and gluconeogenesis (note that glucagon secretion increases after injury, further stimulating hepatic glycogenolysis and gluconeogenesis). Serum albumin falls after trauma because production by the liver decreases and loss into damaged tissue increases due to the action of cytokines and prostaglandins on vessel permeability. The accompanying fluid shift out of the intravascular compartment contributes to dysfunction in various organs. There is also an increase in the release of growth hormone and prolactin.

Q   **What are the overall effects on the metabolic rate due to the stress response?**

A   The overall effect of the various metabolic and hormonal responses is a marked increase in the metabolic rate, a rise in oxygen consumption, a rise in carbon dioxide production, salt and water retention and increased potassium loss from the kidneys. The intense catabolism that follows leads to mobilisation of fatty acids. Amino acids are converted to carbohydrate and there can be quite a marked negative nitrogen balance.

Case 3.9 Sepsis and septic shock

Q What do you understand by the term systemic inflammatory response syndrome?

A Systemic inflammatory response syndrome (SIRS) is a generalised inflammatory response by the body resulting from a variety of clinical insults such as shock, trauma, burns, infection (bacterial, viral, fungal), pancreatitis and tissue ischaemia. For a clinical diagnosis of SIRS to be made, at least two of the following criteria should be satisfied:
- temperature >38°C or <36°C
- heart rate >90 bpm
- respiratory rate >20 or $PaCo_2$ <4.3 kPa
- WCC >12 or <4×10^9/L.

Q What is the relationship between SIRS and septic shock?

A Sepsis is defined as SIRS with documented infection, i.e. the systemic response to an infection. Septic shock is sepsis with refractory arterial hypotension (systolic blood pressure <90 mmHg or mean arterial pressure <60 mmHg or need for inotropes despite adequate fluid resuscitation (40–60 ml/kg of crystalloids)

Q What is the most common cause of sepsis?

A Bacterial infection is the most common cause of sepsis. Although Gram-negative bacteria were considered to the major cause of sepsis, it has been recognised that Gram-positive bacteria account for the same percentage of cases as Gram-negative bacteria. Together they account for more than 95% of cases of sepsis; the rest being fungal or viral.

Q What are cytokines?

A Cytokines are very potent low molecular weight proteins or glycoproteins secreted by a variety of cells. They have a short half-life and are the local factors involved in the inflammatory and immune responses. They act via complex and interactive pathways, with positive feed-back and amplification, similar to the complement cascade. There are more than a hundred different cytokines identified so far. Chemotactic cytokines are called chemokines.

Q What is the role of cytokines in the aetiology of SIRS and sepsis?

A Cytokines are responsible for the inflammatory response observed in SIRS and sepsis. Initially, a local inflammatory response is triggered by the cytokines leading to the induction and release of neutrophils and macrophages. Then the inflammatory response becomes progressively more systemic and uncontrolled, leading to an overwhelming response involving IL-6, IL-8, IL-1 and TNF-α. The cytokines are responsible for a whole host of local and systemic effects, including vasodilatation, increased capillary permeability, impaired oxygen utilisation and myocardial depression.

Q   **How would you recognise a septic patient?**

A   A septic patient would appear generally unwell. In the early stages, the patient may present with SIRS, tachycardia, hypotension, tachypnoea (maybe with accompanying hypoxia) with warm bounding peripheral pulses as a result of peripheral vasodilatation. This is related to the hyper-dynamic circulation associated with decreased systemic vascular resistance and peripheral vasodilation and an increased cardiac output. This type of shock was previously referred to as 'warm shock' since this type of clinical picture is in contrast to the decreased cardiac output and periph-eral vasoconstriction 'cold shock' observed in other types of shock. In addition, hyperthermia may be seen or more rarely and a poor prognostic sign, hypothermia. In the later stages of septic shock, the patient may be hypotensive with peripheral vasoconstriction, especially if the patient is hypovolaemic or myocardial function is compromised. Other pertinent clinical signs and symptoms include oliguria, drowsiness and confusion. With progression of sepsis, individual organs such as the lung, liver, kidney become affected leading to multi-organ dysfunction syndrome, which carries a high mortality.

Q   **What initial investigations would you do in a patient with suspected septic shock and what might these results show?**

A   I would ask for a full blood count, coagulation screen, urea and elec-trolytes, liver function tests, arterial blood gas analysis and request a chest radiograph if the patient is manifesting any evidence of respiratory compromise or early signs of ARDS. Samples of blood, urine, sputum and other suspected sepsis sources should be sent for direct microscopy, culture and sensitivity analysis to allow early identification of pathogens and to guide antibiotic therapy.

Typically, a full blood count would show a high WCC, with neutrophilia, although there might be neutropenia in overwhelming sepsis. The platelet count may be decreased. The coagulation screen may reveal an increased INR (international normalised ratio of prothrombin time) and/or prolonged activated partial thromboplastin time (APTT), due to septic coagulopathy and disseminated intravascular coagulation (DIC), although in the late stages of septic shock an altered coagulation picture might be due to hepatic involvement (dysfunction). Urea and electrolyte results may show varying degrees of renal impairment, or indicate an element of dehydration if urea and sodium are raised disproportionately compared to the creatinine. Arterial blood gas analysis may reveal a metabolic acidosis with or without compensatory respiratory alkalosis (due to hyperventila-tion leading to a reduced $PaCO_2$). The lactic acid levels may be elevated due to tissue hypoxia and anaerobic metabolism. A chest radiograph may reveal some haziness in the lung fields (mostly bilaterally) due to the inflammatory response and early ARDS or frank signs of pulmonary oedema. In the later stages, there may be associated pleural effusion and consolidation of one or more lung fields due to pneumonia.

Q   **Can you briefly outline the principles of managing a septic patient?**

A   Elimination of the predisposing cause and treating the source of infection (source control) is the central principle of management. The other supportive therapies include oxygen, adequate haemodynamic support and appropriate antibiotics. Chest physiotherapy and saline nebulisers are useful to prevent atelectasis and development of ARDS or pneumonia. In advanced cases, the treatment goals will vary according to clinical needs and to support the failing organs with appropriate therapy, i.e. ventilation, dialysis, managing coagulopathy, inotropic support and nutrition; admission to HDU or ITU may be indicated in such circumstances.

Case 3.10 Fluid balance and fluid replacement therapy

Q   **How does the anti-diuretic hormone regulate water balance?**

A   Direct control of water excretion by the kidneys is controlled by the anti-diuretic hormone (ADH) (also known as vasopressin), a peptide hormone secreted by the hypothalamus. ADH facilitates the insertion of water channels into the membranes of cells lining the distal tubules and collecting ducts, allowing water reabsorption to occur. Without ADH, reabsorption of water in the distal tubules and collecting ducts is limited which leads to the excretion of dilute urine. Deficiency of ADH results in diabetes insipidus.

Q   **What factors regulate ADH secretion?**

A   Several factors regulate ADH secretion. These include:

- special receptors (osmoreceptors) situated in the hypothalamus – these are sensitive to increasing plasma osmolarity (when the plasma gets too concentrated). These stimulate ADH secretion

- stretch receptors (baroreceptors) situated in the atria of the heart – these are sensitive to blood volume. They are activated by an increased volume of blood returning to the heart from the venous system. This causes inhibition of ADH secretion since the body attempts to maintain physiological volume by removing excess fluid circulating within the system

- stretch receptors situated in the aorta and carotid arteries – these are stimulated when the circulating volume decreases and the blood pressure falls. These stimulate ADH secretion since the body attempts to maintain sufficient volume to generate the blood pressure necessary to deliver blood to the tissues and vital organs

- head injury, burns or prolonged hypoxia can also stimulate ADH secretion resulting in oliguria and hyponatraemia.

It should be noted that all factors stimulating ADH secretion also stimulate thirst.

Q **How do you distinguish diabetes insipidus from compulsive water drinking?**

A A water deprivation test is used to differentiate diabetes insipidus from compulsive water drinking. Measurements are made of urine and plasma osmolality. In normal subjects (as in compulsive water drinkers), when the plasma osmolality reaches about 295 mmol/kg, the body, by secreting ADH, will attempt to conserve water by concentrating the urine. This increases the urine osmolality. In patients with diabetes insipidus, an increase in plasma osmolality fails to correspondingly increase the urine osmolality.

Q **How does aldosterone help in sodium balance?**

A Aldosterone is a steroid hormone produced by the adrenal cortex. Aldosterone causes increased reabsorption of sodium and excretion of potassium in the distal convoluted tubules and collecting duct. This causes a reduction in the urine volume. Aldosterone is primarily secreted when the plasma osmolality falls; a rise in plasma potassium concentration can also stimulate aldosterone release. Aldosterone secretion is controlled in two ways: (1) the adrenal cortex directly senses plasma osmolarity. When the osmolarity rises, aldosterone secretion is inhibited. The lack of aldosterone causes less sodium to be reabsorbed in the distal tubule, thus decreasing plasma osmolality. In this setting, however, ADH secretion will increase to conserve water, thus complementing the effect of low aldosterone levels to decrease the osmolarity of bodily fluids. The net effect on urine excretion is a decrease in the amount of urine excreted, with an increase in urine osmolality. If the plasma osmolality falls, aldosterone secretion is increased causing increased reabsorption of sodium from the distal tubules and collecting duct; (2) the kidneys sense hypovolaemia (which results in lower filtration rates and lower flow through the tubule). To conserve blood volume, the juxtaglomerular cells in the afferent and efferent arterioles secrete renin, a peptide hormone that initiates a hormonal cascade that ultimately produces angiotensin II (the renin-angiotensin system). Angiotensin II stimulates the adrenal cortex to produce aldosterone.

Case 3.11 Respiratory system mechanics

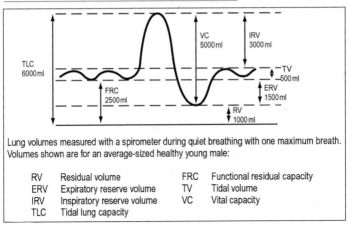

Lung volumes measured with a spirometer during quiet breathing with one maximum breath. Volumes shown are for an average-sized healthy young male:

RV	Residual volume	FRC	Functional residual capacity
ERV	Expiratory reserve volume	TV	Tidal volume
IRV	Inspiratory reserve volume	VC	Vital capacity
TLC	Tidal lung capacity		

Fig. 3.11.1 Lung volumes.

Q **Briefly describe the mechanism of normal breathing.**

A The basic principle which determines both inspiration and expiration is a variation in the pressure gradient within the thoracic cavity (since a pressure gradient is required to generate flow). During spontaneous normal breathing, the inspiratory flow is achieved by creating a negative sub-atmospheric pressure in the alveoli (of the order of $-5\,cm$ of H_2O) by an increase in the volume of the thoracic cavity under the action of the inspiratory muscles. Expiration occurs when the intra-alveolar pressure becomes higher than the atmospheric pressure resulting in gas flow towards the upper respiratory tract. Expiration is aided by the action of the diaphragm.

Q **What are the normal lung values you know of?**

A The tidal volume (Fig. 3.11.1) is the total volume of air that is moved in and out of the lungs with every normal breath. In normal healthy adults, this volume is approximately 500 ml. Minute volume is tidal volume × respiratory rate; this is 500 ml × 14 (normal breaths/min) which equates to approximately 7000 ml/min. However, not all the tidal volume takes part in respiratory exchange, as this process does not commence until the air or gas reaches the respiratory bronchioles. Above the level of the bronchioles, the airways function solely as conduits, conducting the gases to more distal parts and the volume of the conducting airways is known as the anatomical dead-space. This volume is approximately 2 ml/kg or 150 ml in an adult, roughly one-third of the tidal volume. Thus the part of the tidal volume which takes part in respiratory exchange is known as alveolar ventilation. This is (tidal volume − anatomical dead-space) × respiratory rate, which is (approximately) $350 \times 14 = 4900$ ml/min.

Q   What is meant by functional residual capacity?

A   The functional residual capacity (FRC) (Fig. 3.11.1) is the volume of air in the lungs at the end of a normal expiration. The point at which this occurs (and hence the FRC value) is determined by a balance between the inward elastic forces of the lung and the outward forces of the respiratory cage (determined by the muscle tone). There is a fall in FRC with obesity, pregnancy, general anaesthesia and when lying supine. Age, however, does not affect FRC.

Q   What do you understand by the different vital capacities of the lung and what is their clinical significance?

A   Vital capacity is the change in volume of air in the lungs from complete inspiration to complete expiration. The inspiratory vital capacity is the maximum volume of air which can be inspired into the lungs during relaxed inspiration from a position of full expiration. The expiratory vital capacity is the maximum volume of air which can be expired from the lungs during relaxed expiration from a position of full inspiration. The expiratory phase is more commonly used to measure the obstructive or restrictive pattern of lung pathology. Forced vital capacity is the maximum volume of air in litres that can be forcibly and rapidly exhaled following a maximum inspiration. This is the basic manoeuvre used in spirometry tests.

Q   What do you understand by the terms FEV_1 and PEFR?

A FEV_1 (forced expiratory volume in first second) is the volume of air expelled in the first second of a forced expiration starting from full inspiration ($FEV_1\%$ is the FEV_1 expressed as a percentage of the total volume). In normal lung function, this should generally be over 75%, i.e. the subject should be able to get at least three-quarters of his/her total air exhaled in the first second of expiration. PEFR (peak expiratory flow rate) is the greatest flow that can be sustained for at least 10 milliseconds of forced expiration starting from full inflation of the lungs. It is measured in litres/minute using a peak flow meter.

Case 3.12 Control of respiration

Q   Where are the respiratory centres situated and how do they function?

A   The respiratory control centres, located in the brain stem, control the inspiratory and expiratory cycles. These centres set the basic rhythm by automatically initiating inspiration with a two second burst of nerve impulses to the diaphragm and the external intercostal muscles. Contraction of the diaphragm and the external intercostal muscles draws air into the lungs. The neurons stop firing for about 3 seconds and the muscles relax. This automatic rhythmic firing of the inspiratory centre results in a normal breathing rate of 12–15 breaths/minute. Expiration is caused by the elastic recoil of the lungs and the chest wall; forced expiration, on the other hand, is caused by the expiratory centre stimulating the internal intercostal and abdominal muscles to contract.

Q **How does respiration alter with changes in the body's physiological status?**

A The normal involuntary nature of the respiratory cycle can be suppressed or altered to meet the changing metabolic demands of the body since the respiratory system tries to maintain the level of oxygen and carbon dioxide in the body within narrow limits. Although the basic rhythm is determined by the respiratory centres in the brain stem, the rate, rhythm and the depth of ventilation may be modified by the input of central and peripheral chemoreceptors which monitor the carbon dioxide, oxygen and pH.

Q **What do you understand by the term 'chemoreceptors'?**

A There are two forms of chemoreceptors – the central chemoreceptors and the peripheral chemoreceptors. Central chemoreceptors act by monitoring the pH/carbon dioxide of the cerebrospinal fluid in the fourth ventricle. Carbon dioxide diffuses from the blood into the cerebrospinal fluid. The carbon dioxide combines with water forming carbonic acid which dissociates into hydrogen ions and bicarbonate. If the carbon dioxide increases, the hydrogen ions increase and hence the pH falls (acidic). At lower pH, the chemoreceptors increase the breathing rate to exhale more carbon dioxide and to increase the pH. Peripheral chemoreceptors, located in the aortic arch and the carotid arteries, monitor the levels of carbon dioxide, pH and oxygen in the arterial blood. Any alteration in these levels causes these centres to send neural impulses to the respiratory centres via the vagus and glossopharyngeal nerves, which appropriately alter their pattern of respiration.

Case 3.13 Fracture healing

Q **Briefly describe the initial events that follow fracture of a long bone.**

A A fracture not just involves a breakage in the bone, but also damage of the surrounding soft tissues. Immediately after injury, there is haemorrhage, both from the fractured ends of the bone and also from the vessels in the soft tissues. Clotting of the blood leads to a haematoma which surrounds the bone ends (fracture haematoma) and the surrounding injured tissues. Within this organised fracture haematoma, bone develops either directly or following the development of cartilage with endochondral ossification.

Q **What are the stages of fracture healing?**

A Within hours, there is an inflammatory response, comprising of polymorphonuclear leukocytes, lymphocytes and macrophages. Later, fibroblasts infiltrate the area. This inflammatory stage may last for 2–3 weeks. This is followed by the stage of new bone formation. Pain and swelling begin to subside during this stage. Initially, the bone that is laid down (soft callus) consists of immature woven bone. This soft callus cannot be visualised by plain radiography. This stage usually lasts for 4–8 weeks after injury. Between 8–12 weeks of injury, the new bone begins to bridge the fracture (hard callus). This bony bridge can be seen on plain radiographs. This hard callus is gradually converted to stable lamellar bone trabeculae as the recanalising Haversian system bridges the bone ends. At this same time, osteoclasts develop and resorb the necrotic bone ends. The final stage of fracture healing is remodeling of the fracture site although the whole process may take several months or even years.

Q **What is a callus and what are the types you know of?**

A Callus is the immature woven bone that is laid down during healing of fractures. Comprised of a combination of connective tissue and cartilage, it temporarily binds and stabilises the bone. There are primarily two types of callus: (1) the external callus, also known as inductive or bridging callus, is derived from the fracture haematoma and surrounding damaged tissue. This callus is formed by the pluripotential cells. A variety of factors, including mechanical and humoral, may induce these mesenchymal cells to differentiate into a cartilage or bone. It ossifies by endochondral ossification to form woven bone and (2) the internal callus, also known as medullary callus, is due to the proliferation of committed osteoprogenitor cells in the periosteum and the bone marrow. These cells directly produce membranous bone and this response is a once-only phenomenon. It forms more slowly and occurs later during fracture healing. A third type, also known as the periosteal callus, has also been recognised. It forms directly from the inner periosteal layer. This type of callus ossifies by intramembranous ossification to form the woven bone.

Q **What are osteoblasts and osteoclasts?**

A The osteoblasts help in the laying down of seams of uncalcified new bone (osteoid). The osteoclasts are multinucleated cells, probably of macrophage lineage, which resorbs the bone and thus helps in the remodelling of the new bone.

Q **What are the factors that influence bone (fracture) healing?**

A Factors which influencing bone (fracture) healing can be divided into systemic and local causes. Local causes include degree and type of local trauma, amount of bone loss, type of bone fractured, associated vascular injury, local infection and degree of immobilisation. Systemic causes include age, functional activity, nutrition, drugs and hormones.

Q **How does the bone receive its blood supply and what is its significance?**

A Blood vessels enter the bone via the metaphyseal region. They supply the epiphysis and the metaphysis and then anastomose with the blood vessels supplying the diaphysis. The main arterial supply to the diaphysis comes via the nutrient arteries. The nutrient arteries divide in the medulla into ascending and descending branches. These ramify within the medullary cavity and constitute the primary resistance vessels of the osseous circulation. Nutrient veins accompany the arteries which continue in the medullary canal as a central longitudinal venous sinus. This drains the medullary sinusoids through radial connecting sinuses.

Case 3.14 Cardiovascular system

Q **What is meant by cardiac output?**

A Cardiac output is the total volume of blood pumped by the ventricle per minute, or simply the product of heart rate (HR) and stroke volume (SV). Cardiac output (litre/min) = heart rate (bpm) × stroke volume (L); (CO = HR × SV). Cardiac output is also sometimes represented as 'Q' (thus: Q = HR × SV). A change in either the heart rate or the stroke volume thus clearly has an impact on the other components.

Q **Define blood pressure.**

A The term blood pressure refers to the arterial blood pressure, the pressure in the aorta and its branches. Systolic pressure is due to ventricular contraction. Diastolic pressure occurs during cardiac relaxation.

Q **What are the factors that affect blood pressure?**

A The four major factors that interact to affect blood pressure are the: (1) cardiac output; (2) blood volume; (3) peripheral resistance and (4) blood viscosity. When any of these factors increase, the blood pressure also increases. Arterial blood pressure is usually maintained within normal ranges by changes in cardiac output and peripheral resistance. Pressure receptors (baroreceptors), located in the walls of the large arteries in the thorax and neck, are important for short-term regulation of blood pressure.

Q **What is meant by pulse pressure and mean arterial pressure?**

A Pulse pressure (PP) refers to the difference between the systolic pressure and diastolic pressure. Mean arterial pressure (MAP) is determined by the cardiac output, systemic vascular resistance and the central venous pressure. Thus MAP = (CO − SVR) + CVP. Because CVP is usually at or near 0 mmHg, this relationship is often simplified to: MAP=CO − SVR. In practice, however, MAP is not determined by knowing the CO and SVR, but rather by direct or indirect measurements of the arterial pressure. It is usually calculated using the formula: MAP= [(2 × diastolic)+systolic] ÷ 3. For example, if the systolic pressure is 120 mmHg and diastolic pressure is 80 mmHg, then the mean arterial pressure will be approximately 93 mmHg. Diastole counts twice as much as systole because two-thirds of the cardiac cycle is spent in diastole. A MAP of at least 60 mmHg is necessary to perfuse the coronary arteries, brain and kidneys.

Q   **What do you understand by the term systemic vascular resistance?**

A   Systemic vascular resistance (SVR) refers to the resistance in blood flow offered by all of the systemic vasculature, excluding the pulmonary vasculature. This is also sometimes referred to as the total peripheral resistance (TPR). SVR is therefore determined by factors that influence vascular resistance in individual vascular beds. Mechanisms that cause vasoconstriction increase SVR and those that cause vasodilation decrease SVR. Although SVR is primarily determined by changes in blood vessel diameters, changes in blood viscosity also affect the SVR.

SVR can be calculated if the cardiac output (CO), mean arterial pressure (MAP) and central venous pressure (CVP) are known.

SVR= (MAP − CVP) ÷ CO

Because CVP is normally near 0 mmHg, the calculation is often simplified to:

SVR = MAP ÷ CO

It should be noted that although SVR can be calculated from MAP and CO, it is however not determined by either of these variables. A more accurate way to view this relationship is that at a given CO, if the MAP is very high, it is because SVR is high. Mathematically, SVR is the dependent variable in the above equations; however, physiologically, SVR and CO are normally the independent variables and MAP is the dependent variable.

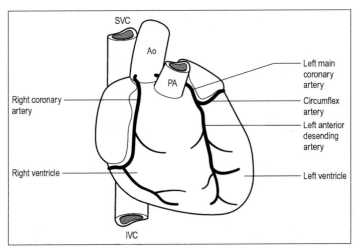

Fig. 3.14.1 Coronary circulation.

Q   **Describe the coronary circulation.**

A   The major vessels of the coronary circulation are the two branches of the left main coronary artery, the left anterior descending and the circumflex and the right main coronary artery. The right provides one-seventh of the circulation, the rest is provided by the left coronary artery. Each feeds the right and the left ventricle, respectively, with a small degree of overlap. The left and right coronary arteries originate at the base of the aorta. The major coronary vessels do not run within the muscle since they lie on the epicardial surface of the heart. They function as low resistance, distribution vessels. However, these epicardial arteries branch into smaller arteries that penetrate the myocardium and become the microvascular resistance vessels that regulate coronary blood flow. These vessels which penetrate the myocardium are of great importance since the wall tension of the myocardium can have a great bearing on coronary blood flow, especially in patients with hypertension. Arterioles give rise to a dense capillary network so that each cardiac myocyte has several capillaries running parallel to the muscle fibre. The high capillary-to-fibre density ensures short diffusion distances to maximise oxygen transport into the cells and removal of metabolic waste products from the cells (e.g. CO_2, H^+).

Case 3.15 Muscle physiology

Q   **What are the different types of muscle?**

A   There are three types of muscles in the human body: skeletal muscle, smooth muscle and cardiac muscle.

Q **Can you briefly describe the general principles involved in muscle contraction?**

A The initial stimulus is an action potential, which travels along the nerve ending to the muscle fibre. In the case of skeletal muscle, acetylcholine is released at the neuromuscular junction causing a large influx of sodium ions into the muscle fibre. This produces an action potential within the muscle, causing depolarisation. This results in the release of large quantities of stored calcium, which initiates the actin and myosin fibres to slide over each other and produce a contraction. The whole process ends by the calcium ions being pumped back into the sarcoplasmic reticulum for storage until the next action potential comes along.

Q **How does this differ in smooth and cardiac muscle?**

A Skeletal muscle contraction has a very rapid onset and a brief duration. Cardiac and smooth muscle, however, have a more prolonged action. They also do not contain motor end plates like the skeletal muscle. In the case of smooth muscle, the contraction is similarly initiated by an influx of calcium ions. This may be produced by nerve stimulation, hormonal stimulation or stretching of the fibres. It is the autonomic nervous system which supplies smooth muscle via the release of acetylcholine and nor-epinephrine, which may be excitatory or inhibitory. Smooth muscle contraction requires far less energy to produce the same tension as skeletal muscle. This is because in the case of organs such as the intestines and gallbladder, tonic muscular contraction followed by relaxation is also approximately 30 times as long. Despite all this however, the force of contraction is often greater than skeletal muscle.

Q **How are skeletal muscles classified in humans?**

A Skeletal muscles in humans are classified into two main types depending on the type of fibre they contain into slow or red fibres and fast or white fibres.

Q **How do these muscle fibres differ from each other?**

A Slow fibres are characteristic of muscles which have or require greater endurance. They have moderate shortening velocities and power outputs and they consume ATP at moderate rates. These have high blood supply (high capillary density), many mitochondria and moderate diameter. Slow fibres are also called red fibres because of their distinctive colour; this is provided by the iron-containing haemoglobin in myoplasm and cytochrome in the mitochondria. If the blood supply is adequate, slow fibres provide great endurance.

The fast fibres are large, pale white in colour and have a more extensive sarcoplasmic reticulum. These cells are pale because they contain little oxygen binding protein. Fast contractions are matched by rapid relaxations. The maximal ATP consumption rate of fast fibres can be met by glycolysis. These fibres fatigue rapidly as glycogen is depleted.

Features of skeletal, smooth and cardiac muscles		
Skeletal	Smooth	Cardiac
• striated • tissue very eosinophilic due to the exceedingly high protein content in the cytoplasm • cells very dense with relatively few nuclei compared with cytoplasmic volume • cells are polygonal in cross-section with peripheral nuclei • usually appears in large bundles • well vascularised by capillaries • high glycogen and mitochondrial content (seen in electron microscopy)	• non-striated • usually 'dense' and eosinophilic • has branching fibres • has central nuclei • presence of intercalated discs • well vascularised • abundant and large mitochondria (seen in electron microscopy)	• striated • eosinophilic • small, elongated, tapered cells • no branching fibres • usually bundled in smaller units than skeletal or cardiac muscle, except when found in very well-organised layers or sheets • not multinucleated • central nuclei, not visible in each cell when cross-sectioned • when contracted, nuclei often assume a corkscrew appearance

Q   **How would you identify a cardiac muscle histologically?**

A   The cardiac muscle have the following features: they are striated, 'dense' and eosinophilic; they have branching fibres; they have a central nuclei, intercalated discs and have abundant and large mitochondria (as seen in electron microscopy) and they are well vascularised.

Q   **Briefly explain cardiac muscle contraction.**

A   Cardiac muscle differs from both smooth and skeletal muscle in that it acts as a syncytium. This is called the 'all or nothing' phenomenon. The heart is composed of an atrial syncytium and a ventricular syncytium separated by specialised conductive fibres. This allows the atria to contract before the ventricles thereby allowing the heart to pump effectively. As with skeletal muscle, the action potential is caused by the opening of fast sodium channels. However, this is also accompanied by the opening of slow calcium channels resulting in a more prolonged period of depolarisation. Cardiac muscle also differs from skeletal muscle in that immediately after the onset of action potential, the permeability of the muscle to potassium ions decreases significantly. This refractory period prevents premature repolarisation of the muscle membrane.

Q   What is Frank–Starling law of the heart?

A   The Frank–Starling law states that the force of myocardial contraction is directly proportional to the initial muscle fibre length. It thus describes the inherent ability of the heart to handle changes in the volume of blood entering (circulating) the heart. When there is an increase in the amount of blood entering the heart (leading to an increased end diastolic volume), the cardiac muscle fibre length increases proportionally thus resulting in an increase in the stroke volume.

Pathology

Case 3.16 Inflammation

Q   What is inflammation?

A   Inflammation is the body's normal response to an insult or injury. It is designed to combat the infection or the insult that caused it. It usually lasts only for a few days although in some instances it may become prolonged leading to chronic inflammation.

Q   What are the signs of inflammation?

A   The clinical signs of acute inflammation are those described by Celsius: redness (rubor – due to dilated blood vessels); increase in temperature or warmth (calor – due to an increase in blood flow to the area); oedema (tumor – swelling of the affected part due to the release of inflammatory mediators); pain (dolor – due to pressure from surrounding oedema) and loss of function. The above features are however seldom present in chronic inflammation.

Q   Can you name some causes for acute inflammation?

A   The causes of acute inflammation may be classified into:
- trauma of any cause, e.g. burns, scalds, wounds, irradiation etc.
- infection: mostly bacterial or viral
- ischaemia
- toxins, e.g. acids, chemicals, corrosives
- allergy, e.g. hypersensitivity reactions.

Q   What molecular and cellular changes occur during acute inflammation?

A   The acute inflammatory response is largely mediated by the degranulation of mast cells which contain histamine granules. The release of histamine results in vascular dilatation and hence increased vascularity to the affected area. Mast cells also degranulate in response to IgE antibody and components of the complement system. The increase in blood supply to the area results in an increase in the release of polymorphonuclear leucocytes (neutrophils). There is extravasation of plasma proteins resulting in the formation of oedema within the damaged tissue. The blood viscosity increases leading to slowing flow or stagnation of blood. This allows neutrophils, which normally travel in the central stream of the blood vessel, to move to the periphery thus making contact with the vessel wall and extravasation into the surrounding tissues guided by adhesion molecules and a chemotactic gradient. Cytokines and lipid mediators (prostaglandins, thromboxane, lipoxins and leukotrienes) are also important components of the response.

Q   **What is the role of neutrophils in acute inflammation?**

A   The neutrophil polymorph is one of the characteristic histological features of acute inflammation. There are about 50 billion neutrophils in the adult human body which are programmed to die in 12 hours. They are drawn to the site of injury in 30 minutes and accumulate in significant numbers by 12 hours. They are attracted to the site of tissue injury by the presence of foreign bodies such as bacteria, other neutrophils, chemotactic inflammatory mediators (interleukin-8, leukotriene B4, platelet activating factor, granulocyte chemoattractant protein-2) and components of the complement system (C5a). They are able to pass through (permeate) the vessel wall because of increased vascular permeability and plasma viscosity (slowing down of blood) with the aid of specific adhesion molecules which are upregulated in inflammation. Their main functions are phagocytosis, elaboration of proteases and free radicals which serve to kill the microorganisms. They also have a limited ability to generate chemokines.

Q   **Name some inflammatory mediators involved in acute inflammation.**

A   ● leukotrienes: derived from arachidonic acid; causes vasodilatation

● prostaglandins: derived from arachidonic acid; cause an increase in vascular permeability and can result in platelet aggregation

● serotonin: released from mast cells; causes vasoconstriction

● lymphokines: released from lymphocytes; attract other inflammatory cells.

Q   **What do you know about the 'cascade systems' that are activated during acute inflammation?**

A   There are also four cascade systems that are activated during the acute inflammatory response. They include:

● coagulation system: activation of this system results in the production of fibrin

● fibrinolytic system: causes fibrinolysis

- kinin system: primarily bradykinin, that causes an increase in vascular permeability and is responsible for the pain associated with inflammation

- complement system: components of this system (mostly C3a and C5a) are essential for chemotaxis of neutrophils and opsonisation of bacteria; they also cause increased vascular permeability.

Case 3.17 Abnormal wound healing

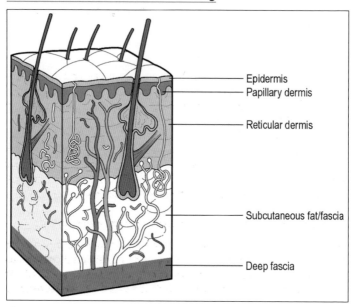

Epidermis
Papillary dermis

Reticular dermis

Subcutaneous fat/fascia

Deep fascia

Fig. 3.17.1 Layers of the skin.

Q   **Describe the structure of normal skin.**

A   The skin is composed of three major tissue layers. The outermost layer is the epidermis, a thin stratified epithelium which varies relatively little in thickness over most of the body surface, except on the palms of the hands and the soles of the feet. Underlying the epidermis is the dermis, a dense fibroelastic connective tissue comprising mainly of collagen and fibroblasts; the dermis forms the major mass of the skin. Found within this structure are extensive vascular and neural networks, excretory and secretory glands and keratinised appendages, such as the hair and nails. The dermis, which can be divided into a superficial papillary dermis and a deeper reticular dermis, merges into a third definable layer, the subcutis or hypodermis, which does not have a clear demarcation. Composed of loose connective tissue and fatty tissue, the functions of the subcutis are to anchor the skin to the underlying structures, to act as a mechanical cushion and to provide insulation against heat loss.

Q   **What is a chronic wound?**

A   A chronic wound usually an ulcer in skin is defined as one in which the normal process of healing is disrupted at one or more points in the phases of haemostasis, inflammation, proliferation, or remodelling. In the majority of chronic wounds, however, the healing process is considered as being 'stuck' in the inflammatory or proliferative phases. Although a strict time frame cannot be imposed, a wound that has failed to heal within 6 weeks of the 'normally expected healing time' is classified as a chronic wound.

Q   **What causes a chronic wound?**

A   Since growth factors, cytokines, proteases and cellular and extracellular elements all play important roles in different stages of the healing process, alterations in one or more of these components could account for the impaired healing observed in chronic wounds. In addition, oxidative damage by free radicals or condition specific factors such as neuropathy in diabetes or ischaemia in peripheral vascular disease may lead to the non-healing nature of chronic wounds. A combination of these cellular and extracellular derangements is implicated in the aetiology of venous, pressure, arterial, diabetic and all other forms of chronic skin ulcers.

Q   **What are the two most common types of excessive scarring?**

A   The two most common forms of abnormal scars are the hypertrophic scars and keloids. They are forms of excessive healing resulting from an overproduction (and/or less degradation) of some components of the healing process including fibroblasts, collagen, elastin and proteoglycans.

Q   **What are the differences between hypertrophic and keloid scars?**

A   There are a number of differences between hypertrophic scars (HTS) and keloids:

- HTS usually develop within weeks after injury but keloids can develop up to 1 year later

- HTS are usually seen in the flexor surfaces, while keloids have a predilection for the sternum, shoulder and earlobes

- HTS do not extend beyond the margins of the origin wound (scar), while keloids are a form of benign dermo-proliferative tumour which extend well beyond the margins of the original wound. In predisposed people, even a trivial injury can predispose to the formation of a keloid.

Q   **What factors predispose to the formation of HTS and keloids?**

A   The incidence of HTS is highest in wounds crossing tension lines, areas of increased skin tension and movement, deep dermal burns and wounds that have been left to heal by secondary intention. In addition, factors causing local inflammation such as persistent irritation, haematoma, infection, wound dehiscence and foreign bodies also predispose to a HTS. Keloids, however, do not have a specific aetiological factor, although there is an almost certain genetic predisposition and is more common in dark skinned races.

Q   **What is the prognosis of hypertrophic scars (HTS) and keloids?**

A   HTS may subside with time and respond to conservative treatment. However, no treatment is proven to be effective in the management of all keloids.

Case 3.18 Cell cycle

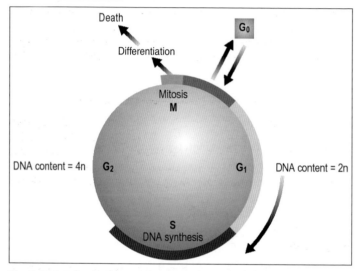

Fig. 3.18.1 Cell cycle.

Q   **How do you define a cell cycle?**

A   A cell cycle is defined as a progressive and orderly sequence of events that occurs within a cell leading to synthesis of DNA and culminates in cell division.

Q   **Can you draw a normal cell cycle?**

A   There are four distinct phases in the cell cycle (Fig. 3.18.1). When the cells are not cycling (dividing), they are in the 'G$_0$' or the quiescent phase. When the cells are stimulated to divide, the cell enters the 'G$_1$' phase, which is also called the first gap phase. This phase is the main determinant of the cell cycle. The next phase is the 'S' phase during which DNA is synthesised. The phase is followed by the 'G$_2$' phase, which is called the second gap phase. This phase can be of varying length. The final phase is the 'M' phase and it is during this phase that there is mitosis (nuclear and cytoplasmic division) prior to cell division.

Q **Can you name some factors that influence the progression of the cell cycle?**

A Some of the factors that influence cell cycle progression include p53, p27, p21, cyclin and cyclin-dependent kinases (CDK) and retinoblastoma and related genes.

Q **Do all cells divide at the same rate?**

A No, the time taken for different types of cells to divide varies. For example, intestinal epithelial cells divide much more rapidly than liver cells. The main determinant of the time taken to divide is the time spent in the 'G_1' phase of the cell cycle whereas the 'S', 'G_2' and 'M' phases are usually of constant length. 'G_2' is a resting phase and permanent cells (e.g. neurons) stay in this phase permanently and do not divide when they reach the end of their lifetime.

Q **How does cell cycling differ from cell differentiation?**

A While cell cycling describes the phases through which the cell progresses before division (see above), cell differentiation is a term that describes the development of a cell with a specialised function that distinguishes it from its parent cell. This occurs as a result of altered expression of selective genes and proteins resulting in the formation of such a cell with a specific function.

Case 3.19 Cellular injury

Q **What is apoptosis?**

A Apoptosis also defined as programmed cell death is a structured disassembly of cellular components on specific cues by an in built mechanism, of which a system of enzymes called caspases is important. This is a normal process occurring during the physiological part of growth and development. It is also a mechanism for removal of cells that contain abnormal DNA.

Q **How is this different from necrosis?**

A Necrosis is cell death occurring as a result of cell injury or exposure to cytotoxic agents. It is therefore pathological and plays no part in normal tissue homeostasis. Necrosis is generally associated with an inflammatory reaction which is not seen in apoptosis. Apoptosis results in the formation of 'apoptotic bodies' which are subsequently removed by phagocytes; this process is not associated with the inflammation seen in necrosis.

Q What are the biological features that are specific to apoptosis?

A In apoptosis, there is loss of plasma membrane asymmetry and attachment, 'blebbed' appearance of the plasma membrane, condensation of the cytoplasm and nucleus, increased mitochondrial permeability, internucleosomal cleavage of DNA (digested into smaller fragments) and the cell eventually shrinks and fragments into 'apoptotic bodies'.

Q What is the physiological importance of apoptosis?

A Apoptosis is an essential part of tissue homeostasis. The constant production of cells by mitosis and removed by apoptosis, allows a continuous cell turnover that is able to cope with environmental changes. Apoptosis, for example, occurs in the endometrium of the uterus as a natural part of the menstrual cycle when levels of hormones fall. It is also responsible for the degeneration of the thymus after childhood.

Q What is the role of apoptosis during embryological development?

A Three types of apoptosis are seen during embryological development and this has important significance: (1) Morphogenic apoptosis occurs when there is structural change in the tissue or organ. This is seen during cell death of the skin separating fingers and cell death in the dorsal neural tube leading to tube closure; (2) Histogenic apoptosis occurs when the tissue or organ undergo differentiation. This occurs in the Müllerian/Wolffian ducts, under hormonal influence, leading to the development of the female/male genital tracts respectively; (3) Phylogenetic apoptosis occurs when the embryological vestigial structures are removed, as occurs in the pronephros.

Q Is it possible to measure or quantify apoptosis?

A It is difficult to accurately measure the process of apoptosis itself as it is generally undetectable when it occurs. It is therefore only possible to identify markers which might indicate that apoptosis has occurred. Generally, apoptosis is assessed by detecting the biological events or morphological features associated with the process of programmed cell death. For example, one of the methods of detecting apoptosis is measurement of 'caspases' induced in apoptosis.

Q Are there any regulators for apoptosis?

A Certain genes may be involved in the regulation of apoptosis. Genes which activate apoptosis include p53 and genes which inhibit apoptosis include c-myc and bcl-2. In addition, hormones such as glucocorticoids can promote apoptosis.

Case 3.20 Vascular disorders

Q A 40-year-old intravenous drug abuser presents with a swelling over his right groin. On examination, the swelling is pulsatile, non-tender and a few inguinal lymph nodes are enlarged. What is the most likely diagnosis?

A This patient has probably developed a pseudo-aneurysm (false aneurysm) of the femoral artery.

Q What is the cause of the enlarged lymph nodes?

A Skin and soft tissue bacterial infections are a common complication of intravenous drug use. This may be due to accidental injection of drugs into the fatty layer under the skin (*skin popping*), leakage of drugs out of the veins during injection (*extravasation*), tissue death (necrosis) due to toxic materials in drugs and increased bacterial colonisation (and/or contamination) on the skin surface. It should however be acknowledged that in intravenous drug abusers there may be persistent swelling of the lymph nodes (due to blocked lymphatic vessels) in the absence of local infection. Discoloration (usually hyperpigmentation) of the skin of the affected area and local scarring may also be commonly observed.

Q Briefly outline the principles of managing this patient.

A Once the patient is stabilised, it is important to make an accurate diagnosis since, at first, it might be difficult to distinguish a false aneurysm from a local haematoma with transmitted pulsations from the femoral artery; re-examination is hence important. A colour Duplex scan is a very useful initial investigation. If detected early and if the defect is small, it may be possible to occlude the site of the leak using the Duplex scanner probe by providing appropriate pressure (+/– injection of fibrin glue into the pseudo-aneurysm). Digital or conventional arteriography can be used to confirm the presence and exact location of the aneurysm. The defect can be repaired electively if simple compression fails. Closure with simple sutures often suffices if the defect is small, but if it is large, a patch or interposition graft may be required. If all the vessels entering the false sac cannot be controlled, the troublesome back bleeding can be prevented by inserting a Fogarty catheter into the relevant branches and inflating the balloons until the repair is completed.

Q What are the borders and contents of the femoral triangle?

A The femoral triangle is a triangular space that lies between the inguinal ligament, the medial border of the sartorius muscle and the medial border of adductor longus. The floor is formed by iliacus, psoas, pectineus and adductor brevis with the anterior division of the obturator nerve lying on it. The contents of the femoral triangle include (from medial to lateral) the inguinal lymph nodes, femoral vein, femoral artery and the femoral nerve.

Q   **Can you give some differential diagnoses for groin swellings?**

A   A swelling in the groin could arise from any of the following anatomical structures in the region:

1. From the skin and subcutaneous tissue: lipoma, epidermoid cyst and local haematoma.

2. From the vein: saphena varix.

3. From the artery: femoral aneurysm.

4. From the lymph nodes: lymphadenopathy due to infection, neoplasm or lymphoma.

5. From the hernial orifices: inguinal hernia and femoral hernia.

6. From the testicular apparatus: hydrocele of the cord or ectopic testis.

7. From the psoas sheath: psoas abscess.

Case 3.21 Disorders of growth, differentiation and morphogenesis

Q   **What is metaplasia and what is its aetiology?**

A   Metaplasia is defined as the transformation of one fully-differentiated cell type into another. Metaplasia usually occurs in response to an environmental stimulus; it is an adaptive process and is usually reversible. It is thought that an underlying genetic process may account for the transformation and that the final differentiated cell type is better able to withstand the new environmental stimulus or challenge.

Q   **Can you give some examples of where such transformation may occur?**

A   Metaplasia can be classified into epithelial and connective tissue metaplasia. Some examples of epithelial metaplasia include: (1) Barrett's oesophagus (replacement of squamous epithelium by gastric epithelium in patients with reflux oesophagitis); (2) breast – apocrine metaplasia; (3) bronchi – squamous metaplasia occurring in the ciliated respiratory epithelium of smokers; (4) bladder and kidneys – squamous metaplasia of the transitional epithelium in the presence of stones and infection such as schistosomiasis and (5) endocervix – squamous metaplasia occurring in response to hormonal surges as in puberty. Connective tissue metaplasia occurs in the bronchial cartilage (tracheopathia osteoplastica), in the vascular system (calcium deposits within atheromatous arterial walls) and in the eye (in response to chronic uveal tract disease).

Q   **Is metaplasia always reversible?**

A   Although it is reversible in most cases, in some instances, a metaplasia may progress to a dysplasia (e.g. bronchial epithelium in smokers) and eventually malignancy. For this progression to occur, however, there should be a persistent environmental stimulus. It is quite unlikely that a metaplastic lesion would progress to malignancy without the persistence of the stimulating factor or a new similar environmental stimulus.

Q   **Is metaplasia clinically significant and if so, why?**

A   Metaplasia can become dysplastic if the agent that caused the meta-plastic transformation persists. Dysplasia can progress to malignancy. Metaplasia can also be misdiagnosed, both clinically and histologically, as a carcinoma.

Q   **So, what is dysplasia?**

A   Dysplasia is a pre-malignant condition characterised by an increase in cell growth, an increase in the number of mitoses, presence of abnormal mitosis, abnormal cellular differentiation, loss of cellular cohesion and cellular atypia including pleomorphism, hyperchromatism and a high nuclear/cytoplasmic ratio. Dysplasia may be caused by prolonged environ-mental stress to the affected tissue, longstanding inflammation and carcinogens. Examples of these include alcohol, smoking, viral infection (e.g. human papilloma virus) and chronic inflammatory conditions. Severe dysplasia essentially resembles a neoplastic lesion apart from the fact that it has not invaded the basement membrane. It may also be referred to as carcinoma-*in-situ* (e.g. cervical intra-epithelial neoplasia).

Case 3.22 Tumours and metastasis

Q   **What is the difference between metastasis and metaplasia?**

A   Metastasis is defined as a pathological state when malignant cells have migrated from a malignant tumour to a site or sites distant from the primary. These malignant cells behave very similar to the primary cancerous cells and have the potential to grow and survive independently of the host (recipient) environment. Metaplasia, on the other hand, reflects a clinical state where one fully differentiated cell type is changed (altered) into another fully differentiated cell type. Whilst metaplasia is usually a transitional (temporary) and benign state (although it could be pre-cancerous in some instances), metastasis is usually a reflection of advanced or spreading malignancy.

Q   **What are the common ways by which metastasis occurs?**

A   Metastasis commonly occurs by one or more of the following routes:

- lymphatic: seen in most carcinomas

- haematogenous: seen in most sarcomas; also follicular cell carcinoma of thyroid

- transcoelomic: seen in carcinoma of stomach, colon, pancreas

- perineural: seen in lymphatic channels in the perineurium; adenoid cystic carcinoma of the salivary gland

- cerebrospinal fluid: seen in medulloblastoma and other tumours of the central nervous system

- iatrogenic: implantation of tumour cells in another area during surgery or as a consequence of surgery

- local metastasis: this can occur when the tumour invades adjacent tissue although many surgeons and pathologists define this as tumour invasion.

Q   **What is the difference between a carcinoma and a sarcoma?**

A   A carcinoma is a malignant tumour of epithelial cells while a sarcoma is a malignant tumour of connective tissue cells. A carcinoma can also arise in organs derived from the mesoderm; examples include carcinoma of the ovary, endometrium and uterine tube and carcinoma of the kidney.

Q   **What are the most common malignant tumours in both sexes?**

A   In men, the most common malignant tumours are of the prostate, lung (broncho-pulmonary), colorectum and the urinary tract. In women, the commonest malignant tumours are of the lung (broncho-pulmonary), breast, colorectum and the urinary tract.

Q   **Can you tell me some of the histological features you might see in a malignant tumour?**

A   Some of the characteristic changes which can be expected in a malignant tumour are: increased mitosis; abnormal mitosis (tripolar, tetrapolar, sunburst or bizarre); an increase in the nuclear-cytoplasmic ratio; pleomorphism (variance of size and shape of tumour cells) and hyperchromatism (increased amounts of DNA leading to dark-stained nuclei). In addition, there may be focal or extensive areas of haemorrhage and necrosis due to abnormal vascularity. The surrounding tissues may also have infiltrative borders with evidence of intravascular or lymphatic spread.

Case 3.23 Tumour markers

Q   **What do you understand by the term 'tumour marker'?**

A   A tumour marker is a substance produced by a tumour which is present in the circulation and can be usually measured in the serum (although there are exceptions such as vanillylmandelic acid (produced by phaeo-chromocytomas) and 5-hydroxy-indole-acetic (5-HIAA) (produced by carcinoid tumours) which are detected in the urine. A tumour marker can aid in diagnosing a tumour and can also be used to monitor the response of the tumour to treatment. After treatment, a rise in the level of the tumour marker may indicate recurrence.

Q   What is a tumour marker comprised of?

A   A tumour marker could be an oncofetal antigen (e.g. carcinoembryonic antigen in colorectal tumours), isoenzyme (e.g. prostate acid phosphatase produced by prostate cancer), or a hormone (e.g. cortisol from an adrenal tumour or ACTH and ADH produced by oat cell lung tumours). In addition, some growth factors may be produced by the tumour to aid their autocrine growth and invasion.

Q   What tumour markers are used in clinical practice?

A   In addition to the carcinoembryonic antigens in colorectal carcinoma and prostate acid phosphatase in prostate cancer mentioned above, some other examples include: α-fetoprotein (AFP), which is produced by primary liver tumours and testicular teratomas; placental alkaline phosphatase (PLAP), which is produced by testicular seminomas and tumours of the pancreas and lung; human chorionic gonadotrophins (HCG) which is seen in choriocarcinomas; vanillylmandelic acid (VMA) which is produced by phaeochromocytomas and 5-hydroxy-indole-acetic acid (5-HIAA) which is produced by carcinoid tumours.

Q   Can you explain, with some examples, how surveillance of tumour progression is undertaken using tumour markers?

A   The measurement of serum levels of carcinoembryonic antigen and α-fetoprotein may be used to monitor the progress of colorectal carcinoma and testicular teratoma, respectively. A sample is usually taken preoperatively although the initial level may not be indicative of the size of the tumour bed. After surgery (e.g. orchidectomy for testicular teratoma), serum levels are monitored frequently until the levels return to normal. Any rise in the carcinoembryonic antigen or α-fetoprotein levels at a later date may indicate tumour recurrence.

Case 3.24 Carcinogenesis

Q   What do you understand by the term carcinogenesis?

A   The process by which a tumour develops is termed carcinogenesis. Although it may imply the development of benign and malignant stages, the term carcinogenesis is usually applied to the development of malignant tumours. The process of carcinogenesis usually begins with a single cell. The cell undergoes mutation as it divides and by a subsequent multi-step process, becomes malignant. This enables it to grow autonomously without the inhibitory effects of the normal cellular growth control. A carcinogen is an agent that induces malignancy. Various carcinogens have been identified by epidemiological evidence and experimental studies.

Q   **What causes the initial mutation?**

A   There are various reasons that may initiate the mutation although it is commonly environmental or genetic. Various risk factors have been identified, including: (1) inherited disease processes such as retinoblastoma and familial adenomatous polyposis; (2) environmental carcinogens such as radiation; (3) exposure to certain chemical carcinogenic agents – nicotine and lung cancer and betel nut chewing and oral cancer; (4) certain viruses such as the relation between human papilloma virus and cervical cancer and Epstein–Barr virus in nasopharyngeal carcinoma; (5) diet, e.g. excessive red meat/fat and colorectal cancer; (6) pre-malignant diseases such as ulcerative colitis; (7) racial predisposition (Chinese and gastric cancer) and (8) inherited risk associated with conditions such as Li–Fraumeni syndrome and multiple endocrine neoplasia syndromes.

Q   **Give me some examples of chemical carcinogens and how do they act?**

A   Chemical carcinogens are usually hydrocarbons which form charged molecules known as 'epoxides'. Epoxides then bind to DNA and RNA finally resulting in a genetic mutation. Some examples of chemical carcinogens include: (1) β-naphthylamine (aromatic amines) used in the rubber/dye industry which causes bladder cancer; (2) Nitrosamines used in fertilisers which cause gastrointestinal tract cancers; (3) Soot (polycyclic aromatic hydrocarbon) which causes scrotal cancer; (4) Aflatoxin (mycotoxin from *Aspergillus flavus*) which causes hepatocellular carcinoma; (5) Azo dyes which cause liver and bladder cancer; (6) Asbestos which causes pleural plaques and mesothelioma; (7) Nickel which causes lung cancer.

Q   **What is the mechanism of genetic mutation?**

A   The carcinogen interacts with the DNA of the cell resulting in functional abnormalities in the genes that it controls. The result is a genetic mutation which causes a dividing cell to act abnormally and grow independently of all normal control and inhibitory mechanisms. Further mutations occur by a multi-step process to allow a malignant tumour to acquire the properties to invade the basement membrane and metastasise.

Q   **What is the difference between 'initiation' and 'promotion'?**

A   Initiation and promotion are both involved in the early stages of carcinogenesis. Initiation is the process by which cellular DNA is altered and hence as the cell divides, it has the potential to become carcinogenic. Promotion is the next step in the process. It includes proliferation of the altered cell and hence the development of carcinoma. Promotion is due to further genetic mutation occurring spontaneously or following exposure to promoters. Initiators and promoters allow the carcinoma to develop to a level where it can grow autonomously.

Q What is an oncogene and what is its role in carcinogenesis?

A Cellular oncogenes are genes which are essential for life. They control normal cell growth and differentiation and it is thought that carcinoma may develop if they have an altered or enhanced expression. Oncogenes may be classified by the function of their gene production: myc – involved in cell proliferation; ras – involved in cyclic nucleotide binding and hence intracellular signalling; bcl-2-involved with apoptosis.

Abnormalities in oncogene expression, therefore, may account for an increased risk of carcinogenesis by producing abnormally functioning oncoprotein and an excessive amount of oncoprotein and loss of usual growth inhibition (tumour suppressor genes). It is thought that abnormal or large amounts of oncoprotein encourage cells to grow of their own accord, to have an increased motility and to have reduced cell-to-cell adhesion. All of the above properties enable the affected cells to develop into a malignant tumour.

Case 3.25 Surgical infections

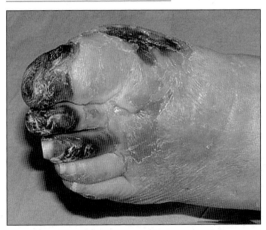

Fig. 3.25.1 Note the presence of a dry gangrene in the tips of the medial three toes with superadded infection in the proximal part of the toes resulting in wet gangrene in a patient with diabetes.

Q What is gangrene?

A Gangrene implies death of macroscopic portions of tissue. A gangrenous part lacks arterial pulsation, venous return, sensation, warmth and function. It can be divided into dry gangrene and wet gangrene.

Q What is the difference between dry and wet gangrene?

A Dry gangrene occurs when tissues are desiccated by gradual slowing of the bloodstream; it is typically the result of atherosclerosis and usually not related to infection. The affected area, commonly the lower limb, becomes black as a result of iron accumulation from degraded haemoglobin. There is a characteristic line of demarcation. The affected part may then undergo mummification and auto-amputate with healing occurring under the affected area. This type of gangrene is commonly seen in gradual atherosclerotic disease with diabetes mellitus, although it may soon become wet gangrene if there is superadded infection.

Moist gangrene occurs when there is venous as well as arterial obstruction, when the artery is suddenly occluded, as by a ligature or embolus and in diabetes mellitus. In moist gangrene, superseded infection and putrefaction are more likely, the affected part becomes swollen and discoloured and the epidermis may be raised in blebs. It is characteristically dusky with a spreading erythema and is frequently malodorous.

Q **What type of gangrene would you expect to see in a patient with diabetes?**

A Diabetic gangrene is due to three factors: trophic changes resulting from peripheral neuritis; atheroma of the small arteries resulting in ischaemia; and excess sugar lowering the resistance to infection. Both dry and wet types of gangrene may be seen in patients with diabetes. However, due to the microvascular disease causing a gradual reduction in the blood flow, dry gangrene is more common; nevertheless, it may soon progress to wet gangrene if appropriate treatment is not instituted and infection supervenes. It should be noted that diabetic gangrene of the toes can occur in the presence of palpable peripheral pulses (absence implies associated major arterial disease).

Q **What other types of gangrene do you know of?**

A Gas gangrene, which is caused by *Clostridium perfringens* (widely found in nature, particularly soil and faeces and causes gas gangrene in about 80% of cases; the other organisms are *Clostridium septicum* and *Clostridium novyi*). Wound infections due to gas gangrene are associated with severe local wound pain and crepitus; gas in the tissues may be noted on plain radiographs. Synergistic spreading gangrene (necrotising fasciitis – Synonyms: Meleney's gangrene of the abdominal wall infections and Fournier's gangrene of the scrotal infections) is usually caused by a mixed pattern of organisms – coliforms, staphylococci, *Bacteroides* species, anaerobic streptococci and *Peptostreptococci*. The extent of subdermal spread of gangrene is always much more extensive than first apparent. Surgical debridement, wide excision and laying open of the affected tissue, combined with broad-spectrum antibiotic therapy and aggressive circulatory support may be necessary to save life; skin grafting, after resolution of acute symptoms, may be needed to cover the large, excised areas. Meleney's gangrene still carries 30–40% mortality. Patients who develop synergistic gangrene usually have a systemic disease such as diabetes mellitus, are on corticosteroids, or may be immunocompromised.

Q   Can you name some other types of clostridial infections?

A   Other clostridial strains causing infections include: *Clostridium difficile* (causes pseudo membranous colitis); *Clostridium tetani* (causes tetanus) and *Clostridium botulinum* (causes botulism).

Case 3.26 Surgical microbiology

Q   Can you give some examples of Gram-positive and Gram-negative organisms?

A   Gram-positive and Gram-negative organisms can be either cocci or rods (bacilli). Examples include:

Gram-positive cocci: *Staphylococcus aureus, S. epidermidis; Streptococcus pneumoniae, S. viridans* (α-haemolytic) *S. pyogenes* (β-haemolytic), and *S. faecalis*

Gram-negative cocci: *Neisseria meningitidis, N. gonorrhoea; and Moraxella catarrhalis*

Gram-positive rods (bacilli): *Corynebacterium diphtheroides; Clostridium tetani, C. perfringens, C. botulinum, C. difficile; and Listeria monocytogenes*

Gram-negative rods (bacilli): *Escherichia coli; Campylobacter; Klebsiella; Yersinia; Enterobacteria; Haemophilus influenzae; Proteus; Legionella; Pseudomonas; Bordetella pertussis; Salmonella; Brucellus; Shigella; Pasteurella multocida; and Vibrio cholera*

Q   What sampling techniques could be used to identify infection in surgical wounds?

A   Various sampling techniques are used to identify wound infection such as wound swabs, tissue biopsy, dermabrasion and absorbent pads, although the first two are the commonly used methods. The ease of obtaining and processing superficial wound swabs, combined with their relative cheap cost and non-invasive nature make them the most used method for wound sampling. However, organisms cultured from a superficial swab reflect the colonising superficial bacterial flora and may not be representative of the organisms in the deeper tissues, as in deep surgical or deep penetrating wounds. Tissue and/or pus should be collected whenever possible, since growth from these samples is more representative of pathogenic flora. These are amenable to quantitative microbiological analysis and other techniques which improve the diagnostic yield. Tissue biopsy should always be carried out when therapeutic debridement of the wound is required, in cases of osteomyelitis and whenever superficial sampling methods have proven ineffective.

Q   What types of microbiological analysis are commonly performed in the laboratory?

A   The two commonly performed microbiological analyses are semi-quantitative and quantitative analysis. Most laboratories perform a semi-quantitative analysis on wound swabs where the bacterial growth is graded as scanty, light, moderate or heavy. Semi-quantitative analysis, however, introduces a bias towards motile and fast growing organisms; fastidious organisms such as anaerobes may be under-represented. Quantitative analysis identifies the number of organisms per gram of tissue. A bacterial load greater than 10^5 organisms or colony forming units per gram of tissue is a predictor of wound infection. However, it should be noted that some wounds which are more heavily colonised might heal spontaneously and, conversely, some organisms are able to cause significant infection at much lower levels of colonisation. The occurrence of wound infection, therefore, depends on the pathogenicity (virulence) of the organism, wound type (and site) and the host response.

Q   **What other types of staining could be used in bacteriological diagnosis?**

A   The Ziehl-Nielsen stain and the auramine stain are other types. The Ziehl-Nielsen stain is used to stain acid- and alcohol-fast bacilli; they are useful to identify Mycobacterium bacilli. The stain involves heating carbol fuchsin, decolorising with acid and alcohol and then counterstaining with methylene blue. If positive for mycobacterium bacilli, they will be seen as red bacilli against a blue background. The auramine stain involves the addition of auramine-phenol, decolorising with acid and then adding potassium permanganate. If positive, the bacilli stain fluorescent yellow against a dark field when viewed under UV light.

Case 3.27 Surgical haematology (1)

Q   **What is the difference between a clot and a thrombosis?**

A   A clot is a solid material formed from the constituents of blood in stationary blood. Thrombus, on the other hand, is a solid material formed from the constituents of blood in flowing blood. Clotting is essentially a function of the intrinsic or extrinsic clotting cascade, while thrombosis is a function of platelets (although the clotting cascade is involved later).

Q   **What are the functions of platelets?**

A   The functions of platelets include: adhesion to a vessel wall; aggregation with contraction to form a dense solid mass in a vessel; release of compounds that contribute towards the clotting cascade such as von Willebrand factor and release of other compounds that have effects on tissue cells such as prostaglandins and thromboxanes.

Q   **What factors contribute to thrombosis?**

A   The factors that contribute to thrombosis are: changes in the vessel wall (atheroma causing a change in the speed and flow though arteries); changes in the blood constituents (thrombocytosis, increase in coagulation factors such as fibrinogen, procoagulant factors released from malignancies, hyperviscosity from hypergammaglobulinaemia and polycythemia and inherited deficiencies of protein C, protein S and antithrombin) and changes in the blood flow (reduction in flow in patients who have compromised venous drainage, such as in the deep veins of the leg, local stasis in aneurysms and turbulence from artificial valves, stents and implanted devices). The above three factors are known as the 'Virchow's triad'.

Case 3.28 Blood transfusion and transfusion reactions

Q   What is the composition of blood?

A   About 55% of blood consists of plasma which is a complex solution of gases, salts, protein, carbohydrates and lipids. The remaining 45% of blood comprises the various cellular elements (red cells, white cells and platelets).

Q   What are the principal blood groups in humans and comment on the antigen and antibody content of each blood group.

A   In humans there are four principal blood groups: O, A, B and AB. 'O' is the most common blood group, accounting for approximately 50% of all groups followed by 'A', 'B' and 'AB'. The plasma contains both antigen and antibody. These are as follows:

Blood group	Antigen present	Antibody present
A	Antigen A	Antibody B
B	Antigen B	Antibody A
AB	Antigen AB	No antibody
O	No antigen	A, B, AB

Q   For what components is the blood tested?

A   All donated blood is tested for blood group antigens mainly, ABO blood grouping system, Rh cde phenotype and red cell antibodies.

Q   What microbes are screened for before accepting a recipient blood?

A   The blood is normally screened for Hepatitis B surface antigen, Hepatitis C antibodies, syphilis antibodies and HIV types 1 and 2 (antibodies).

Q   What other products are obtained when blood is donated?

A   The other blood products include platelets (stored at −32°C), fresh frozen plasma (stored at −30°C), clotting factors, i.e. factor VIII and albumin.

Q   **What are the types of transfusion reactions you are aware of?**

A   Transfusion reactions can occur as a result of any blood incompatibilities. This may be a result of ABO agglutinin incompatibility (usually results in a severe, immediate transfusion reaction), Rhesus incompatibility, HLA antigen as a result of multiple transfusions and haemolytic disease of the newborn which occurs as a result of Rhesus mother carrying a Rhesus positive baby (father's group). The mother develops antibodies to Rhesus positive cells which may cause agglutination of fetal blood during future pregnancies.

Q   **What is the significance of the Rhesus D antigen?**

A   Rhesus D antigen is prevalent within the population and is considered to be the most antigenic of all the Rhesus antigens: C, D, E, c, d and e. Patients are grouped as Rh positive or negative according to the presence of the D antigen.

Q   **What happens if you were to transfuse a Rhesus negative person with Rhesus positive blood?**

A   Although there would be no immediate 'transfusion reaction', anti-Rhesus antibodies would develop over a period of 2–4 weeks. In some instances, this might be sufficient to result in agglutination of transfused cells within the circulation. This is known as a delayed transfusion reaction. When the person receives Rhesus positive blood again, anti-Rhesus antibodies react with the donor cells resulting in an immediate transfusion reaction. This usually has a rapid onset and can be severe (fatal).

Q   **What are the complications of blood transfusion?**

A   The major complications of blood transfusion are anaphylactic reactions, leading to hypotension, DIC and renal failure and transmission of pathogens causing diseases. The important pathogens include viruses causing Hepatitis B, AIDS, syphilis and protozoal infections such as malaria. Mild immunological reactions can occur in patients who have had multiple transfusions; this may present as rigors, low-grade temperature and urticaria. Furthermore, antibodies within the donated blood may react with the patient's white blood cells causing pulmonary oedema. Antibodies in the donor blood to the patient's antibodies may lead to thrombocytopenic purpura.

Q   **How would you suspect a transfusion reaction?**

A   Transfusion reactions occur as a result of incompatibility of one or more antigens/antibodies present in the donor/recipient blood. Although un-common now because of rigorous testing, it is still encountered. The patient may become extremely unwell very quickly. They may complain of gastrointestinal symptoms, dizziness and palpitations. They may develop anaphylaxis and become haemodynamically unstable. This may lead to renal failure. In delayed transfusion reaction, the patient may become jaundiced or suffer renal abnormalities a few days following the blood transfusion.

Case 3.29 Surgical haematology (2)

Q   **Define blood clotting.**

A   Blood clotting is defined as the conversion of fibrinogen to fibrin by thrombin. The clot that is formed by the reaction consists of a dense network of fibrin strands in which blood cells and plasma are trapped.

Q   **What are the main coagulation pathways?**

A   There are two blood coagulation pathways: (1) the extrinsic and (2) the intrinsic pathway. These two pathways converge on the activation of factor X, which catalyses the cleavage of prothrombin to thrombin. Blood clotting via the extrinsic pathway is initiated by the tissue damage and the release of tissue thromboplastin. Blood clotting via the intrinsic pathway, on the other hand, is initiated by exposure of the blood to a negatively charged surface. This occurs in blood vessels when the endothelium is damaged and blood comes into contact with collagen.

Q   **What do you understand by the term prothrombin time?**

A   Prothrombin time is the time taken for the plasma to clot after adding thromboplastin and calcium chloride. The result is expressed as a ratio (the prothrombin time ratio of patients to a control plasma clotting time); this is usually 12–15 seconds.

Q   **Where is prothrombin time commonly used?**

A   Prothrombin time is commonly used to monitor the effects of therapy with warfarin or similar vitamin K antagonist. It is however not very sensitive to monitor the effects of heparin. Prothrombin time is also a useful test of liver function and an important test of haemostatic integrity.

Q   **What is thrombin time?**

A   Plasma will clot directly on the addition of thrombin. The thrombin time is thus the time taken for the plasma to clot on adding thrombin. The normal adjusted time is 12–15 seconds.

Q   **What is the advantage of knowing thrombin time?**

A   Thrombin time may be used to monitor heparin therapy.

Q   What investigation would you ask for in a patient with a history of bleeding disorder?

A   Patients with a history suggestive of von Willebrand's disease and a normal platelet count should have a bleeding time (which is usually prolonged) and a clotting screen including an activated partial thromboplastin time and factor VIII assay.

Patients with prolonged bleeding time and normal clotting time are likely to have a specific platelet defect. A normal activated partial thromboplastin time may, however, be found in patients with mildly low levels of factors VIII, IX, XI or XII.

Case 3.30 Respiratory system

Q   What do you understand by the term 'respiratory failure'?

A   Respiratory failure is a clinical condition when there is impaired gaseous exchange leading to inadequate oxygenation and carbon dioxide accumulation (due to failure of elimination). A patient is said to be in respiratory failure when the PaO_2 is <8 kPa while breathing normal atmospheric air (at rest), with or without a $PaCO_2$ of >6.5 kPa.

Q   What are the types of respiratory failure you know of?

A   Respiratory failure is commonly divided into type 1 or type 2 depending on the severity of impaired gaseous exchange. It can also be divided into acute and chronic. Acute respiratory failure can develop over minutes to hours.

Type 1 failure (hypoxaemic/hypoxic respiratory failure) primarily represents a failure of oxygenation (low PaO_2 [<8 kPa] with a normal or low $PaCO_2$). It is seen in most acute lung diseases such as pneumonia, pulmonary oedema or lung contusion. Fluid in the lung space or collapse of the alveolar units leads to low oxygenation resulting in ventilation and perfusion (V/Q) mismatch.

Type 2 failure (hypercapnic respiratory failure) primarily represents a failure of ventilation. It is characterised by a low PaO_2 (<8 kPa) and a high $PaCO_2$ (>6.5 kPa). This type of failure is seen in conditions such as asthma, acute exacerbations of COPD, opioid overdose and depressed brain stem function causing coma. Respiratory acidosis is commonly seen in acute type 2 failure whereas it is seldom seen in chronic type 2 failure. This is because chronic failure develops over days thus allowing renal compensatory mechanisms to normalise the pH by retention of bicarbonate.

Q What is the relevance of respiratory failure in surgical patients? How is the type of surgery related to postoperative respiratory failure?

A Respiratory failure can occur in previously fit patients or as an acute exacerbation of chronic respiratory disease. Lower respiratory tract infection, collapse of the basal segment of the lung secondary to inadequate pain control or inadequate gaseous exchange due to opioid overdose may also contribute towards respiratory failure in postoperative patients. Postoperative morbidity and mortality are increased in patients with pre-existing chronic lung disease and those with acute respiratory failure (preoperatively). Death from pulmonary complications occurs in about 10% of surgical patients with moderate to severe pulmonary disease undergoing major surgery, particularly emergency surgery and long procedures (typically >4 hours). In addition, postoperative pulmonary disease (and morbidity from it) can occur in up to 40% of patients with mild to moderate lung disease undergoing major surgery. This is further worsened in patients who are obese, and in smokers. An adequate level of pre- and postoperative care, such as in an ITU or HDU, is essential for patients with known respiratory problems.

The effect of general anaesthesia plays a role in postoperative pulmonary complications. General anaesthesia leads to alveolar collapse from reduced FRC and causes reduced lung compliance. Opiate drugs cause respiratory depression. Thoracic and abdominal surgery increases the risk further by decreasing postoperative FEV_1 and FVC by up to 50%. Some surgical procedures by their very nature (e.g. pulmonary resection) cause a reduction in the patient's respiratory function and reserve.

Q Outline your preoperative assessment of a patient who is a life-long smoker with emphysema due for an elective open abdominal aneurysm repair.

A Preoperative assessment will consist of relevant history, examination and appropriate investigations. History will ascertain the severity of the patient's respiratory disease and whether there is any evidence of an acute exacerbation at present. Restricted exercise tolerance, dyspnoea at rest or minimal exertion, the need for regular home bronchodilators or nebulisers and home oxygen therapy are indicative of severe disease. Recent deterioration in exercise tolerance with escalation of nebuliser usage may point towards an acute exacerbation of the disease such as due to lower respiratory tract infection. A history of previous admissions to HDU or ITU for ventilatory support is also important. The cardio-vascular system should be assessed for orthopnoea, paroxysmal nocturnal dyspnoea and peripheral oedema which may further compromise the respiratory compliance.

Clinical indicators of acute respiratory failure include confusion or drowsiness, central cyanosis, tachycardia and tachypnoea. Peripheral oedema and hepatomegaly may be due to cor pulmonale from longstanding disease.

Appropriate investigations include: full blood count for anaemia or polycythemia; biochemistry; liver function tests could be deranged due to cor pulmonale; trace elements such as magnesium and phosphate, deficiency of which might aggravate respiratory failure. Electrocardiogram – to look for any evidence of cor pulmonale or co-existing cardiac disease. Chest radiograph may reveal the cause of any acute element to respiratory failure as well as serving as a useful baseline study in a patient with chronic chest disease. Arterial blood gases will assist in diagnosis between the types and severity and guide therapy. Further tests may include echocardiography to assess ventricular function and lung function tests to assess the severity of disease and any degree of reversibility.

Q **How do you manage an acute deterioration of respiratory function in a patient 4 days after an abdomino-perineal resection?**

A Treatment is divided into supportive measures to improve oxygen delivery, as well as measures to treat the underlying causes and contributing factors. Oxygen therapy, however, should be titrated to achieve adequate oxygen saturation in patients with a history of chronic type 2 failure, who may be reliant on their hypoxic drive (although in emergency and critically ill patients high-flow oxygen should be administered since hypoxia is much more lethal than hypercapnia). Mechanical means of improving oxygenation in type 1 failure include continuous positive airway pressure (CPAP). Pharmacological treatments include the use of bronchodilators ($\beta2$ agonists and theophyllines) to reduce airway resistance, systemic corticosteroids to reduce airway inflammation, antibiotics if there is evidence of pneumonia and improved analgesia if pain is limiting ventilation. Chest physiotherapy including breathing and coughing exercises, ambulation and postural drainage should be performed by specialist physiotherapists.

Q **What are the indications for mechanical ventilation?**

A Mechanical ventilation (i.e. Intermittent Positive Pressure Ventilation [IPPV]) is indicated in the presence of: (1) gross hypoxia, e.g. PaO_2 <8 kPa$_2$ on 60% FiO_2; (2) worsening hypercarbia; (3) worsening respiratory or metabolic acidosis despite adequate treatment; (4) patient exhaustion, restlessness, or an inability to clear sputum. IPPV is used to increase PaO_2, lower $PaCO_2$ and relieve respiratory muscle fatigue, while therapy directed at the underlying cause of the respiratory failure continues. It needs to be acknowledged that IPPV in itself is not a curative treatment but rather a supportive measure.

Case 3.31 Breast disorders and surgical anatomy

Q A 66-year-old woman presents with a painless lump in the upper-outer quadrant of her left breast. On examination, the lump is rubbery and fixed to the adjacent breast tissue. What is the most likely diagnosis?

A The most likely diagnosis is carcinoma of the breast.

Q What type of carcinoma could it be?

A Although the precise type cannot be determined without histology, infiltrating lobular carcinomas, representing 15% of all breast cancer, generally present in the upper outer quadrant of the breast as a subtle thickening. They are difficult to diagnose by mammography. Infiltrating lobular can be bilateral. Microscopically, they exhibit a linear array of cells (Indian filing) and grow around the ducts and lobules.

Q What is the incidence and aetiology of carcinoma of the breast?

A Carcinoma of the breast is the most common cancer in women, affecting 1 in 12 adult women during their lifetime. This disease is the leading cause of death in women between the ages of 40 and 50 years. The aetiology is not clear but genetic, endocrine and dietary factors have been implicated. Although a positive family history (thus implying a genetic link) is a strong determining factor, its development is probably multifactorial.

Q Give some differential diagnosis for breast lumps.

A Lumps in the breast could be either benign or malignant. Benign breast lumps include fibroadenomas, papillomas and cysts. Malignant breast lumps can be divided into: carcinoma-*in-situ* (lobular carcinoma-*in-situ* (LCIS) and ductal carcinoma-*in-situ* (DCIS)); infiltrating ductal carcinoma (IDC); infiltrating lobular carcinoma (ILC); medullary carcinoma; colloid carcinoma; tubular carcinoma; adenoid cystic carcinoma and inflammatory breast cancer. Fibroadenomas are common between the ages of 20–30, cystic diseases and intra-ductal papillomas are common between 30–60 years of age, whilst duct ectasia, plasma cell mastitis and fat necrosis can occur with any age.

Q Describe the lymphatic drainage of the breast.

A The lymph from the lateral part of the breast (upper and lower outer quadrant) drains into the axillary and infra-clavicular nodes. Lymph from the medial part (upper and lower inner quadrant) of the breast drains through the intercostal spaces into internal thoracic (parasternal) nodes.

Q How does the breast receive its blood supply?

A The blood supply to the breast is mainly derived from the lateral thoracic artery by branches that curl around the border of pectoralis major and by other branches that pierce the muscle. The internal thoracic artery also sends branches through the intercostal spaces beside the sternum; those of 2nd and 3rd spaces are largest. Pectoral branches of the thoracoacromial artery supply the upper part of the breast.

Case 3.32 Cardiovascular system

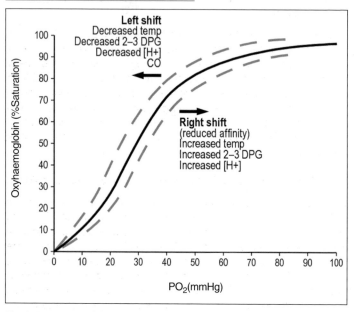

Fig. 3.32.1 Haemoglobin–oxygen equilibrium

Q What do you understand by the haemoglobin–oxygen equilibrium (dissociation) curve? Please draw the haemoglobin–oxygen equilibrium.

A The binding of oxygen to haemoglobin is directly dependent on the partial pressure of oxygen (PO_2) with which the haemoglobin is equilibrated. This relationship is called the haemoglobin–oxygen equilibrium curve.

Q What factors determine the status of the haemoglobin–oxygen curve?

A The normal haemoglobin–oxygen curve in humans is at equilibrium when the hydrogen ion [H+] concentration is 40 mmol/litre (pH: 7.40), the $PaCO_2$ is 6 kPa, the 2-3-diphosphoglycerate (2-3 DGP) concentration is 15 µmol/gHb and the temperature is 37°C. When any of these four physiological factors are altered, there is a corresponding change in the affinity of the haemoglobin for oxygen. For example, an increase in the temperature, increase in CO_2 concentration, a rise in pH or an increase in 2-3 DPG can cause a deviation of the haemoglobin–oxygen equilibrium curve to the right and a corresponding reduction in the affinity of haemo-globin for oxygen. Likewise, a decrease in temperature, a decrease in CO_2 concentration, a fall in pH, or a decrease in 2-3 DPG can shift the curve to the left which increases the affinity of haemoglobin for oxygen.

Q   **What is the clinical significance of the haemoglobin–oxygen dissociation curve?**

A   Because of the sigmoid shape of the haemoglobin–oxygen dissociation curve, when the PO_2 falls in the early stages there is very little change in the percentage saturation of oxyhaemoglobin (i.e. pulse oximeter reading). However, when the oxygen saturation reaches about 80%, it implies that there has been a significant drop in the PO_2 (approximately <6.5 kPa). This results in the clinical signs and symptoms of hypoxaemia including cyanosis, difficulty or laboured breathing and use of the accessory muscles of respiration. Hence, immediate action is warranted when the saturation begins to drop to anything below 90%.

Q   **What do you understand by the terms ventilation and perfusion?**

A   Ventilation (V) is the amount of air (gas) received by the lungs and perfusion (Q) is the amount of blood that flows through the lungs which facilitates gaseous exchange. In normal physiological situations, the ventilation received by an area of lung would be sufficient to provide full exchange of oxygen and carbon dioxide with the blood perfusing that area. The distribution of ventilation across the lung, however, is not homogeneous. The bases receive more ventilation than the apices. This is because ventilation is related to the position of each area on the compliance curve at the start of a normal tidal inspiration (the point of the functional residual capacity). The bases are on a more favorable part of the compliance curve than the apices and hence they receive a greater degree of ventilation. Likewise, perfusion throughout the lung is largely related to the effects of gravity. Therefore, in the upright position the perfusion pressure at the base of the lung is equal to the mean pulmonary artery pressure (15 mmHg or 20 cm of H_2O) + the hydrostatic pressure between the main pulmonary artery and lung base (approximately 15 cm of H_2O). At the apices, however, the hydrostatic pressure difference is subtracted from the pulmonary artery pressure with the result that the perfusion pressure is very low and may at times even fall below the pressure in the alveoli leading to vessel compression and intermittent cessation of blood flow. Although the inequality between bases and apices is less marked for ventilation than for perfusion, in normal situations there is overall good V/Q matching and efficient oxygenation of the blood passing through the lungs.

Q   What is ventilation–perfusion mismatch?

A   A disturbance in either ventilation or perfusion or both could lead to V/Q mismatching. For an area of low V/Q ratio, the blood flowing through it will be incompletely oxygenated, leading to a reduction in the oxygen level in arterial blood causing hypoxaemia. This can normally be corrected by increasing the FiO_2 which restores the alveolar oxygen delivery to a level sufficient to oxygenate the blood fully, provided there is some ventilation in the area of low V/Q.

Case 3.33 Gastrointestinal system and surgical anatomy

Q   **A 69-year-old male smoker presents with dull epigastric pain radiating to the left upper quadrant. The patient gives a history of loss of appetite and recent loss of weight. On examination, he is icteric with mildly enlarged liver and a palpable gallbladder. What is the most likely diagnosis?**

A   The most likely diagnosis is carcinoma of the pancreas.

Q   **What are the signs and symptoms of pancreatic carcinoma?**

A   The most common physical findings are obstructive jaundice, hepatomegaly, loss of appetite, loss of weight and abdominal pain or tenderness. The pain, usually dull-aching or boring in nature, depends on the tumour site and extent: the pain associated with carcinoma of the body and tail of the pancreas is felt in the epigastric region or the back, sometimes radiating to the left upper quadrant, while pain arising from carcinomas of the head of the pancreas radiates to the right upper quadrant. The pain is steadily progressive with increased severity at night. It is aggravated with meals and by recumbency. A palpable gallbladder is found in 12–37% of cases, while thrombophlebitis occurs in less than 10%.

Q   **What investigations would you do to confirm your diagnosis?**

A
- ultrasonography can identify over 90% of pancreatic tumours

- a contrast enhanced triple phase helical CT scan of the pancreas usually defines the tumour and whether it is operable or not

- endoscopy identifies the presence or absence of duodenal involvement and confirms whether or not the tumour is ampullary in origin

- the exact site of obstruction can be determined by endoscopic retrograde or magnetic resonance cholangiopancreatography (ERCP or MRCP).

Q   What are the anatomical relations of the head of pancreas?

A   The head, the broadest part of the pancreas, is moulded to the C-shaped concavity of the duodenum, which it completely fills. It lies over the inferior vena cava and the right and left renal veins at the level of the L2 vertebra. Its posterior surface is deeply indented and sometimes tunnelled, by the terminal part of the bile duct. The lower part of the posterior surface is prolonged, wedge shaped to the left, behind the superior mesenteric vein and artery, in front of the aorta; this forms the uncinate process of the head.

Critical care

Case 3.34 Monitoring and the cardiovascular system

Q   What is meant by central venous pressure?

A   Central venous pressure (CVP) is considered to be a direct measurement of the blood pressure in the right atrium and the superior vena cava. CVP is used as a standard guide for assessing the ability of the right side of the heart to accept fluid load. It is measured by inserting a central venous catheter into the subclavian or jugular vein. The tip of the catheter is intended to rest in the lower third of the superior vena cava. The pressure monitoring assembly is attached to the distal port of a multi-lumen catheter. The normal CVP is 2–6 mmHg.

Q   Name a few conditions that increase or decrease the CVP.

A   Some of the conditions that elevate CVP include: (1) overhydration or increased fluid within the intravascular fluid compartment which increases the venous return; (2) over-resuscitation of hypovolaemia; (3) heart failure, pulmonary artery or tricuspid valve stenosis which limit venous inflow; (4) positive pressure ventilation and (5) excessive straining. Conditions which decrease the CVP include: (1) any cause for a decreased volume within the intravascular fluid compartment; (2) hypovolaemic shock; (3) dehydration, including diarrhoea and (4) negative pressure breathing or mechanical negative pressure ventilation.

Q   Name some indications for central line insertion and CVP measurement.

A   A central venous catheter is commonly inserted for two reasons: (1) to assess cardiac function and monitor treatment, particularly fluid administration and (2) when conventional intravenous access cannot be obtained. Some of the indications for CVP measurement include: (1) to monitor fluid replacement therapy during treatment of hypovolaemic shock; (2) to accurately measure the effect of vasoactive drugs, particularly vasodilators, on venous capacitance and (3) to aid diagnosis of right ventricular failure, when a high pressure will be seen in the presence of poor cardiac output.

Q   **What complications may result from central venous line insertion?**

A   Complications of central line insertion are numerous and relate to the damage to the veins themselves and adjacent structures. Complications include rupture of vessels and haemorrhage with haematoma or haemo-thorax, tension pneumothorax (particularly if the patient is on positive pressure ventilation), air embolism, extravascular catheter placement, catheter misplacement, neurapraxia, arterial puncture, lymphatic puncture and tracheo-bronchial tree puncture. Local infection and sepsis are also important but later complications.

Q   **How would you monitor changes in the CVP?**

A   Isolated CVP values are of limited use since there are variations in the condition and status of the heart in individual patients and the baseline CVP varies from patient to patient. Likewise, some patients such as young adults and athletes have a remarkable ability to compensate and CVP can be normal or even transiently elevated even in the presence of severe hypovolaemia. Hence, continuous monitoring of the CVP is essential not just to monitor the fluid resuscitation status (particularly in patients with hypovolaemic shock), but also to assess the functional ability of the heart. Likewise, patients with compromised cardiac function will not tolerate rapid bolus of fluid infusion and over-enthusiastic resuscitation would exacerbate cardiac failure; careful monitoring of the fluid status is hence essential.

Q   **What is the limitation of CVP monitoring?**

A   CVP monitoring takes into account only the pressure and function of the right side of the heart. There can be a marked disparity between the function of the left and the right ventricles; indeed one can fail inde-pendently of the other. Likewise, pulmonary vascular disease may render the CVP a very poor guide to filling pressures of the left heart. In such cases, it may be useful to measure the left ventricular end diastolic pres-sure (LVEDP) or more accurately the pulmonary capillary wedge pressure (PCWP) from which the left atrial pressure can be inferred.

Q   **What is pulmonary artery wedge pressure?**

A   The pressure in the pulmonary capillaries can be measured by wedging a catheter into a small pulmonary artery, from which the left atrial pressure can be inferred. The normal PCWP is 6–12 mmHg. It should ideally be kept below 15 mmHg to minimise the risk of pulmonary oedema. Values derived from endoscopic Doppler ultrosound (i.e. cardiac output, cardiac index) are now replacing PCWP measurements.

Q   **What are the indications for pulmonary artery catheterisation?**

A   The indications for pulmonary artery catheterisation include: (1) preopera-tive assessment in high-risk surgical patients, e.g. a recent myocardial event or severe respiratory disease; (2) assisting the fluid management of patients with massive haemorrhage, polytrauma, SIRS, sepsis or organ failure; (3) patients requiring infusion of vasoactive drugs to manipulate preload, after load or oxygen transport; (4) diagnosis of non-cardiogenic pulmonary oedema, as in ARDS; (5) management of patients with intra- or postoperative myocardial event and (6) management of cardiogenic shock.

Case 3.35 Acute respiratory distress syndrome

Q   **What is acute respiratory distress syndrome?**

A   Acute respiratory distress syndrome (ARDS) is an acute, diffuse inflammatory process resulting from direct or indirect pulmonary injury. It is also defined as non-cardiogenic pulmonary oedema with a normal pulmonary artery wedge pressure and characterised by stiff lungs, respiratory hypoxia and diffuse pulmonary infiltrates on chest radiograph.

Q   **What are the causes for ARDS?**

A   ARDS is most commonly seen in patients with sepsis but can also occur after trauma, burns, inhalation injuries, shock and pancreatitis. In postoperative surgical patients, abdominal sepsis or central line sepsis should be considered.

Q   **Briefly describe the pathophysiology of ARDS.**

A   Indirect or direct lung injury initiates an abnormal response and movement of neutrophils, platelets and macrophages. Neutrophils and platelets attach to capillary endothelium causing capillary leakage. This leads to oedema of lung tissue and movement of neutrophils and erythrocytes into the lung parenchyma. Lung lymph flow is increased with thickening of the alveolar-capillary membrane. This results in impaired oxygen diffusion and reduced lung compliance as the alveolus is surrounded by fluid. In addition, some of the fluid in the pulmonary parenchyma may leak into the alveoli, giving the characteristic appearance of a hyaline membrane.

Q   **What are the features associated with ARDS?**

A   ARDS is characterised by refractory hypoxaemia (PaO_2 <8 kPa at FiO_2 >0.4), alveolar inflammation and oedema, reduced total compliance (<30 ml/cm water) and a PaO_2 (in mmHg)/FiO_2 ratio of <200 (normal is approximately 500). Pulmonary fibrosis in the later stages of the disease leads to a decrease in the functional residual capacity, further decrease in lung compliance and an increase in the shunt effect. Pulmonary signs are often minimal or non-specific, the patient simply being breathless, progressively tachypnoeic, hypoxic and then cyanotic. Chest radiograph may be normal in the early stages but later shows bilateral diffuse pulmonary infiltration.

Q What are the principles of managing ARDS?

A Treatment, in addition to eliminating the precipitating aetiology, involves ventilating the patient in intensive care. Some general and systemic measures include: (1) providing respiratory support (mechanical ventilation, PEEP, permissive hypercapnoea, prevent barotrauma and inverse ratio ventilation to help alveolar recruitment); (2) avoidance of pulmonary oedema by restricting fluid and diuretics; (3) keeping the tidal volume low (approximately 6 ml/kg); (4) maintaining a low pulmonary capillary wedge pressure (high exacerbates pulmonary oedema); (5) nursing the patient in a prone position in severe ARDS to redirect blood flow to minimise shunting; (6) physiotherapy (although not useful in the early stages but effective in the later stages to remove secretions); (7) inhaled nitric oxide to improve ventilation–perfusion ratio with pulmonary vasodilation and (8) aerosolised surfactant and prostacyclin has also been used but the evidence is limited. Despite appropriate treatment, the mortality of this condition is as high as 50–70%.

Case 3.36 Endotracheal intubation and tracheostomy

Q What are the indications for endotracheal intubation?

A Some of the clinical situations or conditions where endotracheal intubation is indicated include:

- to maintain an airway when there is an impending upper airway obstruction, either mechanical or from an airway pathology

- to protect the airway in patients who are at risk of aspiration, such as in unconscious patients, patients with head injuries with a deteriorating Glasgow Coma Scale and patients with other central nervous system derangements

- where there is a need for assisted ventilation in patients with acute hypoxaemic or hypercapnic respiratory failure, or impending respiratory failure

- to aid hyperventilation by mechanical ventilation in patients with acute intracranial hypertension to reduce the intracranial pressure

- elective endotracheal intubation is performed to anaesthetise patients for many operative procedures and, at times, to facilitate certain diagnostic procedures, e.g. CT scanning.

Q What are the signs of potentially difficult airways?

A Signs of potentially difficult airway include:

- difficulties in positioning the neck as in arthritis, trauma, or previous surgery

- maxillo-facial injuries including Le Fort type fractures

- trauma to the larynx or trachea

- limitation in opening the oral cavity due to whatever reason, e.g. trauma

- stridor or upper airway inflammation as in epiglottitis, laryngeal infection or inhalation burns

- anatomical variations such as small mouth, large tongue, bull neck, receding lower jaw, high arched palate or marked obesity

- congenital malformation/deformities of face and head and neck.

Q   **What are the complications of endotracheal intubation?**

A   Some of the potential complications of endotracheal intubation include:
- oesophageal intubation
- perforation or laceration of upper oesophagus, vocal cords or larynx
- laryngospasm or bronchospasm
- dental and soft-tissue trauma
- aspiration of oral or gastric contents
- intubation of the right bronchus thus causing collapse of the left lung
- dysrhythmias
- hypertension or hypotension.

Q   **What are the indications for tracheostomy?**

A   Some of the indications for tracheostomy include:

- complete obstruction of the upper respiratory tract, e.g. foreign body, tumour

- injury to the head and neck including fractures

- bilateral paralysis of the vocal cords

- oedema of the upper respiratory tract caused by burns, infection or anaphylaxis

- long-term mechanical ventilation for respiratory failure

- to allow pulmonary toileting, e.g. insufficient cough reflex, inability to deal with secretions

- to prepare for large-scale procedures involving the head or neck

- severe sleep apnoea.

Q   **Describe how to perform an open tracheostomy.**

A   Open tracheostomy is performed by positioning the awake patient sitting or in semi-recumbent position and the unconscious patient supine with their shoulders raised slightly and the neck extended (avoid over-extension). The site is selected by marking the thyroid notch, sternal notch and cricoid cartilage. Local anaesthetic is infiltrated below the cricoid cartilage and a

3 cm vertical incision made. Any subcutaneous fat is excised using diathermy. The incision is deepened until the midline of the strap muscles is seen. Tie off or cauterise any blood vessels. Separate and retract laterally the strap muscles (it is essential to continue dissecting only in the midline to avoid damaging adjacent local structures). It might be necessary to divide the thyroid isthmus before it retracts so that it does not rub on the tracheostomy tube. Dry the field and dissect away the remaining peri-tracheal fascia. In previously intubated patients, prepare to swap the circuits and deflate the endotracheal cuff. Lift the cricoid away superiorly to help entry into the trachea. The main choices for entering the trachea are a T-shaped opening (2 cm long transverse incision between the tracheal rings to allow a vertical, midline incision through the lower 2 rings) in thin patients or a U- or H-shaped incision (tracheal flaps are turned back and sutured to the skin) in obese patients. A permanent tracheostomy may be fashioned by cutting a rectangular opening and removing a small part of the trachea.

Case 3.37 Management of head injuries

Q   A 33-year-old male motorcyclist is admitted to the Emergency Unit following a high speed RTA. How are you going to assess this patient?

A   The patient should be assessed according to the advanced trauma life support (ATLS) protocol. The airway should be assessed for patency, blood clots, loose teeth or foreign bodies. If the airway is obstructed, an oropharyngeal (Guedel) or a nasopharyngeal airway should be inserted (nasopharyngeal airway is contraindicated in patients suspected to have basal skull fractures since the nasopharyngeal tube may inadvertently enter the brain). The breathing should be assessed next by looking for chest movements, position of the trachea, percussion of the chest and auscultation to listen for bilateral air entry. The circulatory status should be assessed next by looking for capillary refill, feeling the pulse (tachycardia, thready pulse, etc.) and monitoring the blood pressure. The neurological status is assessed next using the AVPU scale (shorter version of Glasgow Coma Scale) and the papillary response.

Q   He is not responding to voice but withdrawing to pain. He is noted to have a periorbital haematoma and bruising over the mastoid process. On examination, a thin fluid mixed with blood is seen coming out of his nostrils. What do you think is going on?

A   It appears as if the patient has suffered a basal skull fracture. Bruising over the mastoid process (retro-auricular bruising – 'Battle's sign') and periorbital haematoma (Raccoon eyes) are classical signs of basal skull fractures. Middle fossa fractures present with rhinorrhoea/otorrhoea (blood mixed with CSF which does not clot), haemotympanum, ossicular disruption and sometimes cranial nerve palsies (usually VII and VIII cranial nerves).

Q   **What are the possible causes of this patient's decreased consciousness and what one investigation would you request to help you most?**

A   The patient could have an intracranial pathology such as a subdural or an extradural haematoma, concussion of the brain, or a diffuse axonal injury. Subarachnoid haemorrhage, although a possibility in young patients, is unlikely in such type of presentations. The most appropriate investigation in this patient is CT scanning.

Q   **What is the difference between a subdural and an extradural haematoma and how do the patients present?**

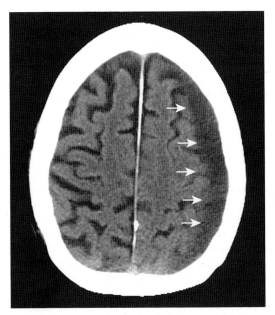

Fig. 3.37.1 Crescenteric collection indicating a subdural haematoma.

A   Acute extradural haematoma should be suspected in a patient with a fluctuating level of consciousness (though not always); the patient may soon recover after a brief loss of consciousness (lucid interval). Acute extradural haematomas are usually associated with trauma and are seen in the young. They are commonly due to a fracture of the temporal or parietal bones causing injury to the middle meningeal artery or vein. Subdural haematomas (Fig. 3.37.1), on the other hand, although seen after trauma, can also occur spontaneously in elderly patients with cerebral atrophy, alcoholics, epileptics and patients on anticoagulants. It is bilateral in about 20% of patients. In chronic subdural haematomas, patients may not become symptomatic for many days or even weeks after head injury (trivial in many cases). They may then present with headache, a fluctuating level of consciousness (not usually seen in acute subdural haematomas), failing intellect and hemiparesis.

Q   **What signs would suggest that this patient is deteriorating?**

A   If bleeding continues and if the developing haematoma is not evacuated, lateralising signs soon develop including an ipsilateral dilated pupil and contralateral hemiparesis. This eventually leads to bilateral fixed pupils and later coma which culminates in respiratory arrest.

Case 3.38 Management of neurological trauma

Q   **A 25-year-old male motorcyclist who was involved in a high-speed RTA is brought to the Emergency Unit by the paramedics. He is fully conscious but says that he is unable to move the fingers of his left hand. What might be the aetiology?**

A   Spinal cord injury is a strong possibility given the mechanism of injury. However, local injury to a nerve or bone could also result in this type of clinical picture.

Q   **Describe the different types of spinal cord injury.**

A   Spinal cord injury could be broadly divided into primary neurological injury and secondary neurological injury. Primary neurological injury is a direct consequence of the initial injury, for example, due to trauma, vertebral fractures or ligamentous damage. There is impingement of the spinal cord by the bone or soft tissue (mainly ligaments). Blunt trauma is more common than penetrating trauma in causing primary neurological injury. Secondary neurological injury is subsequent to or as a consequence of primary neurological injury, particularly if there is a delay (or inappropriate) management. This is due to hypoxia, reduced spinal perfusion, poor immobilisation of the cord, oedema around the damaged cord, haemorrhage into or around the cord, electrolyte abnormalities such as hyper- or hypoglycaemia and hypercalcaemia.

Q   **What clinical features may lead you to suspect spinal cord injury in a trauma patient?**

A   The possibility of a spinal cord injury should be suspected if the patient was involved in a high-speed RTA, fall from a height and major trauma of any cause. Clinically, a spinal cord injury should be suspected in a patient with multiple injuries including multiple long bone fractures, head injury, abnormal breathing pattern (diaphragmatic breathing), abnormal reflexes such as abdominal, anal and bulbocavernous reflexes and priapism.

Q   At what level of spinal cord injury do you expect respiratory difficulties?

A   A spinal injury occurring at or above C5 will result in paralysis of the diaphragm (the phrenic nerve which supplies the diaphragm arises from C3–C5). Any injury at the level of the thoracic vertebrae (up to T12) will affect the intercostal muscles and interfere with breathing. Also, patients with a spinal cord injury may also have associated chest injuries, e.g. rib fractures, which further worsen respiratory efforts.

Q   Define spinal shock.

A   Spinal shock is a clinical state seen in patients with spinal cord injuries. It may occur immediately after the injury and may last for approximately 4–6 weeks, although in some patients it can last indefinitely. This state is characterised by flaccid paralysis, priapism, autonomic dysfunction, gastric dilatation and diaphragmatic breathing (in high cervical cord lesions). With time, this state resolves, as some areas of the spinal cord may recover. Permanently damaged areas may, however, become spastic.

Case 3.39 Compartment syndrome

Q   What is meant by compartment syndrome?

A   Compartment syndrome is an increase in the interstitial fluid pressure within an osseofascial compartment of sufficient magnitude to cause a microcirculatory compromise leading to myoneural necrosis.

Q   What are the causes for compartment syndrome?

A   A compartment syndrome is a devastating early complication usually seen after fractures, particularly of the long bones and crush injury. Up to 45% of all cases of compartment syndrome are caused by tibial fractures, more common in open tibial fractures compared with closed tibial fractures, probably reflecting the severity of the injury. The other causes include deep thermal burns, electrical injuries, restricting tourniquets, gunshot injuries, fluid extravasation (e.g. intravenous regional anaesthesia) and snake envenomation.

Q   What signs and symptoms would make you suspect compartment syndrome in a patient?

A   Severe pain in response to passive stretch of the ischaemic muscles is by far the most dramatic and reliable clinical sign. Early in its development, the peripheral pulses are normal as are digit colour, temperature and capillary refill since it is the microvasculature which is initially affected. Loss of peripheral pulses is usually a late and sinister sign, suggesting imminent tissue ischaemia. Thin cutaneous nerve fibres are more susceptible to ischaemia than the motor fibres and distal paraesthesia occurs before motor loss. The limb becomes tense and swollen and if not treated, the muscle weakness progresses to paralysis; irreversible muscle damage occurs within about 8 hours of developing compartment syndrome.

Q   **What biochemical abnormalities would you expect to see in a patient with compartment syndrome?**

A   Areas of muscle may infarct giving rise to rhabdomyolysis, hyperkalaemia, hyperphosphataemia, high uric acid levels and metabolic acidosis. Serum creatinine kinase levels may be elevated. If the compartment syndrome is untreated, worsening muscle necrosis and the release of toxic metabolites could lead to acute renal failure.

Q   **What investigation would you do to make the diagnosis and how do you manage this condition?**

A   Classically compartment pressures are measured using a slit catheter device. The normal resting pressure within the compartment tissues is approximately 3–4 mmHg. Compartment pressures in excess of 30–35 mmHg in a normally perfused patient suggested the need for open compartment fasciotomy. Recent evidence, however, suggests that fasciotomy should be undertaken if the difference between the diastolic pressure and the measured compartment pressure is less than 30 mmHg. However if clinical suspicion persists (increasing pain on passive movement of the affected group of muscles), even if the pressures are normal, fasciotomies of the affected compartments should be performed.

Q   **Which nerve is most likely to be affected in fractures of the forearm bones and why?**

A   In compartment syndromes affecting the anterior forearm, the commonest neurological damage is to the median nerve. This is because it is located in the centre of the muscle mass to be infarcted, whereas the ulnar nerve lies along the periphery of the compartment and is therefore subject to less ischaemia and damage.

Operative surgery

Case 3.40 Excision of toenails

Q   **Describe the pathology of onychocryptosis (in-growing toenails).**

A   Persistent contact between the edge of the nail plate and the skin of the nail fold results in, pressure necrosis, ulceration and subsequent suppuration of the skin secondary infection by *Staphylococcus aureus*.

Q What treatment options are available?

A Treatment is either conservative or surgical. Conservative measures include trimming of the nail-plate transversely in a straight line as opposed to a curve, daily bathing and drying and advice on footwear. Surgery is indicated when symptoms persist despite conservative measures. Simple nail plate avulsion is performed to relieve pus. Complete excision of the nail bed (Zadek's procedure) ± phenolisation removes the germinal matrix therefore preventing regrowth of the nail and recurrence.

Q Describe how you would perform a Zadek's procedure.

A The procedure is performed under local ring block using plain local anaesthetic (NB no adrenaline – as this could result in irreversible digital ischaemia) or general anaesthetic.

The foot is prepared with antiseptic and draped. If local anaesthetic is used, a rubber 'band' tourniquet is placed around the proximal phalanx. A tourniquet may also be applied when a general anaesthetic is used as it results in an avascular field. Plain lidocaine or xylocaine is then infiltrated on the medial and lateral aspects of the toe at the level of the distal inter-phalangeal joint to block the neural bundles. Dissecting scissors are inserted under the nail plate and opened, which causes the nail plate to lift. The nail plate can then be avulsed by attaching a heavy clip and rotating medially or laterally. Small vertical incisions are then made on the medial and lateral skin covering the matrix of the nail. This results in a flap when elevated exposing the germinal matrix. The germinal matrix is then excised as a block ensuring adequate medial and lateral dissection. The skin incisions are then loosely approximated with non-absorbable sutures.

Q Describe the frequent complications which result from this procedure.

A
- Wound infection can result following the procedure and usually settles with antiseptic dressings

- Recurrence is uncommon if an adequate dissection of the germinal matrix is performed. Recurrence can present as a nail spike, these are treated by a repeat excision or by the application of phenol.

Case 3.41 Abdominal incisions and closure

Q Describe the principles required to make a good abdominal incision.

A The incision should be long enough for good exposure for the procedure to be performed safely and efficiently, but short enough to avoid unnecessary complications. The incision should be easy to extend and allow secure closure. Skin should be incised in Langer's lines, while muscle should be split in the direction of its fibres whenever possible.

Q   **Describe the anatomical structures encountered when performing a midline abdominal incision.**

A   The midline incision passes through skin, subcutaneous tissues, the linea alba, transversalis fascia, extraperitoneal fat and peritoneum.

Q   **How would you perform a midline incision?**

A   A midline incision is used when wide exposure to all four quadrants is required. The skin incision is made in the midline and curved around the umbilicus. The skin incision is deepened until the linea alba is exposed. Bleeding points are picked up with toothed forceps and cauterised. The linea alba and transversalis fascia are incised to expose the peritoneum. The peritoneum is picked up and incised slightly to the left to avoid the ligamentum teres. Two fingers are inserted to allow safe division of the peritoneum upwards and downwards.

Q   **Why should the midline incision pass around the umbilicus?**

A   To avoid the ligamentum teres and the unclean umbilicus.

Q   **How do you close a midline incision?**

A   Using a mass closure technique all layers of the wound excluding skin are closed with a non-absorbable suture. The suture material should be at least four times the length of the wound with bites being taken at least 1 cm apart and 1 cm deep (Jenkins' rule). The skin is closed with skin clips or subcuticular sutures (absorbable or non-absorbable).

Q   **What are the potential complications of a midline abdominal incision?**

A
- wound haematoma: results from poor haemostasis and can result in an abscess or wound infection

- wound infection (superficial surgical site infection, SSSI): rates vary with the type of procedure performed (5% for clean-contaminated surgery, e.g. elective gastrectomy, up to 25% after contaminated cases despite adequate antibiotic prophylaxis, e.g. colonic resection)

- superficial/full thickness dehiscence: a superficial dehiscence involves the separation of the skin and subcutaneous layers only and usually presents when the skin sutures are removed and is probably related to an SSSI. A full thickness dehiscence involves a complete disruption in whole or part of its length. A full thickness dehiscence usually occurs before the tenth postoperative day and is usually heralded by blood stained serous fluid (the 'pink' sign) and presents with the protrusion of a loop of bowel or omentum. It relates to poor surgical technique and not infection. It carries a 30% mortality rate and following repair 30% of patients develop an incisional hernia

- incisional hernia formation: results from the gradual separation of all layers of the abdominal wall with the exception of the skin and probably represents an unrecognised dehiscence

- stitch sinuses: can be avoided by using a synthetic monofilament absorbable material.

Case 3.42 Inguinal hernia

Q **Describe the layers encountered when performing an inguinal hernia repair.**

A
- skin and subcutaneous fat

- superficial (Camper's and Scarpa's) fascia

- superficial layer of fascia of the external oblique muscle

- the anterior wall consisting of the external oblique aponeurosis including the external ring medially and the arching fibres of the internal oblique muscle laterally

- the spermatic cord in the male or the round ligament of the uterus running in the inguinal canal, with the floor formed by the inguinal (Poupart's) ligament laterally and the lacunar (Gimbernat's) ligament medially and the roof formed by the lower edge of internal oblique and transversus abdominus muscle

- the posterior wall is usually formed laterally by the transversus abdominus aponeurosis and transversalis fascia with the remainder being transversalis fascia which is reinforced by internal oblique muscle medially; the deep inguinal ring is a normal defect in the transversalis fascia.

Q **What types of herniation can occur within the inguinal canal?**

A
- indirect inguinal hernia in which the hernial sac leaves the abdomen through the internal ring and passes down the inguinal canal antero-laterally to the spermatic cord or round ligament

- sliding indirect inguinal hernia in which some or the entire posterior wall of the sac is composed of herniated viscus. (NB no complete peritoneal sac)

- direct inguinal hernia in which the medial hernia sac, covered by transversalis fascia, passes through Hesselbach's triangle, an area bordered by the inferior epigastric artery, the inguinal ligament and the lateral border of the rectus abdominus muscle.

Q **How would you perform the repair of a non-recurrent unilateral inguinal hernia in a 28-year-old man?**

A Using a tension-free prosthetic mesh repair as described by Lichtenstein with prophylactic antibiotic cover.

The procedure is preferably performed under general anaesthetic but may also be performed under regional or local anaesthetic with the patient in the supine position. A skin crease transverse incision 2–3 cm above the inguinal ligament is made. The superficial epigastric, circumflex and external pudendal veins are identified and ligated as the incision is deepened. The external oblique aponeurosis overlying the spermatic cord is divided in the line of its fibres and retracted by applying artery clips to the edges. The spermatic cord is elevated with a hernia ring following identification, elevation and retraction of the ilioinguinal nerve. The indirect sac (if present) is identified on the spermatic cord by splitting the investing layers in the line of the cord. The sac is elevated to the level of the internal ring, opened and any viscus or omentum reduced. The sac is then twisted and transfixed at the level of the internal ring and the sac distal to the ligature excised. The posterior wall is palpated to identify any direct herniation. A polypropylene mesh is cut into a 'fish-like' shape with a defect near the tail to accommodate the spermatic cord. The mesh is placed under the cord with the 'head of the fish' being sutured with non-absorbable material to the fascia overlying the pubic tubercle and the body to the internal oblique aponeurosis, conjoint tendon superiorly and the inguinal ligament inferiorly. The 'tails' are then crossed over the cord and sutured laterally. The external oblique aponeurosis, fascia and skin are closed in layers with absorbable sutures.

Q **What are the potential complications of this surgery?**

A
- acute urinary retention
- haematoma formation
- seroma formation
- superficial wound infection (SSI)
- abscess formation
- mesh infection
- hydrocele (when the distal sac is left in place)
- nerve injuries, e.g. ilioinguinal, genitofemoral
- damage to the vas deferens
- ischaemic orchitis and testicular atrophy
- recurrence rates have been reported to be as low as 0.77%
- injury to viscus (bladder/bowel) with sliding hernias.

Case 3.43 Femoral hernia

Q **What are the boundaries of the femoral canal?**

A
- anterior: inguinal ligament

- lateral: femoral vein which is covered in a thin septum

- medial: aponeurotic insertion of the transversus abdominus muscle and transversalis fascia

- posterior: pectineal (Cooper's) ligament, the pubic bone and the fascia over the pectineus muscle.

Q **Describe the aetiology of a femoral hernia.**

A Femoral hernias are acquired. Normally the iliopsoas and pectineus muscles bulge into the femoral canal, thus acting as a barrier to the development of femoral hernia. Muscle atrophy in old age allows raised intra-abdominal pressure to push the peritoneum and extra-peritoneal fat into a weakened canal and the space beyond. Femoral hernias are also more common after an inguinal hernia repair on the ipsilateral side.

Q **How would you repair a femoral hernia in a 75-year-old woman, where the hernia is tense, tender red and irreducible?**

A Several approaches are possible including the low approach (Lockwood), inguinal approach (Lotheissen) or the high approach (McEvedy or Henry). The high approach is performed in the emergency situation by making a transverse unilateral Pfannenstiel type incision, which can be extended in order to perform a laparotomy if necessary. The incision is deepened to the rectus sheath which is also incised. The rectus muscle is retracted medially; if necessary, the muscle layer laterally may be incised for a short distance. The now exposed transversalis fascia is incised transversely exposing the preperitoneal space. The hernia sac is identified and released by first manipulating from above or below and then if necessary by incising the medial margin of the femoral ring. The sac is opened and the contents inspected.

The bowel is assessed for viability, if doubt remains, the bowel is wrapped in warm saline soaked swabs and left for 5 minutes. If the bowel is considered to be non-viable a resection is performed, otherwise the sac is ligated and excised. The femoral ring defect is repaired by suturing the iliopubic tract to the posterior margin of the pectineal ligament using a non-absorbable suture. A prosthetic mesh plug may be inserted into the defect but is at risk of becoming infected if inserted in the emergency situation. The wound is closed in layers using a non-absorbable suture for the rectus sheath and an absorbable suture for the other layers.

Q **What are the potential complications of this surgery?**

A
- acute urinary retention
- haematoma formation
- seroma formation
- superficial wound infection
- abscess formation
- mesh infection
- damage to the accessory obturator artery
- bladder perforation
- stenosis of the femoral vein
- recurrence.

Case 3.44 Para-umbilical hernia

Q   **Describe the anatomy of a para-umbilical hernia.**

A   The round ligament, the remnants of the urachus and umbilical arteries insert into the umbilical cicatrix usually on the superior rim thus creating a weak area in the abdominal fascia. The lowest tendinous insertion of the rectus abdominus muscle inserts into the linea alba at the level of the superior umbilical rim resulting in a further weakness. Herniation results from the disruption of the linea alba and usually occurs above the cicatrix.

Q   **What factors predispose to the formation of a para-umbilical hernia?**

A   Para-umbilical hernias are acquired and can occur at any age. Factors predisposing to herniation include:
- obesity
- multiple pregnancies
- raised intra-abdominal pressure, e.g. ascites.

Q   **How do para-umbilical hernias differ from umbilical hernias in the adult?**

A   Acute abdominal distension (e.g. ascites, continuous ambulatory peritoneal dialysis) may result in the umbilical cicatrix giving way resulting in an umbilical hernia. Management of umbilical hernias should be conservative as most of these patients have serious underlying pathology. However, surgical repair is indicated if the hernia becomes incarcerated.

Q   **How do para-umbilical hernias tend to present?**

A   Para-umbilical hernias tend to increase in size over time. Intermittent abdominal pain is a frequent symptom, which results from omentum becoming trapped by a narrow neck. Bowel may become trapped and result in obstruction. Para-umbilical hernias do not resolve spontaneously and have a high incidence of incarceration and strangulation, therefore surgical repair is always indicated.

Q   **Describe how you would perform a para-umbilical hernia repair.**

A   A curved incision above or below the umbilicus (depending on the site of the hernia) is made from the '9 to the 3 o'clock position' (if the skin is degenerate the umbilicus should be excised by means of an elliptical incision). The sac is separated from the fat by sharp dissection down to the rectus sheath and freed by clearing the rectus sheath around the hernial defect. The sac is opened and the contents inspected. The contents if viable are reduced back into the peritoneal cavity. The sac is transfixed and excised. The rectus is repaired either transversely or longitudinally depending on the defect, with interrupted non-absorbable sutures or a mesh. If there is a large dead space a suction drain should be placed. The skin is closed with subcuticular absorbable sutures.

Q   **What complications can occur with this surgery?**

A
- seroma
- haematoma
- wound infection
- respiratory infections as these patients tend to be obese.

Case 3.45 Surgical management of peptic ulcer disease

Q   **Describe the different acute presentations of peptic ulcer disease.**

A   Peptic ulcer disease may present with pain, perforation or bleeding. Classically gastric peptic ulceration presents with epigastric pain which comes on with eating, relieved by vomiting and associated weight loss; whereas duodenal peptic ulceration presents with hunger pain relieved by eating. Rarely patients give such a clear description, while the pain may be mild through to severe. Erosions of the stomach or duodenum may deepen resulting in a perforation. The classic presentation of a perforation (most commonly a duodenal ulcer) is of sudden onset, severe upper abdominal pain and guarding after previous dyspepsia. In the elderly, perforations may be asymptomatic (silent). Peptic ulceration accounts for 35% of cases of upper gastrointestinal bleeding. Peptic ulcers bleed because of erosion of blood vessels within the ulcer, the most common being a posterior erosion into the gastroduodenal artery. The severity of bleeding is related to the size of the vessel affected. Bleeding may present with haematemesis (commoner in gastric ulceration); and melaena or rectal bleeding ± hypovolaemic shock (commoner in duodenal ulceration).

Q   **Name two common aetiological factors associated with perforated peptic ulceration.**

A   Chronic use of non-steroidal anti-inflammatory drugs (NSAIDs) and *Helicobacter pylori* infection.

Q   **Describe the surgical management of perforated peptic ulcer disease.**

A   Initial management includes fluid resuscitation, passage of a nasogastric tube, analgesia and administration of broad-spectrum antibiotics. A small-perforated duodenal ulcer may be closed with simple interrupted sutures and reinforced with an omental patch laid on top. However, a larger ulcer requires an omental patch laid into the defect and then sutured in place with interrupted sutures. Sutures tied too tight result in the omental patch becoming infarcted. A perforated gastric ulcer on the greater or lesser curves is excised with a sleeve of mesenetry and sent for histology to exclude malignancy. The fresh edges are brought together with interrupted sutures with an omental patch sutured on top. Large perforated ulcers of the stomach or duodenum or those of the pylorus are unsuitable for a simple repair and require a partial gastrectomy. A Billroth II (Polya) partial gastrectomy involves resecting the distal two-thirds of the stomach, closing the duodenum distal to the duodenum (distal to the ulcer) and an end-to-side gastrojejunal anastomosis. A full peritoneal lavage with copious amounts of saline should be performed following any procedure for a perforated peptic ulcer. Postoperatively the patient should be commenced on a proton pump inhibitor and undergo *Helicobacter pylori* eradication if necessary

Q   **What are the indications for surgery in bleeding peptic ulcers?**

A   Surgical intervention is required if (1) there is massive bleeding (i.e. 6 unit blood loss in a patient >60 years or 8 units in a patient <60 years); (2) active bleeding not controlled endoscopically or (3) if bleeding recurs following endoscopic haemostasis.

Q   **Describe the surgical management of a bleeding duodenal ulcer.**

A   The majority of bleeding duodenal ulcers requiring surgical intervention are located on the posterior wall of the first part of the duodenum and involve the gastroduodenal artery. The ulcer is approached via a longitudinal duodenotomy that may be extended into the pylorus to gain better access. A finger is placed on the bleeding point if haemorrhage is excessive. If access is still difficult, the duodenum is mobilised laterally (Kocher's manoeuvre). Blood and clot is then suctioned to obtain a better view. The vessel in the base of the ulcer is identified and is under-run above and below with a small round-bodied needle (to avoid injury to underlying common bile duct) with a No. 1 suture material (absorbable and of a moderate strength duration, e.g. Vicryl). The duodenotomy is closed transversely with interrupted sutures ± omental patch. Postoperatively, the patient should be commenced on a proton pump inhibitor and undergo *Helicobacter pylori* eradication if necessary.

Case 3.46 Cholecystectomy

Q   **Describe the port placement at laparoscopic cholecystectomy.**

A   Four ports are required, two 10 mm and two 5 mm. The first 10 mm port is placed by making a small subumbilical incision either transversely or longitudinally. The linea alba is identified and is drawn up into the wound by the placement of a clip. The rectus sheath is incised and a stay-suture on a J-needle is passed through each edge and a finger passed through the defect into the peritoneal cavity. A 10 mm Hassan cannula is then passed through the defect into the peritoneal cavity and is held in place with the stay suture. The trocar is removed from the Hassan cannula, a pneumoperitoneum created and a 10 mm laparoscope passed.

The three further ports are then placed under direct vision. The second 10 mm port is placed one-third of the way from the xiphisternum to the umbilicus in the midline. The two 5 mm ports are usually placed in the right flank in the anterior and mid-axillary lines.

Q **Briefly describe the operative technique of laparoscopic cholecystectomy.**

A Following passage of the ports, the patient is placed in a head up position and is rotated towards the surgeon standing on the left of the patient. To enable dissection of Calot's triangle (formed by the base of the liver above, the common hepatic duct to the left and the cystic duct below), a grasper is placed through the extreme right port and attached to the fundus of the gallbladder, which in turn is passed towards the patient's right shoulder over the right lobe of the liver. A second grasping forceps is passed through the right medial port and is attached to the neck of the gallbladder and retracted laterally to expose Calot's triangle. Dissection of Calot's triangle is performed with a Petelin curved forceps passed through the epigastric 10 mm port. The cystic duct and cystic artery are identified and a window opened between the gallbladder and the liver. If there is any doubt over the anatomy an on-table cholangiogram should be performed through the cystic duct. When the surgeon is certain of the anatomy; the cystic duct and artery are triply clipped (with two clips on the proximal end) and divided. The fundus of the gallbladder is then dissected from the liver, placed in a retrieval bag and removed via one of the 10 mm ports. The peritoneal cavity is washed if any bile or stones are spilt. A small suction drain may be placed in the gallbladder fossa via a 5 mm port site.

Q **What are the complications of laparoscopic cholecystectomy?**

A
- wound infection rate <2%
- bleeding and haematoma formation
- bile duct injury 0.2–0.4%
- bile leak (usually due to the unrecognised division of an accessory bile duct or dislodgement of the cystic duct clips) resulting in a bile collection.

Q **Describe the conversion from laparoscopic to open cholecystectomy.**

A Approximately 5% of elective cholecystectomies require conversion to open procedure, rising to up to 50% in the emergency situation. Four incisions may be employed: midline, paramedian, right transverse or right subcostal. A right subcostal is usually used as the right lateral and medial ports and proximal 10 mm port incisions may be incorporated into the incision. The liver is then retracted superiorly while the colon and duodenum are retracted inferiorly by the assistant's left hand using a wet pack. A retracting forceps is placed on the neck of the gallbladder to facilitate dissection of Calot's triangle. The cystic duct and artery are only ligated and divided when the surgeon is confident that they have been positively identified. An on-table cholangiogram should be performed if there is any doubt over the anatomy or if stones are thought to be in the common bile duct. The gallbladder is then dissected from the liver from the fundus first or from the cystic duct end first.

Case 3.47 Pancreatectomy

Q   **What preoperative investigations are necessary to assess resectability of a head of pancreas tumour?**

A
- plain chest radiograph to exclude lung metastases

- abdominal ultrasound scan to identify the tumour and assess for liver metastases

- CT abdomen to assess for local invasion and lymphadenopathy as well as to assess the liver

- endoscopic ultrasound to more accurately assess local invasion

- ERCP ± stent placement may be necessary to relieve obstruction and to obtain brushings for cytology

- staging laparoscopy.

Q   **What curative procedure is required for a head of the pancreas tumour?**

A   Pancreaticoduodenectomy is performed as embryologically, anatomically and surgically the head of the pancreas, the common bile duct and the duodenum are an inseparable unit. Their shared blood supply necessitates removal of the duodenum if the head of the pancreas is removed. A modern alternative to the original pancreaticoduodenectomy as described by Whipple is to preserve the pylorus to improve gastric emptying postoperatively (pylorus preserving pancreaticoduodenectomy).

Q   **Describe a pancreaticoduodenectomy as performed for cancer.**

A   Pylorus preserving pancreaticoduodenectomy is performed for pancreatic cancers localised to the head, neck or uncinate process. Access is obtained with two joining subcostal incisions (rooftop) or combined upper midline and transverse incisions. Attention is paid to the presence of ascites, peritoneal seedlings and liver metastases. A full laparotomy is performed to assess resectability. The duodenum is mobilised medially (Kocher's manoeuvre) to assess the head of the pancreas posteriorly. The neck is also mobilised to identify the superior mesenteric vein along the inferior border of the neck of the pancreas as it joins the portal vein. If the portal vein is clearly involved, the tumour is unresectable and a bypass procedure is employed. Resection starts with division of the first part of the duodenum between non-crushing clamps or a GIA stapler. The gastro-epiploic artery and the gastroduodenal artery are ligated and divided. The gallbladder and bile duct are then mobilised and the common hepatic duct divided close to origin of the cystic duct. The superior mesenteric vein is dissected free and the pancreatic neck divided. The duodenojejunal flexure is mobilised and the jejunum is divided with a GIA stapler 15 cm distal to the ligament of Treitz. The upper jejunum is advanced through the mesocolon and the entire specimen is removed and sent for histology. Three anastomoses are then formed: two-layered, end-to-end pancreatico-duodenal, single layer, end-to-side choledochojejunostomy (common hepatic to jejunum) and a two-layered end-to-side duodenojejunostomy. All anastomoses are performed with absorbable sutures.

Q **What common complications may occur following pancreatico-duodenectomy?**

A
- delayed gastric emptying
- pancreatic fistula
- bleeding
- abscess formation following anastomotic leak
- pancreatic exocrine insufficiency
- diabetes (rare)
- general complications (e.g. surgical site infection, cardiovascular events, pneumonia).

Q **What curative procedure should be performed for a tail of pancreas cancer?**

A Tail of pancreas tumours usually present late and are rarely amenable to curative resection. The procedure of choice is distal pancreatectomy ± splenectomy in which the pancreas is divided as it crosses the portal vein. A large drain is placed in the pancreatic bed.

Case 3.48 Splenectomy

Q **Describe the anatomical relations of the spleen.**

A The spleen is situated in the left hypochondrium between the gastric fundus and left hemidiaphragm. It is usually a domed shaped tetra-hedron with its shape dictated by the impressions of the stomach, left kidney, pancreas and colonic splenic flexure. In the adult it is approximately 12 cm long, 7 cm broad and 4 cm wide. The spleen lies between the 9th and 11th rib with the long axis lying along the 10th rib and is therefore vulnerable to injury when the lower ribs are fractured. The lower pole does not extend beyond the mid-axillary line. Enlargement of the spleen occurs along the 10th rib, with the spleen only becoming palpable when at least three times its normal size.

Q What investigations are required if a ruptured spleen is suspected?

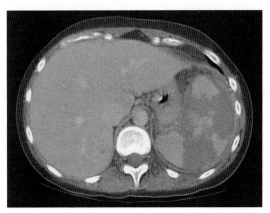

Fig. 3.48.1 Splenic haematoma with free intraperitoneal blood.

A Injury to the spleen may result from trauma or due to an iatrogenic cause during another abdominal operation, e.g. gastrectomy or splenic flexure mobilisation. Presentation within 48 hours of the initial injury is described as 'early' or as 'delayed' if the clinical signs develop more than 48 hours after the injury. Splenic injuries most frequently result from blunt trauma to the upper abdomen. Suspicion is raised if fractures of the left lower ribs are present on the chest radiograph. Spontaneous rupture may also result due to trivial injury in a diseased spleen (e.g. infectious mononucleosis). Patients present with varying degrees of hypovolaemia depending on the degree of rupture. If the patient is stable, a CT (Fig. 3.48.1) or ultrasound scan should be performed by an experienced radiologist. If the patient is unstable, an urgent laparotomy should be performed. Previously, diagnostic peritoneal lavage (DPL) was performed in the stable patient. However, this procedure makes interpretation of CT or ultrasound scan difficult and is very unreliable.

Q Describe the operative management of a ruptured spleen.

A A laparotomy is performed through a midline incision to identify the source of bleeding. The assistant retracts the left side of the abdominal wall and the left hand of the operator is passed over the spleen, which is then drawn forward and the peritoneum lateral to and above the spleen are divided. This in turn allows the spleen to be drawn forward towards the surgeon. The splenic artery and vein are identified as they enter the splenic hilum. These are clamped and divided as they pass from the tail of the pancreas into the hilum. The short gastric arteries and vein are identified individually and divided. Any remaining peritoneal attachments are divided in order to remove the spleen. Haemostasis is confirmed by pouring warm saline into the splenic bed and observing for signs of bleeding.

Q   **When may splenic preservation be an option?**

A   A decision to observe patients with splenic trauma may be taken if the patient is haemodynamically stable, has no signs of splenic capsule disruption or free intraperitoneal blood on the CT scan and has no other major intra-abdominal injuries. These patients must be observed closely in hospital for at least 1 week and require a laparotomy if they develop signs of hypovolaemia. An early laparotomy is required if there are signs of hypovolaemia ± signs of free intraperitoneal blood on CT. Preservation of some or all of the spleen is commonly practised in children due to the risk of overwhelming post-splenectomy sepsis (OPSI). Preservation at operation is performed using fibrillary collagen glues, suturing, omental patches or absorbable mesh bags. These patients must be observed closely in the postoperative period and require a further laparotomy if they develop signs of bleeding.

Q   **What therapies are required postoperatively?**

A   All patients who have undergone splenectomy, but in particular children and young adults, are at risk of OPSI due to *pneumococci* and other encapsulated organisms. In particular, patients under going emergency splenectomy require prophylactic antibiotics to be administered at in-duction. Postoperatively, they require broad-spectrum antibiotics until vaccinated with *Haemophilus influenzae* type B, influenza, *meningococcal* group C, *pneumococcal* vaccines and established on prophylactic phenoxymethylpenicillin.

Case 3.49 Appendicectomy

Q   **What is the aetiology of acute appendicitis?**

A   Bacterial infection of the appendix results from blockage of the lumen by faecoliths or from enlargement of lymphoid aggregates within the wall of the appendix. Inflammation advances through the wall to involve the omentum and adjacent organs. Occlusion of the appendicular artery results in tissue necrosis, gangrene and eventually perforation. Perforation results in a localised abscess or generalised peritonitis.

Q   **What are the clinical features of acute appendicitis?**

A   The presentation of acute appendicitis varies. The most discriminating clinical variables are: the patient complains of central colicky abdominal pain for less than 24 hours, which shifts to the right iliac fossa; on examination, there is a low-grade pyrexia with guarding in the right iliac fossa. Signs and symptoms of appendicitis are influenced by the position of the appendix in relation to the caecum.

Q   What are the differential diagnoses for acute appendicitis?

A   Gynaecological conditions in young women (of childbearing age) are commonly mistaken for appendicitis. Acute appendicitis is slightly more common in young men (peak incidence 30 years of age); however, more appendicectomies are performed in young women due to gynaecological conditions mimicking acute appendicitis. Gynaecological causes include: salpingitis, Mittelschmerz, ovarian cyst torsion, ruptured ectopic pregnancy (a pregnancy test must be performed in all women of child-bearing age presenting with right iliac fossa pain). Other causes include mesenteric lymphadenitis, gastroenteritis, perforated peptic ulcer and urinary tract infection.

Q   Describe the operation of conventional open appendicectomy.

A   A skin crease incision is made over the point of maximal tenderness, which usually lies on a line one-third of the way between the anterior superior iliac spine and the umbilicus (McBurney's point). The incision is deepened through the subcutaneous fat and fascia to expose the external oblique aponeurosis. The external oblique aponeurosis, the internal oblique muscle and transversalis fascia are split in the lines of their respective fibres. The peritoneum is picked up and divided between clips in the line of the skin incision. A bacteriology swab is taken for microscopy, culture and sensitivity. The caecum is delivered into the wound in order to locate the base of the appendix. If it is not possible to deliver the caecum, the incision is extended to facilitate better access to the appendix (the appendix should never be flicked into the wound as it may come away from the caecum). The mesoappendix is divided between clips and ligated. The base of the appendix is identified, ligated near the base with a 0 or 1 absorbable suture and divided between clips to prevent spillage. If the appendix is obviously inflamed, local peritoneal lavage is performed (if pus is present) and the wound closed at this point. A normal appearing appendix is removed in a similar fashion with a search for the cause performed thereafter. The distal small bowel is delivered into the wound to identify a possibly inflamed Meckel's diverticulum. The presence of bile, blood or bowel contents necessitates a formal laparotomy. The wound is closed in layers with absorbable sutures. Prophylactic antibiotics should be given to all patients.

Q   What potential local complications may occur following open appendicectomy?

A   Surgical site infections (SSIs) are common following open appendicectomy with the rate being higher in patients with inflamed appendicitis. Most frequently, these are superficial incisional infections characterised by superficial cellulitis that respond well to systemic antibiotics. A small number of patients may develop deep incisional infections, which are characterised by purulent discharge and may result in a superficial dehiscence.

Some patients, especially children, are at risk of developing an organ space infection (pericaecal collection), which are characterised by localised low-grade pyrexia, abdominal discomfort and a fluctuant mass on abdominal or rectal examinations. Most pericaecal collections are amenable to radiological guided drainage. Later some patients may develop adhesional bowel obstruction.

Case 3.50 Colectomy

Q **What preoperative investigations are required prior to a colonic resection for a bowel tumour?**

A Bowel cancer presents as an emergency (obstruction, perforation or rarely excessive bleeding) or with chronic symptoms (anaemia, change of bowel habit, colicky abdominal pain or rectal bleeding). Patients presenting with symptoms suspicious of colorectal cancer require either a rigid sigmoidoscopy and double-contrast barium enema or a flexible sigmoidoscopy/colonoscopy. Colonoscopy is the method of choice as this technique allows a biopsy and histological confirmation of a colonic cancer. CT scanning of the abdomen and a chest radiograph are required to screen for liver and lung metastases. A CT scan may also show intra-abdominal spread and is increasingly used to identify intraluminal lesions in the colon when treated with bowel preparation prior to scanning (CT colography). In the emergency situation, a plain abdominal radiograph shows the typical features of large ± small bowel obstruction. A caecum >12 cm in diameter requires an urgent laparotomy, as there is a high risk of perforation. Before committing the patient to an emergency laparotomy, the patient should undergo a water-soluble contrast study to identify the level of obstruction and to exclude pseudo-obstruction.

Q **What preparations are required prior to performing a colonic resection?**

A Assessment of fitness is obtained through a full history and examination; full blood count, urea and electrolytes and electrocardiogram. Blood should be taken for group and save or cross-match depending on the procedure performed. Preparation for colonic resection requires full informed consent and venous thromboembolism prophylaxis. The day prior to surgery the bowel is mechanically prepared with oral sodium picosulphate (the patient may require intravenous fluids if becoming dehydrated). At induction, prophylactic antibiotics are administered intra-venously and carried on for 3–5 days postoperatively if there is contamina-tion at the time of surgery. A urethral catheter is passed following induction to decompress the bladder and to assess the perioperative urine output.

Q   **Describe the vascular pedicles that are required to be identified when performing the various segmental colonic resections.**

A   Radical excision of a colonic tumour along with the appropriate vascular pedicle and accompanying lymphatic drainage is necessary to obtain a curative resection or local control of disease. Division of a vascular pedicle renders the associated colon ischaemic and necessitates its segmental removal. Right hemicolectomy requires the division of the ileocolic and right colic pedicles. A left hemicolectomy requires division of the left colic pedicle. An extended left or right hemicolectomy requires division of the middle colic pedicle in addition to the above pedicles. These pedicles must be divided near their origins with the superior and inferior mesenteric arteries respectively.

Q   **Describe a standard right hemicolectomy as performed for a caecal carcinoma.**

A   The procedure is performed through a midline incision. A full laparotomy is performed to assess the extent of disease. The right colon is retracted towards the midline and the peritoneum in the right paracolic gutter is divided from the caecal pole to the right hepatic flexure. The lesser sac is then entered and the greater omentum divided to the mid-third of the transverse colon (the intended division of the transverse colon). While the assistant retracts the right colon towards the midline, the surgeon dissects the colonic mesentery off the posterior wall making sure not to damage the duodenum, ureter or gonadal vessels. The ileocolic and right colic pedicles are identified and ligated. The sites of division on the terminal ileum and transverse colon are identified and divided be-tween soft and crushing clamps or with a linear stapling (GIA) device. The anastomosis is then created end-to-end, end-to-side or side-to-side. The cut ends of the ileum and transverse colon should be approximately the same diameter. The diameter of the small bowel may be extended by incising the anti-mesenteric side of the small bowel. The anastomosis is performed preferably in two layers (all layers placed seromuscularly) or using a single layer of interrupted absorbable sutures. The anastomosis may also be completed using a linear stapling device (if the terminal ileum and colon have been divided using a GIA stapler) by placing the ileum and transverse colon side-to-side and passing each limb of the stapling device into small enterotomies. The remaining defect is closed with the GIA stapler. The mesenteric defect is closed with interrupted sutures to prevent internal herniation.

Case 3.51 Small bowel resection

Q What indications would require a segmental resection of the small bowel?

A
- congenital atresia, intussusception
- Meckel's diverticulum causing perforation or bleeding
- trauma to the bowel or mesentery
- inflammatory conditions, e.g. Crohn's disease
- devascularisation secondary to hernia strangulation, volvulus or mesenteric embolus
- fistulas secondary to previous surgery or inflammatory conditions
- tumours of the small bowel, e.g. lymphoma, carcinoid or gastro-intestinal stromal tumours.

Q Describe a wedge excision of a Meckel's diverticulum.

A A Meckel's diverticulum is a true diverticulum as it involves all layers of the bowel. When present it arises from the antimesenteric surface of the ileum approximately 50 cm (range 15–167 cm) from the ileocaecal valve in the adult. The length of the diverticulum is usually 1–5 cm in length. The tip may be free or its tip may be attached to the umbilicus by a persistent vitellointestinal duct, this may be patent occasionally (omphalo-ileal fistula). The mucosa is usually ileal but ectopic gastric, duodenal or pancreatic mucosa may be present. This ectopic mucosa may cause erosions resulting in bleeding or perforation.

A wedge excision is performed by first milking back the contents of the terminal ileum and then applying light non-crushing clamps to keep the field free of contamination. The diverticulum is excised by applying crushing clamps obliquely so their tips are touching and then cutting the specimen using a scalpel against the clamps. The resulting enterostomy is closed transversely in two layers using interrupted absorbable sutures or in a single layer with sutures placed seromuscularly. A wedge excision is not suitable if the diverticulum is large and a formal small bowel resection should be performed.

Q Describe a stricturoplasty as performed for small bowel Crohn's disease.

A Small bowel Crohn's disease can result in obstructive lesions throughout the small bowel and may be multiple. Multiple small bowel resections increase the risk of short bowel syndrome. Stricturoplasty results in maximum conservation of bowel length. This technique is ideally suited to short fibrotic strictures, while longer strictures with active inflammation are better managed with resection of the affected bowel.

The procedure is performed by milking back the contents of the proximal bowel and then applying light non-crushing clamps to either side of the stricture. The stricture is divided longitudinally and sutured transversely with interrupted seromuscular absorbable sutures. To ensure no strictures have been missed a Foley catheter is passed along the small bowel prior to the last suture being placed. The balloon is inflated and then drawn back through the bowel. See 4.49 Crohn's disease.

Q   **Describe a segmental small bowel resection as performed for a small bowel tumour.**

A   A full laparotomy is performed through a midline incision to assess the extent of the disease. Soft non-crushing clamps are placed approximately 10 cm proximal and distal to the tumour. A triangle of peritoneum is incised on either side of the bowel from where it is divided proximally and distally to the root of the mesentery. The mesentery is then held up to the light to identify the vessels in order to clip and divide them individually. Crushing clamps are applied at the point where the bowel is to be divided and the specimen excised by using a scalpel to cut the bowel against the clamps. The two cut ends of the bowel are aligned with no tension and preferable anastomosed in one layer with interrupted seromuscular absorbable sutures. The anastomosis is commenced by placing the corner sutures first. Alternatively, the anastomosis may be completed side-to-side with a GIA stapler in a similar fashion to a right hemicolectomy.

Case 3.52 Rectal surgery

Q   **Describe Dukes' classification of colorectal cancers.**

A   Dukes' staging is based on histological examination of the resected specimen. This system is easy to remember, reproducible and may be used in conjunction with the TNM classification system.

Dukes' staging

A   Invasive carcinoma not breaching the muscularis propria
B   Invasive carcinoma breaching the muscularis propria, but not involving the local lymph nodes
C1   Invasive carcinoma involving the regional lymph nodes (apical node negative)
C2   Invasive carcinoma involving the regional lymph nodes (apical node positive)
D   Distant metastases

Q   **What are the benefits of performing a total mesorectal excision?**

A   A total mesorectal excision is removal of the entire rectal mesentery and rectum including that distal to the tumour as an intact unit. This is performed as part of a low anterior resection or abdominoperineal resection and is the optimal surgical treatment for a rectal cancer. Total mesorectal excision requires precise sharp dissection in the areolar plane outside the visceral fascia that envelopes the rectum and mesentery. This technique results in less damage to the autonomic nerves and a lower local recurrence rate. However, care must be taken, as careless dissection may cause more damage to the autonomic nerves.

Q   **What are the treatment options for a low rectal cancer?**

A   A poorly differentiated rectal cancer requires a distal margin of 2 cm from the lowest point of the tumour. The lower the tumour the more difficult it will be to preserve sphincter function. It is generally accepted that tumours of the upper rectum should be treated by anterior resection (resection of the rectum and anastomosis of the remaining rectum/anus to the colon), while tumours 5 cm or less from the anal verge should be treated by abdominoperineal excision (resection of the rectum and anus and formation of a permanent colostomy). Anastomotic leakage after anterior resection is high and therefore most surgeons form a temporary ileostomy, which is reversed 3–6 months later when healing has occurred.

Q   **Describe the operation of anterior resection.**

A   Preoperatively, the bowel is mechanically prepared and thromboembolic prophylaxis administered. The stoma therapist will have marked for an end colostomy and temporary ileostomy. At induction, prophylactic antibiotics are administered. The patient is placed in the Lloyd–Davies position and a urinary catheter inserted. A laparotomy is performed through a lower midline incision to assess the extent of disease. A self-retaining retractor is placed and the small bowel packed into the right upper quadrant. The sigmoid colon is retracted towards the midline by the assistant and the lateral peritoneum incised. The peritoneum on the medial side of the sigmoid is then incised and held to the light to identify the inferior mesenteric pedicle with the artery and vein ligated close to their origin. The peritoneal incisions are extended down into the pouch of Douglas to where they meet. As the sigmoid is mobilised the left ureter and gonadal vessels are identified and preserved. The presacral plane is opened by incising the peritoneum posterior to the rectum (avoiding damage to the sacral veins). A total mesorectal excision is performed as above.

A Roticulator transverse stapling device is placed 5 cm below the tumour with the rectum stretched and fired. A non-crushing and crushing clamp are placed across the sigmoid colon, which is divided with a scalpel and the specimen removed. The proximal end of the circular end-to-end stapling gun (CEEA) is placed in the proximal cut bowel and held in place with a purse string suture. The stapling gun is then passed by the assistant into the rectal stump and the spike deployed through the stump adjacent to the staple line. The spike is removed and the ends of the gun attached, approximated and fired. A circular knife within the instrument removes two doughnuts of bowel, which are inspected for completeness after the gun has gently been removed. A temporary loop ileostomy is then formed in the right iliac fossa. See 4.48 Obstructing rectal lesion.

Case 3.53 Haemorrhoids

Q **Describe the aetiology and pathology of haemorrhoids.**

A Haemorrhoids are an abnormality of the vascular cushions of the anal canal. There are classically three cushions, which provide a conforming seal when the internal sphincter muscle is contracted. Degeneration of the supporting smooth muscle and fibroelastic tissue results in prolapse and the symptoms of haemorrhoids. The formation of haemorrhoids is commoner in patients who suffer with constipation or strain at stool. Patients with symptomatic haemorrhoids usually present with bleeding at stool, prolapse, perianal discomfort pruritus or minor soiling. Patients may present with an exacerbation of pain due to acute haemorrhoidal thrombosis.

Q **Can haemorrhoids be classified?**

A The symptoms of haemorrhoids are classified according to degrees. They do not necessarily progress from one degree to another. Haemorrhoids that present with bleeding only are classified as first degree. Haemorrhoids that with prolapse but reduce spontaneously are classified as second degree, while those that prolapse but do not reduce spontaneously are classified as third degree. Examination requires a careful external examination and proctoscopy to exclude other diseases particularly cancer.

Q **Describe the conservative management of haemorrhoids.**

A Patients with mild discomfort, pruritus or bleeding are advised to use bulk laxatives or increase dietary fibre ± self-medicated topical preparations. Patients who are more symptomatic may undergo an outpatient procedure, which include: injection sclerotherapy, rubber band ligation or infrared photocoagulation. Injection sclerotherapy is performed by injecting 3–5 ml of a 5% solution of phenol in an oily medium into the submucosa of each haemorrhoid, well above the dentate line using a 'Gabriel' needle and syringe. Rubber band ligation is performed by grasping the mucosa of a non-prolapsing haemorrhoid above the dentate line using a suction device. The rubber band is then released from the ligator on to the base of the haemorrhoid. Infrared photocoagulation is performed by applying an infrared probe onto the surface of the haemorrhoid and delivering a pulse of infrared light.

NB Rectal bleeding cannot be written off as haemorrhoidal bleeding until adequately investigated.

Q   **Describe the operation of open haemorrhoidectomy.**

A   Operative intervention is indicated if non-operative measures fail to control symptoms particularly those of prolapse. Preoperatively, the rectum is prepared with enemas or rectal washouts. The patient is placed in the lithotomy position. The skin is shaven, prepared with chlorhexidine and draped. The anal canal is inspected and palpated using a Parks bivalve anal speculum. Local anaesthetic and adrenaline are injected at the planned sites of incision to aid haemostasis. The apex of the first (largest) haemorrhoid is grasped with an artery forceps and a triangular incision is made into the perianal skin and mucosa using scissors or cutting diathermy. A plane of dissection is then developed between the haemorrhoid and the internal sphincter muscle until the pedicle is identified. The pedicle may be divided with diathermy or ligated. This process is repeated for the remaining haemorrhoids and haemostasis secured. If there is a large external component it is imperative that adequate skin bridges are left between excision sites to prevent stenosis.

Q   **What are the complications of surgery?**

A
- bleeding
- stenosis
- recurrence
- urinary retention
- pain
- constipation.

Case 3.54 Malignant breast lump

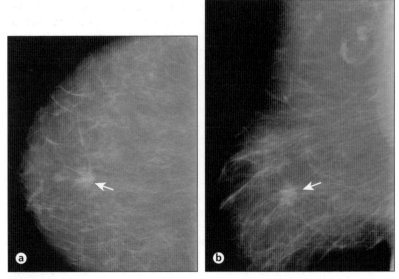

Fig. 3.54.1 (a) The CC (cephalocaudal) view shows a spiculated lesion in the left breast. **(b)** The lateral oblique view has been windowed to enhance the lesion.

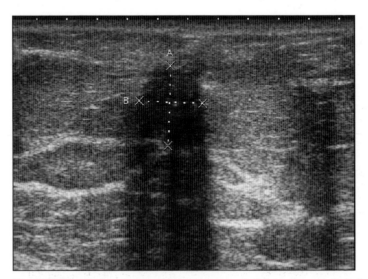

Fig. 3.54.2 The ultrasound scan of the lesion shows an indistinct edge, with the lesion having a lower echogenicity compared with the surrounding breast tissue and post acoustic shadowing. These findings are classical of a breast cancer.

Q   How should a breast malignancy be confirmed?

A   A breast lump should be assessed by triple assessment: clinical examination, cytology/histopathology and radiological assessment. The majority of women presenting with a breast cancer present with a palpable breast lump. Classically the lump is hard, painless, immobile ± fixed to skin and pectoral muscle. Patients may also present with bloody nipple discharge, skin changes (peau d'orange – due to axillary lymphatic obstruction causing oedema of the skin) and palpable axillary lymphadenopathy. Samples for cytology are obtained by fine needle aspiration (FNA), but a core biopsy is required for histopathological assessment. The advantage of FNA for cytology is that it causes less discomfort to the patient than a core biopsy but has the disadvantage of being more difficult to assess than histopathology. Mammography (Fig. 3.54.1a,b) is the most commonly used radiological assessment. However, in women less than 35 years of age an ultrasound scan (Fig. 3.54.2) is performed (as the denser ductal tissue in younger women is more difficult to assess with mammography). Abnormalities identified on breast cancer screening are assessed in a similar fashion. Suspicious lesions identified radiologically but with normal histopathology, should undergo stereotoctic biopsy or, an open wire guided biopsy, where a barbed wire is placed radiologically in the lesion prior to surgery.

Q   How is breast cancer classified?

A   Breast cancer is assessed using the TNM classification:

T = Tumour
T1:   2 cm diameter or less. No fixation or tethering
T2:   2–5 cm diameter (or <2 cm) with tethering or nipple retraction
T3:   5–10 cm diameter (or <5 cm) with infiltration, ulceration or peau d'orange over the tumour, or deep fixation
T4:   Any tumour with infiltration or ulceration wider than its diameter; tumour >10 cm.

N = Nodes
N0:   No palpable axillary nodes
N1:   Mobile palpable axillary nodes
N2:   Fixed axillary nodes
N3:   Palpable supraclavicular nodes. Oedema of the arms.

M = Metastases
M0:   No evidence of distant metastasis
M1:   Distant metastasis.

Q   Describe the removal of the axillary lymph nodes.

A   Axillary node assessment and tumour grade (1, 2 or 3; with grade 3 being the most biologically active cancers) are necessary to aid prediction of prognosis. Previously, it was necessary to perform a block dissection of the axillary fat and lymph nodes. Today axillary node sampling (sentinel node biopsy) is performed. Sentinel node biopsy works on the principle that any single area in the breast has primary lymphatic drainage to one or two regional lymph nodes. These sentinel nodes can be identified by injecting a radiolabelled dye into the edge of the tumour. A gamma camera is used to identify three nodes, which are excised, labelled and sent for histopathological assessment. This technique much reduces the risk of arm lymphoedema postoperatively but is considered to be inappropriate for tumours greater than 4 cm in diameter.

Q   **What operative intervention should be offered to a 55-year-old woman with a 2 cm malignant breast lump?**

A   Operative treatment is the only choice to achieve cure in an early breast cancer. The patient (preferably in the presence of their partner) should be given the choice of mastectomy or breast conserving surgery. The most commonly performed mastectomy is a total mastectomy in which all of the breast tissue and nipple-areolar complex is removed leaving the pectoralis fascia intact. Patients keen to preserve tissue should be given an option of breast conservation (wide local excision) in which the tumour is removed with a 1 cm rim of normal breast tissue. There is no difference in survival between breast conservation therapy and mastectomy. There is however an increased risk of local relapse with breast conservation surgery. Therefore, most patients undergoing breast conservation will require radiotherapy to the breast in all but early tumours.

Q   **Describe the operation of total mastectomy.**

A   Informed consent should be obtained (preferably in the presence of the partner). The patient is placed supine with the patient's arm at right angles to the trunk on an arm board. A transverse elliptical incision is made to include the nipple-areolar complex. Tissue forceps are applied to the upper skin edge. The plane between the skin and breast tissue and the flap are developed with diathermy until the pectoralis fascia is identified. The tissue forceps are then attached to the inferior skin edge and the inferior flap developed in a similar fashion. The dissection is completed medially and the breast tissue removed from the pectoralis fascia from medial to lateral. The perforating muscular vessels should be identified and ligated. The lateral dissection is completed by removing the axillary tail off serratus anterior. A sentinel biopsy is performed early in the procedure as described above. A suction drain is placed in the pectoral area and a second drain is placed in the axilla with both drains taken out through the inferior flap and labelled. The subcutaneous tissue is closed with interrupted absorbable sutures making sure to avoid dog-ears. The skin is then closed with an absorbable subcuticular suture.

Case 3.55 Parotidectomy

Q   **What are the indications for superficial parotidectomy?**

A   Superficial parotidectomy is performed rarely for chronic parotitis secondary to an inaccessible calculus, sicca syndrome (an autoimmune condition interfering with parotid function and producing enlargement of the parotid, lacrimal and other salivary glands due to duct system dilatation) and most commonly performed for adenomas and well-differentiated carcinomas. Superficial parotidectomy is curative for most benign adenomas and well-differentiated tumours. Total parotidectomy is indicated for poorly differentiated tumours. When performing a total parotidectomy every attempt should be made to preserve the facial nerve unless grossly invaded by tumour.

Q   **Describe the anatomical relations of the parotid gland.**

A   The parotid gland lies between the sternocleidomastoid and the ramus of the mandible. Anteriorly it overlies the masseter, its duct emerges from this anterior extension and runs across the remaining masseter, then turns medially to pierce the buccinator and opens into the mouth opposite the second molar tooth of the upper jaw. The external carotid artery penetrates the parotid and divides into the superficial temporal and maxillary artery as it exits. The posterior facial vein accompanies the external carotid artery. The facial nerve enters the gland on its posteromedial surface and runs anteriorly dividing into five branches: temporal, zygomatic, buccal, mandibular and cervical.

Q   **What structure is at risk and what must be done to this structure?**

A   The facial nerve is at risk of injury. Its five branches must be identified and protected early in the procedure. A nerve stimulator is frequently used to aid identification of the nerve and its branches.

Q   **Describe the operation of superficial parotidectomy.**

A   Preoperatively, the patient is consented and warned of damage to the facial nerve and its branches. The patient is positioned prone with head-up tilt provided by a head ring and faced away from the surgeon. When draping it is important to leave the pinna and mandible clearly exposed. An S-shaped incision is made starting in front of the pinna extending towards the mastoid process and then into the upper skin crease of the neck. The three parts of the incision are deepened individually securing haemostasis as the procedure progresses. The anterior branch of the greater auricular nerve is identified and preserved as the superficial part of the incision is deepened. The facial part of the incision is deepened until the junction of the cartilaginous and bony external auditory meatus is identified. The mastoid part of the incision is deepened to the insertion of the sternocleidomastoid muscle. The facial nerve is identified and preserved running deep to the stylomastoid artery, which is ligated and divided. The parotid tissue is now dissected superficial to the main trunk of the facial nerve and its branches. The anterior skin flap is retracted to expose the parotid duct at the anterior margin. The duct is ligated and divided at the anterior border of the masseter. A suction drain is left in the parotid bed and wound closed in layers with absorbable sutures.

NB If any part of the facial nerve is transected during the operation, an immediate end-to-end repair should be performed. If it is not possible to approximate the two ends then a nerve graft using the anterior branch of the greater auricular nerve is performed.

Case 3.56 Vascular–distal bypass

Q   **What is intermittent claudication?**

A   Patients with chronic lower limb vascular disease classically describe intermittent claudication. This is a cramp like pain usually experienced in the calf muscles (but may also be experienced in the buttock and thigh) on exercising. The pain is not experienced at rest. It is important to determine how long the patient has experienced the pain, how far they can walk before the pain comes on with exercise and the impact on their quality of life. It should also be determined whether the symptoms have deteriorated and over what time scale.

Q   **Define critical ischaemia.**

A   Critical ischaemia is described as rest pain (a pain initially experienced at night, which requires the patient to dangle their foot out of bed to relieve the pain, which eventually becomes constant), tissue loss ± gangrene and an ankle systolic blood pressure of <50 mmHg. These patients are at risk of limb loss in the short term.

Q   **What investigations are required in a patient presenting with a chronically ischaemic limb?**

A   Patients should be questioned to identify the impact of intermittent claudication on their quality of life. Patients who are mildly or moderately affected should be assessed by ankle brachial pressure index (ABPI) and an arterial Duplex performed if <0.9. Patients with mild or moderate disease should be advised on smoking cessation, weight loss and diet, control of hypertension and hypercholesteroaemia, prescribed an antiplatelet agent and given a structured exercise programme. Patients severely affected by intermittent claudication or with symptoms of critical ischaemia should be offered arteriography (digital subtraction intra-arterial, CT or MR angiography), with a view to performing an endovascular (angioplasty ± stent placement) or to plan a bypass procedure.

Q   Describe the operation of femoro–distal (anterior tibial artery) bypass.

A   A femoro–distal bypass is indicated if there is a long occlusion extending distal to the popliteal artery or if there are multiple stenoses proximal to the popliteal artery in patients experiencing critical ischaemia. Preoperatively, the long saphenous vein should be mapped and marked with Duplex for use as a bypass graft as this provides greater longer patency rates than a synthetic graft. The arteriogram should be reviewed with a vascular radiologist to identify the most suitable vessel to anastomose to distally. The patient should be assessed for comorbidities (ischaemic heart disease, renal impairment, diabetes mellitus) and have their medical management optimised. The patient should have their limbs and groins and legs shaved immediately before coming to theatre and be grouped and saved or cross-matched according to local protocols. The patient is positioned supine with the skin of both legs, groins and anterior abdominal wall prepared and draped with an adhesive transparent drape. A longitudinal incision centred over the femoral pulse is deepened to expose the junction of the common femoral, superficial femoral and profunda femoris arteries. These arteries are then slung and clamped. A longitudinal arteriotomy is made over the anterior surface of the common femoral artery and extended to the superficial femoral artery (approximately 2 cm). The inflow is assessed by briefly opening the proximal clamp. The long saphenous vein is identified at its junction with the common femoral vein and is ligated and divided. The vein is then dissected distally (ligating tributaries as they are identified) to the medial malleolus where it is divided. The vein is marked with ink, to avoid twisting, and reversed. A second longitudinal incision is made over the chosen site of the distal artery to be anastomosed (usually the lower third) and deepened to identify the anterior tibial artery deep in the anterior compartment, which is then assessed for suitability. The anterior tibial artery is then slung and clamped proximally and distally and a vertical arteriotomy made. A subsartorial tunnel is then formed using a plastic tunneler and finger dissection. The reversed non-twisted graft is pulled into the anterior compartment and the tunneler removed. The graft is then anastomosed end-to-side proximally and distally with a double-ended 5/0 and 6/0 Prolene suture, respectively. The clamps are removed and the graft flow assessed by hand-held Doppler. The wounds ± suction drains are closed in layers with absorbable sutures and skin clips.

   NB Immediate re-exploration of the graft is required if the patient's foot does not become pink at the end of the procedure or the foot becomes white/mottled in the postoperative period.

Case 3.57 Orchidopexy

Q **Describe the development and descent of the testis into the scrotum.**

A The testis develops from the genital ridge (coelomic epithelium and mesoderm) on the posterior wall of the coelomic cavity in the 5th week of fetal life. The genital ridge joins with the mesonephric duct (which forms the epididymis and vas deferens) and descends to the level of the internal ring at 7 months' gestation; external ring at 8 months and enters the scrotum by birth. The descent of the testis relies on the gubernaculum which is attached to the inferior pole. As the testis descends, it carries with it a fold of peritoneum which forms the tunica vaginalis as it passes along the inguinal canal. This is known as the processus vaginalis if the tunica fails to obliterate normally. The testis may leave its normal course at any point and eventually may arrest in an abnormal position (ectopic testis).

Q **Why is it important for undescended/ectopic testis to be placed surgically in the scrotum?**

A The incidence of imperfect descent of a testis at birth is approximately 2%. At 1 year, the incidence is 1%. It is important to differentiate these conditions from retractile testes, which are normally lying testes with an overactive cremaster muscle. A testis not placed in the scrotum by the age of 12 months results in testicular hypoplasia (early degeneration of testicular germ cells occurs in the first 6–12 months of age and may result in tubular dysplasia) and defective spermatogenesis (sterility if bilateral). Therefore, early surgery is now advised to hopefully prevent these changes. The risk of testicular malignancy is 4–10 times more common in these patients.

Q **Describe the operation of orchidopexy as performed for un-descended or ectopic testis.**

A The child is placed supine and the groins and scrotum prepared and draped. A skin crease groin incision is centred over the deep ring which is at the mid point of the inguinal ligament. The testis and cord are identified using blunt dissection. Laparoscopy is useful for locating the impalpable testis. Ectopic testes are either in the superficial inguinal pouch, femoral triangle or perineum and are always easily palpable. The cord is inspected to identify a possible indirect hernial sac. The cord is mobilised and the lateral bands divided. A sub-Dartos pouch is then fashioned by passing a finger through the groin incision down into the scrotum and dividing the scrotal skin overlying the tip of the finger. A pocket is developed beneath the skin with an artery forceps (large enough to accept the testis). A clip is then passed up through the scrotum through the scrotal incision. The clip is attached to the loose tissue overlying the testis and is then drawn down and out through the scrotal skin and then passed into the prepared pouch. The external oblique and Scarpa's fascia are closed prior to closing the skin with subcuticular absorbable sutures or tissue glue.

Q **Describe the diagnosis and treatment of testicular torsion.**

A Testicular torsion is either extravaginal (occurring in neonates) or intra-vaginal (occurring in older children due to a high investment of the tunica vaginalis allowing excessive mobility of the testis). Neonatal torsion is usually painless and presents with a hard, non-tender scrotal mass at birth, with the torsion usually being a prenatal event. Torsion in older children results in sudden severe scrotal pain often associated with nausea and vomiting. The main differential diagnoses are: epididymo-orchitis (usually of longer duration and is usually associated with a urinary tract infection) and torsion of a testicular appendage (hydatid of Morgagni). If there is any doubt, an emergency exploration of the scrotum must be performed. The testis is approached through a transverse incision on the lateral side of the affected hemiscrotum. The tunica is opened to reveal a dusky-blue testis. The testis is detorted and its viability assessed. If the testis remains black, despite detorsion and warming, an orchidectomy is performed. If viable, the testis is fixed to the tunica with three sutures to prevent recurrence. There is now a move to avoid suture fixation and instead employ a sub-dartos pouch. If the testis is torted, then the contralateral hemiscrotum is opened and the testis fixed in a similar manner.

Case 3.58 Nephrectomy

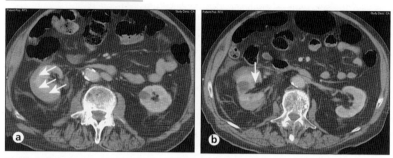

Fig. 3.58.1 (a,b) Large laceration through the hilum and body of the right kidney.

Q   **Describe the operation of left nephrectomy for a non-functioning kidney.**

A   The patient is placed in the right lateral position and the table broken (head and feet ends lowered) to increase access between the ribs and pelvic rim. An incision is made running parallel to the 12th rib in the subcostal space. This incision provides good access but injury may occur to the subcostal nerve. The incision is deepened to expose the 12th rib. The tip of the 12th rib is removed using rib cutters. The muscles are divided in layers with diathermy. Anteriorly the colon is seen covered by peritoneum and posteriorly the perinephric (Gerota's) fascia. The perinephric fat is entered inferiorly with finger dissection until the ureter (the ureter can be differentiated from other structures as it shows peristalsis when touched with forceps) and gonadal vessels are seen. The ureter is doubly ligated and divided. The kidney is now mobilised with a mixture of sharp and blunt dissection to leave the kidney only attached by its pedicle. The vein lies anterior to the artery in the pedicle. The vein and artery are clamped (three clamps) individually and doubly ligated before dividing. A suction drain is placed in the renal bed and the wound closed in layers with absorbable sutures.

Q   **How should this procedure be modified for a renal cell carcinoma?**

A   A radical nephrectomy performed through a midline abdominal incision is performed if metastases are not present. This procedure involves removal of the kidney together with the upper ureter, adrenal gland and surrounding perinephric fat within Gerota's fascia, plus any enlarged para-aortic lymph nodes or thrombus extending into the renal vein or inferior vena cava.

Q   **What procedure should be performed for a transitional cell carcinoma of the renal pelvis?**

A   A nephro-ureterectomy would be performed as for a standard nephrectomy as described above. Following mobilisation of the kidney and division of the artery and vein, the kidney is then pushed towards the iliac fossa and the loin closed as above. The patient is then placed supine and a lower midline incision is made and the lower ureter approached extra-peritoneally. The ureter is mobilised and the kidney delivered into the wound. The ureter is divided from the bladder, which is then oversewn in two layers. A non-suction drain is placed and brought up through a separate stab wound and left for ten days.

Q   **How should blunt renal trauma be managed?**

A   Blunt renal trauma is classified as Types I–V: Type I: microscopic/gross haematuria, contained subscapular haematoma, treated with bed rest until gross haematuria settles (Fig. 3.58.1a). Type II: non-expanding perirenal haematoma ± cortical laceration <1 cm requires bed rest and prophylactic antibiotics. Type III: laceration >1 cm deep without extravasation, Type IV: laceration >1 cm with extravasation and Type V: multiple lacerations ± pedicle injury (Fig. 3.58.1b). Types III–V all require surgical intervention. The kidney is approached through a midline incision. A full laparotomy is performed to assess associated injuries. When exploring the kidney, it is important to control the renal pedicle before exploring the retro-peritoneal haematoma. Lacerations to the renal parenchyma can usually be repaired. Injuries to the pedicle usually necessitate nephrectomy. Before performing a nephrectomy, the contralateral kidney should be carefully inspected.

Case 3.59 Transurethral resection

Q   **Describe the pathophysiology of benign prostatic hypertrophy.**

A   Bladder outflow symptoms of hesitancy, poor stream and nocturia result from benign prostatic hypertrophy, although the actual size of the gland and severity of symptoms are unrelated. The prostate gland is composed of distinct zones (central, peripheral and transition). Under the action of androgens, the glandular spaces increase in size. Enlargement of the transition zone (inner group of glands) causes compression and atrophy of the peripheral zone (peripheral group of glands) forming a pseudocapsule. This results in an endoscopic appearance of lateral lobe intrusion into the prostatic urethra and the formation of middle lobe protruding into the bladder through the bladder neck. See 4.52 Prostate cancer.

Q   **How are the bladder outflow symptoms objectively assessed?**

A   A detailed history and full examination including rectal examination of the prostate are performed. A mid-stream urine sample is sent for microscopy and culture. Blood is sent for urea and electrolytes. Patients should complete a frequency/volume chart for the previous 2 weeks to establish the diagnosis. The degree of symptoms may be objectively measured by the urine flow rate, in which the patient voids into a machine when a full bladder is achieved. A peak urine flow of less than 10 ml/second (with a minimum voiding of 150 ml) strongly suggests obstruction. A bladder ultrasound probe is used to estimate the residual bladder volume at the end of the procedure. Pressure/flow cystometry (pressure transducers placed in the rectum and bladder) may be necessary to distinguish between outflow obstruction and detrusor failure.

Q **What medical managements are available to treat bladder outflow symptoms?**

A Highly selective alpha-blockers (α_{1c} e.g. tamsulosin) act on the smooth muscle of the prostate producing an increased flow rate. 5-α-reductase inhibitors (e.g. finasteride) blocks conversion of testosterone to its inactive metabolite dihydrotestosterone resulting in a reduction of prostate size over several months. Adverse effects include retrograde ejaculation and postural hypotension.

Q **Describe the operation of transurethral prostatectomy.**

A The patient is advised of the risk of incontinence, impotence and retrograde ejaculation at the time of consenting. A cystoscopy is performed first to assess the size of the prostate and to exclude a prostatic tumour. Tumour is a contraindication due to the risk of implantation of tumour cells in the raw prostatic bed. The resectoscope and working elements are inserted into the urethra. During the procedure, irrigating fluid (isotonic glycine) is delivered and removed via the resectoscope. Under direct vision, a diathermy loop is moved backwards and forwards removing slices of tissue until the capsule is visible (the capsule is identified by circular fibres). Haemostasis is achieved by placing the loop on bleeding points and pressing the coagulation pedal. Resection is performed in a set fashion starting at the 6 o'clock position, resecting the middle lobe to the level of the veru montanum (seminal colliculus, which is seen as a small swelling). Resection must remain proximal to the veru montanum to avoid injury to the external urethral sphincter which is distal to it. The lateral lobes ('2 and 11 o'clock') are then resected to the level of the capsule. Bleeding points are coagulated with the loop and the chippings are washed out with an Ellick's evacuator. It is important to remove all chippings as they may block the catheter postoperatively. A three-way catheter is inserted at the end of the procedure to allow irrigation.

Q **What other surgical management may be offered to younger men with bladder outflow symptoms?**

A A bladder neck incision (transurethral incision of the prostate) may be performed by passing an endoscopic diathermy knife and cutting the prostate at the '5 and 7 o'clock positions'. The incisions extend from beyond the bladder neck to the level of the veru montanum to the depth of the prostatic capsule. These incisions form grooves along which urine may pass. A transurethral prostatectomy is required if this procedure fails to improve symptoms.

Case 3.60 Methods of fracture fixation

Q **Describe the normal healing of a fracture.**

A Normal healing requires: good apposition of the bony ends, adequate blood supply, immobility and freedom from infection. The stages of bone healing are as follows:

- haematoma forms at fracture site following trauma (0–4 days)
- granulation tissue forms with mobilisation of macrophages and osteo-clasts (remove dead bone) and invasion of osteoblasts (form new bone) (0–14 days)
- a bridge between the bone ends is formed by osteoid tissue (forming a firm mass of callus). Callus forms both outside the bone as subperiosteal callus and inside as endosteal callus. The pH of the tissue increases at this stage and calcium is deposited (2–6 weeks)
- ossification of skin bridge (6–12 weeks)
- callus matures (3–6 months)
- gap between cortical ends bridged (6–12 months)
- remodelling and architecture restored (12–24 months).

Q **Describe the principles of fracture treatment.**

A Treatment of a fracture requires reduction (traction, manipulation or open reduction), holding the fracture fragments (traction, casting, internal or external fixation devices), preservation of joint movement and function (early joint movement ± weight bearing) and rehabilitation (physiotherapy and occupational therapy).

Q **What are the possible complications of fracture healing?**

A Immediate complications of a fracture are associated with other injuries, which occurred at the time of trauma, e.g. neurovascular injury, trauma to other organs/limbs. Early complications are divided into general (e.g. fat embolism, venous thromboembolism, pneumonia) and local (skin necrosis, wound infection). Late complications include: delayed wound healing (usually due to infection), delayed or non-union of the fracture (usually due to mobility – requires better reduction and mobilisation ± bone grafting), malunion (the fracture unites in an unsatisfactory position), growth disturbance of the bone (due to injury in the growth plate in children), avascular necrosis (e.g. scaphoid), reflex sympathetic dystrophy (pain, altered sensation, abnormal blood flow, sweating and trophic changes in surrounding soft tissues).

Q   Describe the principle of fracture fixation.

A   Anatomical reduction is difficult to maintain in intra-articular and forearm fracture with casts. Therefore, AO (*Arbeitsgemeinschaft für Osteosynthese fragen*) techniques are used to maintain reduction using standardised screws and plates. AO screws are cylindrical and either self-tapping (sharp-ended) or round-ended. Screws are either cortical (fully threaded) or cancellous (partially threaded). The core of the screw corresponds to the size of the drill bit to be used. The grip of the screw depends on the width of the thread and the distance between threads. Plates are of two types: neutralisation or dynamic compression.

Preoperatively the radiographs are reviewed and a treatment plan formulated (excessive comminution is a contraindication). A radiographer and image intensifier are required in theatre. The patient is positioned to allow access to the fracture site and potential bone grafting sites. The limb is exsanguinated and a tourniquet is inflated. An incision should be planned over the fracture site, which allows the minimum of dissection. The bone ends are identified and held temporarily in place with reduction forceps. A lag screw technique may be used to produce stabilisation causing interfragmentary compression, i.e. the effect is produced by the screw crossing the fracture where the threads firmly grip the far side of the cortex. A buttress (antiglide) plate and screws is usually necessary in an oblique fracture. Transverse fractures of a long bone require offset screws and a dynamic compression plate. A radiograph of the treated fracture is taken, the tourniquet released and haemostasis secured. Muscle and skin are closed in layers with absorbable sutures and a splint applied.

Case 3.61 Hemiarthroplasty

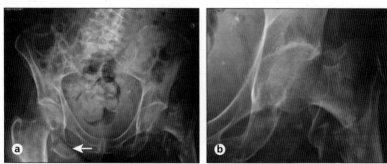

Fig. 3.61.1 (a) Left hip intertrochanteric fracture and right pubic ramus fracture. **(b)** Close-up view of left intertrochanteric fracture.

Q   Classify fractures of the femoral neck.

A   Fractures of the proximal femur are subdivided into extracapsular, intra-capsular and fractures of the femoral head. Intracapsular fractures are at greatest risk of non-union and avascular necrosis. Intracapsular fractures are classified by Garden's classification (Stage I–IV with IV having the greatest risk of avascular necrosis), which is based on the A–P radiograph. Intracapsular fractures have the greatest risk of avascular necrosis, as the high cervical fracture is most likely to interrupt the blood supply to the femoral head. Non-displaced or impacted fractures in the elderly may be treated conservatively or with AO screws. However, displaced fractures require prosthetic replacement (Thompson or Austin–Moore prosthesis) to achieve early mobilisation and to avoid fracture non-union.

Extracapsular fractures (Fig. 3.61.1a,b) are less likely to result in avascular necrosis as the blood supply to the femoral neck tends not to be affected. Fracture non-healing is less of a problem as the surface areas of the fracture tend to be larger and there is less movement of the femoral head. They are classified by the Boyd–Griffin classification. This classification aims to identify those fractures, which are unstable and more likely to collapse. Undisplaced fractures may be treated with multiple fine pins or crossed AO screws.

Trochanteric fractures are divided into pertrochanteric (through both trochanters), intertrochanteric (between the trochanters), subtrochanteric or avulsion of the greater trochanter. These fractures tend to be unstable and are not usually affected by non-union. A dynamic hip screw and plate (Fig. 3.61.2) creates compression between the fracture surfaces (acts like a plaster cast).

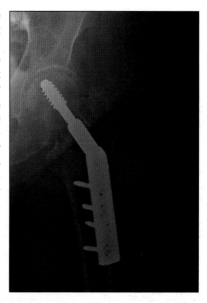

Fig. 3.61.2 The same fracture treated with a dynamic hip screw (DHS).

Q **Describe the operation of hemiarthroplasty as performed for a fracture of the femoral neck.**

A Patients with a displaced subcapital fracture (Garden grades III and IV) are at high risk of avascular necrosis and are best treated with a hemiarthroplasty. The patient is positioned supine with a sandbag under the affected hip. A longitudinal incision approximately 15 cm long is centred over the greater trochanter. The incision is deepened to the fascia lata which is divided in the line of the incision. A plane is developed between the gluteus medius and minimus. The insertion of gluteus medius into the lateral border of the femur is divided exposing the joint capsule, which is incised in a T fashion. The femoral neck is exposed and cut at an angle by crossing the leg over the contralateral leg and using a trial prosthesis as a template. The femoral head is next removed using a corkscrew device. The removed femoral head is measured with callipers in order to pick the most appropriate sized prosthesis. The femoral canal is now enlarged laterally using a box chisel. A bone spike is passed down the shaft to form a tract which is then enlarged using broaches. The prosthesis is inserted into this tract making sure it is seated firmly on the calcar. The acetabulum is cleared of any debris and the prosthesis reduced using traction in the line of the femur. The stability of the prosthesis is checked and the wound closed in layers with absorbable sutures. Postoperatively the patient should be encouraged to mobilise early with full weight bearing.

Q   **Describe the operation of dynamic hip screw as performed for subtrochanteric fractures of the femur.**

A   The patient is positioned supine and reduction of the fracture is attempted using the image intensifier, the leg is then maintained in this position. The skin is incised distally from the greater trochanter. The fascia lata is incised and the vastus lateralis is detached from the fracture site using a periosteal elevator. A lag screw is inserted to maintain the reduction (making sure that its position will not subsequently interfere with placement of the plate). The dynamic hip screw is inserted using a guide wire. The plate is then attached to the dynamic hip screw and then held in place with cortical screws. The position of the plate is checked with the image intensifier and the wound closed in layers. The patient should mobilise postoperatively with partial weight bearing.

Principles of surgery

Case 3.62 Basic principles of anastomosis

Q   **What is a surgical anastomosis?**

A   An anastomosis is the operative union of two tubular structures.

Q   **What basic principles are required in bowel anastomosis.**

A   The bowel may be anastomosed end-to-end, end-to-side or side-to-side. Prior to joining two ends of bowel, it is important to make sure that both cut ends of bowel have a good blood supply. Contamination of the cut ends should be kept to a minimum by using non-crushing clamps. There should be good approximation of the two ends (disparity in size can be reduced by incising longitudinally along the anti-mesenteric border of the smaller of the two lumens effectively increasing the circumference). Following anastomosis there should be no tension in the anastomosis. The defect in the mesentery should be closed to prevent internal herniation.

Q   **What techniques are available to anastomose the bowel ends?**

A   The bowel can be joined by either a hand-sewn technique or by the use of a stapling device. Hand-sewn techniques may be formed in one or two layers and sutured using a continuous suture or interrupted sutures. Sutures should be placed seromuscularly from outside to in, using the submucosal grooves as landmarks for the needle to emerge from. Some surgeons include the mucosal layer in the suture, as this will form a gas-tight barrier. Suture material should be absorbable and the needle round-bodied.

Q   **What is the aim of a vascular anastomosis?**

A   The aim of a vascular anastomosis is to produce a watertight join of the two vessels, without tension and maintaining the normal lumen.

Q   **Describe the technique of vascular anastomosis.**

A   The vessels are anastomosed either end-to-end or end-to-side. An artificial conduit (graft) is joined in a similar manner. It is imperative when performing a vascular anastomosis to handle the vessels gently and avoid touching the vessels with forceps. Sutures should be small (≤3/0), non-absorbable, double-ended and on round-bodied needles. The needle is always inserted from inside to out on the lower vessel (to avoid raising an intimal flap) and outside to in on the upper vessel.

Case 3.63 Day-case surgery

Q   **Define ambulatory surgery.**

A   Ambulatory surgery is the selection of patients for a planned surgical procedure, returning home within 24 hours of their procedure.

Q   **What facilities are required for ambulatory surgery?**

A   Ambulatory surgery requires a dedicated ambulatory care unit, which may be free-standing or integrated within the main hospital. The unit should contain operating theatres, recovery area and a nearby ward to allow for a quick turnaround of patients.

Q   **Describe patient selection for ambulatory care.**

A   Suitability for ambulatory care surgery is dependent on social factors, age, medical factors and body mass index. Social factors which may preclude ambulatory surgery include: long travel distances home, or no accompanying adult able to stay in the patient's home for the required 24 hours. There is no upper age limit, however older patients tend to be more frail and suffer more co-morbidities. Medical problems which preclude ambulatory care include: heart disease (uncontrolled hypertension or angina), asthma (steroid-controlled) and diabetes (poor glycaemic control). The upper limit of body mass index varies between units but is usually in the range of 30–35 kg/m^2.

Q   **Who should perform ambulatory care pre-assessments?**

A   Patients who are deemed suitable for day-case surgery should be sent to the ambulatory care unit for assessment. Ambulatory care pre-assessment should be nurse-led, with the pre-assessment team rather than the surgeon making the final decision regarding suitability for ambulatory care, or the need for in-patient admission.

Q   **What is the criterion for discharge home from the ambulatory care unit.**

A   A checklist of criteria for discharge is completed by the nurse and includes: vital signs within normal limits for greater than 1 hour following surgery, patient coordinated and orientated, good analgesia with a supply to take home, drinking, no incisional bleeding and the accompanying person has arrived. Written and verbal instructions should also be supplied regarding postoperative care and follow-up. A telephone number to ring in case of emergency should also be supplied.

Clinical

Clinical case scenarios

QUESTIONS & ANSWER

Superficial lesions

Case 4.1 Lipoma

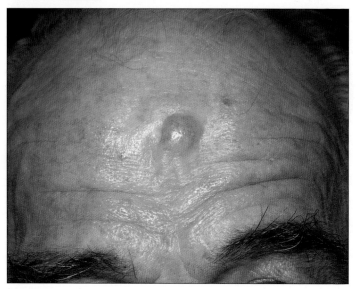

Fig. 4.1.1

Q   **Describe what you see.**

A   There is a 1.5 cm hemispherical swelling with a well-defined edge on the mid forehead. The skin that overlies the lump is normal (it may sometimes be a little stretched and hence have a glazed, transparent appearance). The shape is often the most obvious diagnostic feature. Classically, they are spherical in shape. However, subcutaneous lipomas which are caught between two resistant tissues (as the skin and the deep fascia) may become flattened. They then appear discoid or hemispherical.

Q   **How are you going to examine this lump?**

A   ***Temperature:***   The temperature of the overlying skin is normal.
        Tenderness: Lipomas are usually non-tender and can be palpated firmly
           without discomfort to the patient.
        Size: Lipomas come in all sizes (measure and mention the size in two or
           three dimensions).
        Surface: The surface usually feels smooth, but gentle pressure may
           reveal a bosselated surface, the bosses being the individual lobules.

Edge: The edge is well-defined, while the margins may be irregular. Because the edge is soft, compressible and sometimes quite thin it slips away from the examining finger. This is called the 'slip sign'.

Consistency: Lipomas are characteristically soft. Most lipomas contain a soft but solid jelly-like fat if they are cut open immediately after removal.

Fluctuation: Most small lipomas feel soft but do not fluctuate. However, large lipomas may fluctuate since the fat may move from one lobule to another.

Transillumination: Large lipomas transilluminant.

Relations: Lipomas may arise within deep structures, such as a muscle and bulge out into the subcutaneous tissues. These lipomata are fixed deeply and may become more prominent if they are pushed out of the muscle.

Lymph nodes: The regional lymph nodes should not be enlarged.

Local tissues: The surrounding tissue is usually normal, but there may be other lipomas nearby.

Q What is a lipoma?

A A lipoma is a cluster or collection of fat cells which have become over-active and so distended with fat that they have become palpable lumps.

Q What are the common sites for a lipoma?

A Lipomas (also called lipomata) are most common in the subcutaneous tissue of the upper limbs, especially the forearm, back, and thighs although they can occur anywhere where there is fat.

Q How would you treat a lipoma?

A Lipomas are usually innocuous and asymptomatic, and thus do not require treatment. However, they can become painful requiring treatment. Patients may also request treatment for aesthetic reasons. Surgery is the treatment of choice. Simple excision and direct closure is usually adequate. If there is infiltration into the surrounding tissues, along with debulking, all the infiltrating fat should be removed. However, it is essential to preserve as much normal tissue as possible since excessive removal could lead to a contour defect and difficulty in wound closure. There may be recurrence if the lipoma and all the affected fat are not removed in entirety.

Q What is Dercum's disease?

A These are multiple, painful lipomas (lipomatosis). They usually arise in adults, more commonly in middle-aged obese women. The aetiology is unclear although a familial inheritance has been implicated.

Case 4.2 Sebaceous (epidermoid) cyst

Q   **Describe what you see.**

A   There is a 2 cm hemispherical
swelling with a punctum on
the right side of the back.

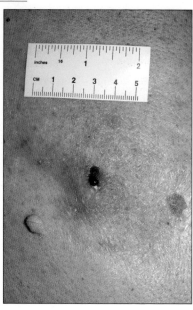

Fig. 4.2.1

Q   **How would you examine a sebaceous (epidermoid) cyst?**
A   ***Position:***   Most sebaceous cysts are found in the hair-bearing parts
of the body. The scalp, scrotum, neck, shoulder and back are the
common sites, but they can occur wherever there are sebaceous
glands. They do not occur in the palms or soles.
Colour: The overlying skin is usually normal.
Tenderness: Uncomplicated sebaceous cysts are non-tender. Pain and
tenderness is a sign of infection.
Temperature: The temperature of the skin over a cyst is normal except
when the cyst is inflamed or infected.
Shape: Most sebaceous cysts are tense and consequently spherical.
Size: They can vary from a few millimetres to 4–5 cm in diameter.
Surface: The surface of the sebaceous cyst is smooth.
Consistency: Most sebaceous cysts feel firm but they may be soft.
Indentation on pressure may be present.
Fluctuation: They are usually fluctuant unless very tense.
Reducibility: Non-reducible.
Pulsatility: Non-pulsatile.
Transillumination: They do not transilluminant.
Percussion: Sebaceous cysts are dull to percussion and do not have a
fluid thrill because their contents are like thick cream.

Relations: Being cutaneous in origin, they are tethered to the skin and the skin is not pinchable separate from the swelling in the region of the punctum. However, they are movable from the deeper and surrounding structures.

Lymph nodes: The local lymph nodes are not normally enlarged.

Q What is the aetiology of a sebaceous cyst?

A The skin is kept soft and oily by the sebum secreted by the sebaceous glands. The 'mouths' of these glands open into the hair follicles. If the 'mouth' of a sebaceous gland becomes blocked, the gland becomes distended by its own secretions and ultimately becomes a sebaceous cyst.

Q What is Cock's peculiar tumour?

A Infection of the cyst wall and the surrounding tissues produces a boggy, painful, discharging swelling with or without ulceration known as Cock's peculiar tumour. This characteristically occurs in the scalp and it may resemble a tumour.

Q How should sebaceous cysts be managed?

A Surgical excision is the treatment of choice. Surgery involves complete removal of the cyst along with its contents, and the cyst wall. Recurrence is likely if a portion of the cyst lining is left behind. Hence, the cyst should be removed intact with an ellipse of skin over the apex containing the punctum.

Case 4.3 Squamous cell carcinoma

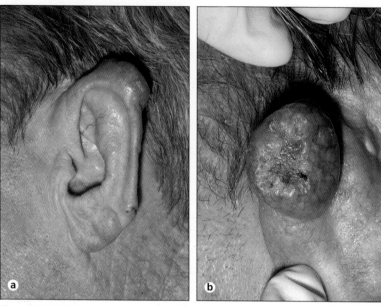

Fig. 4.3.1a,b

Q   **Describe what you see.**

A   There is a red-brown, ulcerated, exophytic lesion on the superior aspect of the pinna of the left ear. This lesion is most likely to be a squamous cell carcinoma (SCC).

Q   **What are the characteristic features of a squamous cell carcinoma of the skin?**

A   It presents as a cauliflower-like, exophytic growth or as an ulcer with everted edges. The base is indurated and the ulcer may be fixed to the underlying tissues. The regional lymph nodes may be enlarged.

Q   **Do you know of any special types of squamous cell carcinoma of the skin?**

A   Marjolin's ulcer is a type of squamous cell carcinoma which rarely develops in a long standing benign ulcer or a scar. The most common underlying cause is a venous ulcer in the leg. The most common scar is a burns scar. Marjolin's ulcers are less aggressive tumours that do not metastasise as readily as the usual SCCs. They may not have the characteristic everted edge and may be associated with more induration in the surrounding tissues.

Q What is the differential diagnosis of a SCC?

A
- actinic keratosis
- amelanotic melanoma
- basal cell carcinoma
- Bowen's disease (intraepithelial carcinoma)
- keratoacanthoma
- pyogenic granuloma
- seborrhoeic wart (keratosis).

Q How should SCCs be managed?

A Histology should be confirmed by an incision biopsy from a non-necrotic area or by excision biopsy if the lesion is small. Definitive management depends on the balance between the site and stage of the disease and the fitness and expectations of the patient.

Surgery is generally the treatment of choice. It is also preferred in areas where radiotherapy is poorly tolerated (lower-third of leg; overlying a bone; scalp (causes alopecia); upper eyelid). Small lesions may be treated by a wide local excision with a margin of 1 cm and primary closure. If the excision is anticipated to leave a large defect, then skin grafting or reconstruction with flaps should be planned in liaison with a plastic surgeon. Flaps are the choice if postoperative radiotherapy is planned. Extensive lesions involving the digits or extremities may necessitate an appropriate, oncologically-sound amputation. Regional lymphadenectomy (ilioinguinal, axillary or cervical block dissection) is indicated only if nodes are involved.

Radiotherapy is an alternative as a primary treatment. Radiotherapy is preferred in areas where surgery may be cosmetically disfiguring or result in a poor functional outcome (nasolabial area, inner canthus of the eye, lower eyelid). Radiotherapy is also useful as an adjuvant; to treat recurrences; to manage nodal disease or for palliation.

Cryotherapy has been used successfully for small and localised lesions.

Case 4.4 Basal cell carcinoma

Q   **Describe what you see.**

A   There is a raised ulcerated lesion on the lateral aspect of the left lower eyelid. There are visible telangiectasia within the skin and the edge of the ulcer is pearly-pink in colour. This lesion is most likely to be a basal cell carcinoma (BCC).

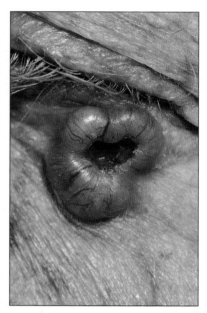

Fig. 4.4.1

Q   **What are the clinical types of basal cell carcinoma?**

A   Five types are recognised clinically:

Nodulocystic: most common type, present as dome-shaped nodules with telangiectasia of the overlying skin which may be thinned giving it an almost translucent appearance.

Ulcerative: rodent ulcer, the raised or rolled pearly edge with central umbilication is characteristic.

Pigmented: pigmentation (brown or black) is seen more commonly in patients with dark skin.

Morphoeic: appears like a flat white or yellowish, scar-like plaque with a central depression.

Superficial (multicentric): thin pink, scaling plaque with well defined edge. Usually occur in the trunk.

Q   **What are the clinical features of a typical ulcerated basal cell carcinoma?**

A   It commonly occurs in the upper part of the face above a line drawn between the corner of the mouth and the lobule of the ear. It classically has a well-defined margin and an indurated, raised (rolled) edge with a pearly glistening beaded appearance at some part of the circumference. Small ulcers may have a central depression (umbilication) with a scab. There is usually no regional lymphadenopathy.

Q   What is the differential diagnosis of basal cell carcinoma?

A   ***Nodular lesions***   should be differentiated from dermal cellular naevi, sebaceous gland hypertrophy, keratoacanthoma, benign skin adnexal tumours, dermatofibroma, malignant fibrous histiocytoma and molluscum contagiosum.

Ulcerative lesions   need to be differentiated from a squamous cell carcinoma (shorter history, more exuberant growth, everted edges and nodal metastasis are characteristic of SCC).

Pigmented lesions   may resemble a melanoma. But they have a brown hue as opposed to a dusky greyish brown colour of melanoma. Seborrhoeic keratosis and compound naevus are other lesions that may appear like pigmented BCC.

Morphoeic lesions   may be mistaken for a scar or scleroderma (morphoea).

Superficial lesions   need differentiation from Bowen's disease, discoid eczema and psoriatic plaques.

Q   What are the various ways of treating a basal cell carcinoma?

A   ***Surgical excision***   is the treatment of choice as most lesions are small and amenable to simple excision and primary closure. A margin of 3–5 mm is considered adequate. Larger lesions with evidence of induration beyond the visible lesion, morphoeic lesions and recurrent lesions require a 1 cm margin. Larger lesions may also need a local rotation or transposition flap to cover the defect.

Curettage and diathermy   is an option for small lesions.

Radiotherapy   is an effective treatment for large lesions, as BCC is a radiosensitive tumour. Morphoeic lesions are an exception in that they are radio-resistant.

Moh's micrographic surgery   involves mapping and serial excision, the completeness of which is confirmed by microscopic examination of wet preparations of tissue in the same session. It allows for ensuring clear margins while at the same time preserving as much of normal tissue as possible. Its value is in vital areas such as the face where tissue preservation is a prime concern, in recurrent lesions and in morphoeic lesions which may extend beyond the macroscopically visible margins.

Cryotherapy   also gives good results.

Cytotoxic agents   applied topically (5-fluorouracil, methotrexate, podophyllin) are useful in small but symptomatic BCCs in bedridden or frail patients.

Case 4.5 Melanoma

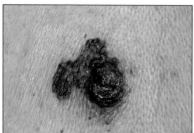

Fig. 4.5.1

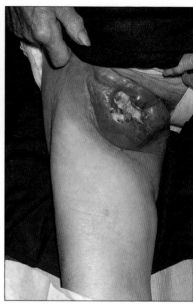

Fig. 4.5.2

Q   **Describe these lesions.**

A   Figure 4.5.1 is a superficial, spreading, pigmented skin lesion, which is raised in part. This lesion is most likely to be a superficial spreading melanoma. Figure 4.5.2 has occurred in an elderly woman who has previously undergone excision of a malignant melanoma from the right lower leg and represents ulcerated metastatic spread to the inguinal lymph nodes.

Q   **What types of melanoma are you aware of?**

A   Clinicopathologically four classical types are recognised, namely:
   Superficial spreading: common in females, on the legs and are usually macular.
   Nodular: common in males and in the trunk.
   Acral lentiginous: occur typically in the palms and soles.
   Lentigo maligna melanoma: occur classically in the sun-exposed areas, especially face.

   Clinical variants which may fall into any of the above types are occasionally seen. Examples are the desmoplastic type (associated with a significant fibrotic reaction), neurotropic type (tends to spread along cutaneous nerve trunks and cause pain), subungual type (occurring under the nails) and amelanotic melanoma (which lacks the dark pigmentation).

Q What is the differential diagnosis of a melanoma?

A
- histiocytoma (dermatofibroma)
- inflamed seborrhoeic keratosis (basal cell papilloma)
- melanocytic naevi
- pigmented basal cell carcinoma
- pyogenic granuloma (for amelanotic melanoma)
- small thrombosed hemangioma
- subungual haematoma (for subungual melanoma)
- thrombosed plantar wart.

Q What features of a melanoma would help differentiation from most of the other lesions that may resemble melanoma?

A Though there is no single feature which is diagnostic, a constellation of characteristics is quite typical of a melanoma.

History: Presence of itching and any recent change in size, shape or colour, are important features.

Examination: Size >7 mm, irregular and asymmetric borders, variable colour within the lesion (which may for example appear as an irregularity of the usual halo around the lesion), bleeding, crusting and oozing are vital clinical pointers to the diagnosis.

Q What are the components of physical examination of a suspected melanoma?

A Melanomas are very aggressive tumours that disseminate by local, lymphatic and haematogenous routes. So, even though the primary lesion appears relatively small, a thorough regional and systemic examination should be performed.

The lesion:
Inspection (use a hand lens if available): site, size and extent with respect to anatomical landmarks, shape especially symmetry, colour, margin, surface, discharge/bleeding, floor (if ulcerated).

Palpation: temperature, tenderness, consistency, compressibility, pulsatility, fixity, induration of the base and surrounding tissues.

The region:
Presence of satellite and in-transit nodules.

Regional lymphadenopathy (bilateral particularly if on the trunk or close to midline).

Evidence of locoregional neurovascular compromise or musculoskeletal invasion (if relevant).

Rectal examination (when relevant) – sometimes the primary could be in the anal canal and asymptomatic with an in-transit lesion on the anterior upper thigh which may be the presenting feature (anal canal drains to the inguinal nodes).

The system:
Examine for possible hepatic metastasis – icterus, hepatomegaly, ascites.
Lung metastasis: pleural effusion, pleural rub.
Soft tissue/skeletal and neurological examination as relevant.

Q **If you are asked to excise this lesion, how would you plan your margins?**

A An initial excision biopsy should be performed with 1–2 mm margins. Definitive treatment in terms of margins would be guided by Breslow thickness (measured by a micrometer from the granular layer of the epidermis to the deepest penetrating cell). The guidelines are:

Thickness <1 mm: 1 cm margin
Thickness 1–2 mm: 2 cm margin
Thickness >2 mm: 3 cm margin (some authorities suggest a 2 cm margin).

Case 4.6 Keratoacanthoma

Q **Describe this lesion.**

A There is a domed-shaped lesion, with a central crater containing keratin, at the lateral angle of the left eye. The lesion is most likely a keratoacanthoma.

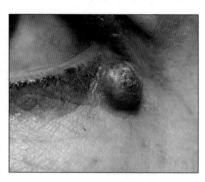

Fig. 4.6.1

Q **Describe the clinical course of a keratoacanthoma.**

A It starts as a nodule in the light exposed skin. It increases in size relatively rapidly over a few weeks after which it remains static for a few weeks before remitting in 3–4 months.

On examination, it is solitary, skin coloured, crateriform nodule with crusting or a small central ulceration with no discharge. It is non-tender, with no rise in basal temperature. It is well-defined, has a rubbery firm consistency with no surrounding induration. It is non-pulsatile, non-compressible and non-fluctuant. There is no regional lymphadenopathy.

Q **What is the differential diagnosis of a keratoacanthoma?**

A Squamous cell carcinoma and basal cell carcinoma should be excluded.

Q **How would you treat keratoacanthoma?**

A Observation is an option if diagnosis is certain, as it tends to involute. Simple excision with primary closure may be performed if it is suspicious and histological proof is necessary. Curettage and diathermy, cryotherapy are the other options. Keratoacanthoma may be a pleasant histological surprise when a lesion thought to be a skin cancer has been excised.

Case 4.7 Ganglion

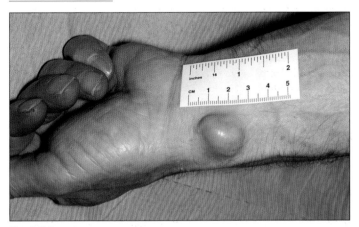

Fig. 4.7.1

Q **Describe this lesion.**

A There is a 2 cm smooth, hemispherical swelling on the plantar surface of the left wrist overlying the radiocarpal joint. The lesion is most likely a ganglion.

Q **What is a ganglion?**

A A ganglion is a cystic soft tissue lesion which is formed by myxomatous degeneration of fibrous tissue. It has a thick capsule, which is not lined by epithelium and contains a clear, gelatinous, 'glassy' fluid. It may be attached to the joint capsule or a tendon, but does not communicate with the joint.

Q **What are the common sites for a ganglion?**

A The carpal area of the dorsum of the hand, volar side of wrist and fingers, lateral aspect of the dorsum of foot, around the ankle and knee areas and along the spine.

Q   **What are the clinical features of a ganglion?**

A   An otherwise asymptomatic swelling occurs in a typical site with normal appearing overlying skin. The swelling is rounded, non-tender, non-pulsatile, usually non-compressible, with a smooth or bosselated surface. Consistency is variable with the larger lesions being soft and fluctuant while the smaller ones feel firm. Mobility may be restricted. The ganglion should be examined with the underlying joint in different positions.

Q   **What is the differential diagnosis of a ganglion?**

A   Bursae and synovial protrusions occurring around joints may present like ganglia.

Q   **Are you aware of any lesions with a similar histology occurring elsewhere?**

A   Cystic encapsulated lesions, which are histologically identical to a soft tissue ganglion, are known to occur in subperiosteal, intraosseous, intraneural locations and in the meniscus of the knee.

Q   **How should a ganglion be managed?**

A   If small and asymptomatic, it may just be observed. Excision is an alternative. Because of its close relation to joints and tendons, the surgery may need to be performed under a tourniquet for safe dissection and complete excision. Fenestration with a wide bore needle has also been described, but may be associated with a high recurrence rate. Recurrence even after surgical excision is as high as 30–50%.

Case 4.8 Pyogenic granuloma

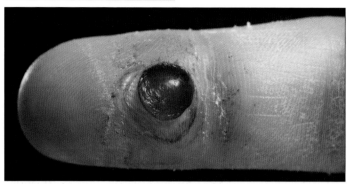

Fig. 4.8.1

Q What is the most likely diagnosis of the lesion shown? What causes it?

A It is a pyogenic granuloma. The exact aetiology is unknown, but it is thought to be a reactive lesion secondary to trauma. The role of infection is uncertain. Despite its name, it is neither pyogenic nor granulomatous.

Q What are the typical findings on clinical examination?

A It is a red, pink or bluish black, pedunculated or sessile lesion, protruding from the skin surface measuring <1 cm (but may occasionally grow to 5 cm in size). It is soft, non-tender, partly compressible, non-pulsatile and bleeds on contact. The surface may be smooth or verrucous and it may discharge or become crusted.

Q What are the common sites of pyogenic granuloma?

A Hands, feet, lips, head and neck are the common areas. It may also occur in the mucosa of oral cavity and anal canal.

Q Can histopathology explain the clinical findings?

A Yes. Pathologically it is a proliferation of small blood vessels, set in a gelatinous stroma, which erupts through a breach in the epidermis. The epidermis forms a collar at the base or may partly envelope the lesion. It lacks collagen but is rich in mucin. Plump endothelial cells are surrounded by mast cells, plasma cells, fibroblasts and when there is a surface erosion, by neutrophils.

Q Are you aware of any histopathologically identical lesions occurring in other areas of the body?

A Yes. The three conditions known, which have an identical histological picture to pyogenic granuloma, are:
- granuloma gravidarum of the oral cavity
- juvenile angiofibroma of nasopharynx
- urethral caruncle.

Q What other lesions should be differentiated from a pyogenic granuloma clinically?

A The diagnosis of a typical pyogenic granuloma is straightforward. However, the following lesions may sometimes closely resemble a pyogenic granuloma:
- ulcerated or nodular melanoma
- inflamed seborrheic keratosis
- angioma
- glomus tumour
- Kaposi's sarcoma
- metastatic carcinoma
- molluscum contagiosum
- viral warts.

Q How are pyogenic granulomas managed?

A
- surgical excision with coring out of the stalk
- diathermy
- cryosurgery.

Case 4.9 Parotid adenoma

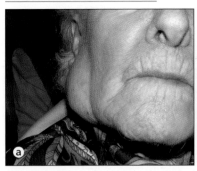 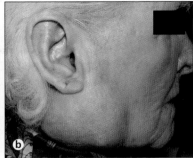

Fig. 4.9.1a,b

Q What abnormality can you see on this patient's face?

A There is enlargement of the right parotid gland.

Q What are the main components of examination of a parotid gland?

A The position and size of the mass should be assessed and described in relation to local landmarks: ear lobule, angle of mandible, masseter muscle.

Other features of a mass in general, such as tenderness, temperature, surface, consistency, fixity, and fluctuation are assessed.

Oral inspection and bimanual examination should be performed to assess the deep lobe and the opening of the parotid duct.

Regional lymph nodes should be examined.

Facial nerve palsy has important prognostic and therapeutic considerations and is vital aspect of parotid assessment.

Contralateral parotid and other salivary glands (submandibular, sublingual) and dryness of the eyes and mouth should also be assessed.

Q What is the differential diagnosis of a unilateral parotid mass?

A The following possibilities may have to be considered in a unilateral swelling in the region of the parotid gland:
- dental cysts
- epidermoid cyst
- hypertrophy of masseter
- lipoma
- lymphangioma
- mandibular tumours
- mastoiditis
- myxoma of masseter
- neuroma of facial nerve
- parotid metastasis
- preauricular lymphadenopathy
- temporal artery aneurysm
- branchial cysts and parasitic cysts (from cystic parotid tumours such as Warthin's tumour and cystic pleomorphic adenoma)
- winged mandible (in the first arch syndrome).

Q What are the indicators of malignancy in a parotid gland?

A Pain, facial nerve palsy and metastasis indicate malignancy. In addition, rapid increase in size, skin tethering and skin ulceration should also arouse suspicion.

Q Are there any tumours unique to the parotid gland?

A Papillary cystadenoma lymphomatosum (Warthin's tumour) occurs only in the parotid gland. It is seven times more common in men and occurs most commonly in the seventh decade. About 10% are bilateral. They are clinically soft and may be fluctuant.

Q **Are there any peculiar features of an adenoid cystic carcinoma?**

A There are three features which distinguish an adenoid cystic carcinoma of the parotid. Perineural spread is common and it may spread along the trunks of the cranial nerves to the brain. About 20% of them present with facial nerve palsy. Haematogenous spread is also common to the lungs. Lastly, despite its dissemination, it is a slow growing tumour and 5-year survival rates are in the region of 60–80%.

Q **What are the salient principles in managing parotid tumours?**

A Incision biopsy is contraindicated for a parotid mass. This is because two-thirds of the tumours are pleomorphic adenomas and biopsy risks extra-capsular seeding which leads to multifocal local recurrences that are difficult to treat. Exceptions are when the skin is ulcerated or when the chance of malignancy is high. Fine needle aspiration cytology is a useful diagnostic tool, which does not carry the risk of seeding.

Preoperative cross-sectional imaging (CT, MRI) should be performed to evaluate the extent of disease and to assess the deep lobe.

For benign tumours involving the superficial lobe only, a superficial parotidectomy is performed with facial nerve sparing. In tumours involving the deep lobe, a total conservative parotidectomy is performed. Recurrences of pleomorphic adenoma may be treated by radiotherapy.

In malignancy, the procedure of choice is total parotidectomy, with facial nerve sparing whenever possible. In adenoid cystic carcinoma, however, the nerves (facial, auriculotemporal, greater auricular) should be excised widely. Facial nerve reconstruction could be considered.

Postoperative radiotherapy is considered if clearance is not adequate. Lymphadenectomy is only performed if nodal spread is proven.

Case 4.10 Wound infection

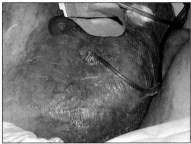

Fig. 4.10.1

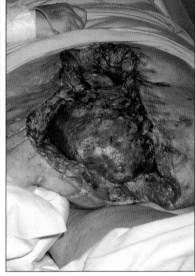

Fig. 4.10.2

Q   **Describe what you see.**

A   • There is a superficial spreading cellulitis of the anterior abdominal wall in a patient who has recently undergone a laparotomy and formation of stoma.

  • There is a dehiscence of a midline laparotomy wound. The bowel is contained within the peritoneal cavity by a layer of granulation tissue.

Q   **How are surgical site infections defined?**

A   A superficial incisional surgical site infection is one which occurs within 30 days of surgery and involves the skin and subcutaneous tissue of the incision. A deep incisional surgical site infection is one which occurs within 30 days of the surgery (or within 1 year if an implant is left *in situ*) and involves the deep soft tissues (fascia and muscle). The defining criteria for an infection itself are variable and there is no universal consensus. Widely accepted criteria include the presence of pus or isolation of a pathogenic organism in the context of local signs of inflammation. Disputed definitions include those that consider the presence of one or a combination of inflammatory signs sufficient (without objective demonstration of a pathogenic organism or the need for the presence of pus); subjective labelling of infection by the health care worker and the surgeon laying the wound open for suspected infection.

Q   **What are the various ways a wound infection might present and what complications may it cause?**

A   *Localised signs:*
- signs of acute inflammation: Calor (heat), rubor (erythema), dolor (pain), tumour (swelling), and loss of function (functio laesa)
- discharge (purulent or non-purulent).

Locoregional complications (usually with the above signs):
- spreading cellulitis
- abscess
- skin or flap necrosis
- wound dehiscence
- gas gangrene (crepitus)
- necrotising fasciitis
- prosthetic infection (e.g. mesh).

Systemic complications:
- otherwise unexplained postoperative pyrexia
- septic shock
- organ failure
- protracted infection over a large area may lead to malnutrition and hypoalbuminaemia (usually related to sepsis)
- may sometimes serve as a source for a distant infection, e.g. seeding of a prosthetic heart valve. This may however be difficult to prove.

Q   **What are the principles in managing a laparotomy wound infection?**

A   Management starts with establishing a diagnosis and making an early assessment of the risk factors; the probability of an underlying serious cause and the severity of infection. In relevant situations, consider and rule out possible prosthetic infection, anastomotic leak and deep wound dehiscence. The presence of any of these complications would need individualised care.

Uncomplicated, localised infections without a spreading cellulitis or evidence of an underlying collection, in the absence of pyrexia may be managed conservatively. Wound swabs and mapping of the wound may be necessary. Removal of sutures or staples to ensure drainage should be undertaken if there is a significant discharge or collection. The wound is left open to heal by secondary intention or may be closed later when clean (secondary suture). Antibiotic treatment is necessary only for locally invasive infection or systemic sepsis.

Wounds with necrotic tissue require debridement. A dressing that preserves moisture and absorbs effluent should be chosen. Multiple dressing changes and irrigation may be necessary. Topical negative pressure therapy (vacuum assisted closure) may be of value in managing large wounds.

Necrotising fasciitis is life threatening and should be treated with urgent wide excision of involved tissues down to healthy bleeding tissue and systemic broad-spectrum antibiotics.

Q **What may an infection occurring in the region of the wound many weeks or months after an operation signify?**

A Infections which present late may have a specific cause related to the surgery or to an underlying disease process in the patient. The causes that need to be explored depend on the site of operation (laparotomy wound versus a breast wound), type of initial surgery (implant or non-implant), the primary pathology which necessitated the surgery (such as Crohn's disease or malignancy) and co-morbidity of the patient (such as diabetes, AIDS).

Foreign bodies (such as non-absorbable suture material, a piece of gauze, a surgical instrument, spilled gallstones) or an implant (mesh, vascular graft, joint prosthesis) may underlie the wound infection and may need special imaging and individualised management including removal.

There may be an ongoing underlying pathology such as osteomyelitis (usually over a leg or foot in a diabetic patient). Crohn's disease may fistulate through a laparotomy wound. Local recurrence after an abdominoperineal resection or radiation for cancer may present as a breakdown and present with a discharge of a perineal wound with or without true infection.

Case 4.11 Pilonidal sinus

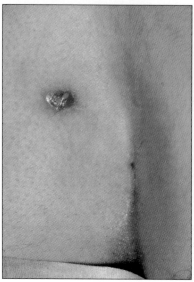 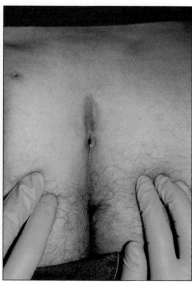

Fig. 4.11.1   **Fig. 4.11.2**

Q   **Describe these lesions.**

A
- There is a punctum (or a pit) in the natal cleft which is most probably the external opening of a pilonidal sinus. There is also an erythematous swelling laterally suggestive of an abscess pointing to the skin

- There is a discharging sinus in the natal cleft of a patient who has previously undergone excision of pilonidal disease.

Q   **What are the clinical and epidemiological associations of sacrococcygeal pilonidal sinus?**

A   *Ethnicity:*   higher incidence in whites
       Age: 80% occur between ages 20–29
       Gender: four times more common in men
       Occupation: hairdressers, drivers
       Body habitus: obesity, being dark haired, being hirsute.

Q   **Does a pilonidal sinus occur elsewhere in the body?**

A   Yes. Though the sacrococcygeal pilonidal sinus occurring in the natal cleft is the most common type, it is also known to occur between the fingers and toes, at the umbilicus and in the axilla.

Q   **What clinical problems does the pilonidal sinus disease pose?**

A   Recurrent inflammation with pain and discharge, abscess formation, protracted healing of the raw areas created in the region either during the natural course of the disease or after surgical treatment; high incidence of wound breakdown due to infection and recurrence of pilonidal disease with simple treatment methods are the major problems.

Q   **What would you find on clinical examination?**

A   There is usually a depressed pit in the midline in the sacrococcygeal region (natal cleft) with or without visible hairs protruding. There may be a spontaneous discharge or a discharge expressible on pressure. There may be evidence of scarring or deep induration. There may be multiple openings in and around the midline. The openings usually do not extend between the coccyx and the anus, which if present should alert one to the possibility of a fistula in ano, or anorectal Crohn's disease.

   If it is inflamed or formed an abscess the abscess component would display all features of a subcutaneous abscess.

Q   **What are the treatment options for a pilonidal sinus?**

A   A number of treatments are available. The principles are to achieve ablation of all the tracts, to choose methods that reduce hospital stay and time to return to work in the short term and to prevent recurrence in the long term.

   In the acute presentation (abscess), incision and drainage and leaving the wound open is standard treatment.

   In an elective presentation, one of many options may be chosen. Methods that avoid a midline closure are associated with the best long-term results.

Non-surgical techniques
Sclerosant injection and cryotherapy have a limited role.

Surgical techniques without significant surrounding tissue recruitment:
Lord's procedure: excision of tracts with small localised incisions and brushing with lateral drainage when necessary.

Wide excision and leave wound open with or without marsupialisation. Wounds take a long time to heal, but use of a vacuum device (vacuum assisted closure) reduces healing times.

Wide excision and simple primary midline closure: various suturing techniques are described, but may have high recurrence rates.

Surgical techniques with tissue mobilisation:
These aim to achieve one or both of: (1) lateralising the main suture line; (2) making the gluteal furrow shallow. They may or may not involve flaps.

Examples are Z-plasty; V–Y-plasty, Karydakis flap; Bascom cleft technique and Limberg flap.

Case 4.12 Fibroadenoma

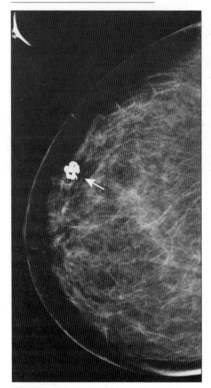

Fig. 4.12.1

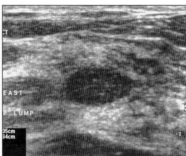

Fig. 4.12.2

Q **What do these radiological investigations show?**

A
- The mammogram shows a stippled 'popcorn' like density in the lateral left breast, these appearances are classical of a calcified fibroadenoma.

- The ultrasound scans show an echogenic lesion with minimal post acoustic shadowing. These appearances are classical of a non-calcified fibroadenoma.

Q **What are the features of a fibroadenoma on clinical examination?**

A On inspection there are usually no visible abnormalities unless the fibroadenoma is large or superficial, when a hemispherical smooth elevation of the contour may be seen. Specifically, there is no distortion, puckering or dimpling of skin or peau d'orange nor is there nipple retraction.

On palpation, there is a smooth, rubbery firm, well-defined, regular, non-tender, non-compressible, non-fluctuant, mobile lump in the breast, typically in the upper outer quadrant (but may occur anywhere). Mobility is the single most characteristic feature ('breast mouse'). Sometimes more than one may be found in the same breast and if more than five are present, then the diagnostic term multiple fibroadenomas is used (this is rare).

Retroareolar fibroadenomas and those in older women may have restricted mobility.

Axillary examination does not reveal any regional lymphadenopathy.

Q   What are the types of fibroadenoma?

A   *Common type:*   measure 1–3 cm
Superficial type: measure up to 4 cm and lie close to the skin
Giant fibroadenoma: measure >5 cm in size.

Q   What is the differential diagnosis?

A   Breast cysts and fibroadenosis are the usual differential diagnoses. In older women, due to calcification and restriction of mobility, features may simulate a carcinoma. Giant fibroadenomas should be differentiated from phyllodes tumours.

Q   How should fibroadenomas be managed?

A   Diagnosis should be confirmed by a combination of assessments: clinical examination, imaging (mammogram or ultrasound) and cytology (FNAC). Small fibroadenomas (<4 cm) may be observed provided the diagnosis is certain, if asymptomatic and the patient is in agreement. In larger lesions, symptomatic cases and those in which there is a suspicion of malignancy, excision biopsy is performed.

Q   What would you tell a patient who is anxious about the natural history of a fibroadenoma?

A   Fibroadenomas are not neoplasms, but are aberrations of normal development and involution (ANDI). After an initial growth phase to reach 2–4 cm, about 70% remain static, 15–30% regress and about 5–10% progress in size. There may sometimes be sudden variation in size such as during pregnancy, as fibroadenomas are responsive to hormonal influences. They may sometimes undergo degeneration.
    The risk of malignant change in a fibroadenoma is very low (<1:1000). If and when it occurs, it is usually a lobular carcinoma, usually an earlier mis-diagnosis.

Case 4.13 Thyroglossal cyst

Q   A 16-year-old male has presented with a thyroglossal cyst. What would you expect when he protrudes his tongue? Why?

A   A thyroglossal cyst moves upwards on protruding the tongue. This is due to a failure of the migratory tract of the thyroid to obliterate.

Q   Where may the cyst occur?

A   The cyst can occur anywhere along the thyroglossal duct from the lingual foramen caecum to the thyroid isthmus.

Q   **What investigation must be performed prior to surgery?**

A   A radioiodine uptake scan I^{123} should be performed since the cyst may contain some or all of the thyroid tissue (rare). If the thyroid is located within the cyst then the cyst should be excised leaving the thyroid tissue behind. Care should be taken to preserve the blood supply of the thyroid.

Q   **Describe the surgical management.**

A   The patient is positioned supine, with the neck extended by 20°, and the table placed in the foot down position. A transverse incision centred over the cyst is made. Superior and inferior flaps are developed. The cyst is dissected out and is excised in continuity with the tract and the body of the hyoid bone. The duct is dissected out proximally to the foramen cecum. The middle portion of the hyoid bone is excised as the cyst usually transverses the body and has a high recurrence rate if left in-situ (Sistrunk's procedure).

Case 4.14 Multinodular goitre

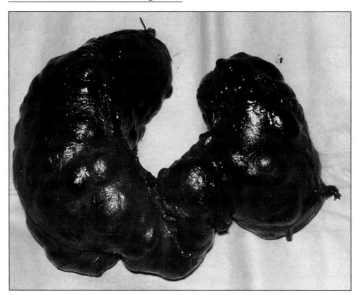

Fig. 4.14.1

Q   **What is this pathological specimen?**

A   Multinodular goitre.

Q How would you proceed to examine an anterior neck swelling suspected to be of thyroid origin?

A *General examination:*
Look for signs of thyroid dysfunction (hypo- or hyperthyroidism).

Thin build, anxious disposition, warm sweaty hands, tremors, eye signs (lid lag, lid retraction, exophthalmos, chemosis, ophthalmoplegia), tachycardia are indicative of thyrotoxicosis. While obesity, apathy, psychomotor retardation, puffiness of face, coarse voice, rough-dry skin and slow reflexes are indicative of hypothyroidism.

In a large goitre with suspected malignancy, observe for Horner's syndrome (ptosis, miosis, enophthalmos and anhidrosis) due to involvement of the sympathetic trunk.

Observe for evidence of superior vena-caval obstruction.

Examination of the neck:
The neck should be examined from the back and the front.

Inspection:
Observe overlying skin: prominent veins, scars.

Confirm it is a thyroid swelling: movement with deglutition (other swellings which move on deglutition are thyroglossal cyst, subhyoid bursitis, pretracheal or prelaryngeal lymph node fixed to trachea and larynx, respectively).

If it is high in the neck, does it move on protrusion of tongue (thyroglossal cyst)?

Extent of the swelling.

Is the lower limit seen?

A small goitre may be made to appear prominent by asking the patient to extend the neck and raising the hands to support the occiput (Pizzillo's method).

A retrosternal goitre causing superior vena-caval obstruction causes facial suffusion and precipitates dizziness when the upper limbs are raised vertically upwards so that the sides touch the ears (Pemberton's sign).

Palpation:

The thyroid
● confirm movement on swallowing
● size, shape and extent, lower limit
● are both lobes enlarged?
● examine each lobe individually when possible
● surface: smooth/nodular/bosselated
● consistency: soft/firm/hard.

The tracheal position. Is there evidence of tracheal softening by chronic pressure: pressure on the goitre directed towards the trachea precipitates stridor (Kocher's test)?

The lymph node basin: anterior and posterior triangles, bilaterally. Note number, size, mobility and consistency.

The carotid arteries: benign swellings push the carotid arteries posteriorly but do not obliterate the pulse, whereas malignancies may engulf the carotid making the pulsations non-palpable (Berry's sign).

Percussion: dullness over sternal-manubrium in retrosternal goitre.

Auscultation: bruit over thyroid in primary toxicosis or stridor in tracheal compression.

Indirect laryngoscopy: to assess vocal cords.

Q **What is the differential diagnosis of a multinodular goitre?**

A History and physical examination usually are sufficient to make a diagnosis of multinodular goitre. However, the following conditions may occasionally present with a nodular gland.

- anaplastic carcinoma
- Hashimoto's thyroiditis
- medullary carcinoma
- multicentric differentiated thyroid cancer
- simple diffuse goitre with haemorrhage into cysts.

Q **How would you treat a patient with multinodular goitre?**

A ***Observation:***   In patients who are not symptomatic and there is no malignancy.

Surgery: Large goitre, pressure symptoms, proof or suspicion of malignancy, retrosternal extension or reduced quality of life (cosmetic).

Both lobes are nodular: Total thyroidectomy with post-operative thyroxine.

Only one lobe is nodular: Lobectomy or hemithyroidectomy (with isthmus).

Radioactive Iodine ablation (10–30 millicuries)   is an alternative in patients who are not surgical candidates, especially if associated with a dominant toxic nodule. It is sometimes useful in recurrences after earlier thyroid-conserving surgery.

Case 4.15 Solitary thyroid nodule

Q **What are the causes of a solitary thyroid nodule?**

A The causes may be grouped into neoplastic and non-neoplastic causes.

Neoplastic causes are:
- carcinoma
  - primary (papillary, follicular, medullary, primary thyroid lymphoma, anaplastic carcinoma)
  - secondary (carcinoma, lymphoma)
- adenoma
  - follicular (colloid, fetal, embryonal, Hürthle cell)
- other rare causes: lipoma, hemangioma, teratoma.

Non-neoplastic causes are:

- dominant nodule in a multinodular goitre (most common cause of an apparent solitary nodule)

- focal thyroiditis

- cysts of the thyroid or parathyroids; thyroglossal cysts

- hyperplasia: agenesis of a lobe with contralateral hyperplasia, remnant hyperplasia (post-surgical, post-radiation therapy).

Q **Short of fine needle aspiration biopsy (FNAB), what features on thyroid evaluation in general would suggest a benign or malignant nature of the underlying pathology?**

A Thyroid lumps are notoriously difficult to predict with accuracy on clinical grounds alone. However, gross judgements about the relative probabilities may be made based on a few useful features.

Features in history: Residence in an iodine deficient area and family history of a simple goitre may suggest a benign cause while a definite exposure to radiation in childhood, a family history of medullary carcinoma or multiple endocrine neoplasia and presence of obstructive symptoms with a relatively small swelling would raise the possibility of a malignant cause. A thyroid lump in a child should be regarded as malignant. Rapid growth (over 4 weeks) is a worrying feature. For a given lesion, older age and female gender would be relatively low risk categories when compared to younger patients and males.

Clinical examination: A solitary, firm to hard nodule, enlarged regional nodes and vocal cord palsy suggests a malignancy compared to a soft lump or a presence of multinodularity in the rest of the gland.

Serology: A high level of autoantibodies may suggest thyroiditis while a raised calcitonin level suggests medullary carcinoma.

Imaging: A hot nodule on a radioiodine scan is unlikely to be malignant whereas a cold nodule has a 20% chance of being malignant. A purely cystic lesion on ultrasonography is likely to be benign.

Q **What is the value of FNAB? Does FNAB in thyroid disease have any shortfalls?**

A FNAB is a useful test in thyroid disease and should be performed in all solitary nodules, in any suspicious nodule in a diffusely enlarged gland and to evaluate palpable lymph nodes. It may also be of therapeutic value in thyroid cysts. Some of the situations where one may choose not to perform it are Graves' disease and an obviously hot nodule on radionuclide scan with no other suspicious features. With a false negative rate of about 5% and a false positive rate of less than 1%, FNAB is the first line investigation in the evaluation of thyroid swelling.

However, FNAB performed blindly may suffer from sampling errors leading to a false negative result. A certain proportion of cytological reports, are indeterminate (C1) and hence are non-contributory. Together, this means that cytology is useful if it identifies a definite malignant lesion but cannot be relied upon if it is negative when there are other indicators (clinical, imaging) of a suspicious lesion.

FNAB cannot differentiate a follicular adenoma from a follicular carcinoma. Similarly, Hashimoto's thyroiditis and Hürthle cell adenomas; certain anaplastic carcinomas and lymphomas may be difficult to differentiate.

Q **What other tests may be helpful?**

A Ultrasonography of the thyroid nodule would differentiate a cyst from a solid mass and is useful in guiding FNAB and aspiration of cysts. Ultrasonography is capable of assessing the rest of the thyroid and find additional nodules not felt clinically. It is also useful in evaluating the neck for any regional adenopathy.

Radioactive iodine scanning (Tc^{99m} or I^{123}) is not routinely indicated, but may be useful in identifying a toxic adenoma and identifying a dominant nodule in a diffuse toxic goitre.

Thyroid hormone assays, antithyroid antibodies and serum calcitonin are other useful tests in relevant situations, but they need not be performed routinely.

Musculoskeletal and neurology

Case 4.16 Ruptured long-head of biceps

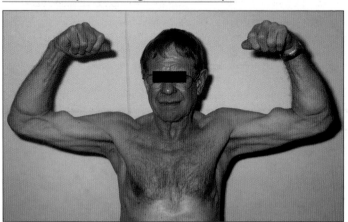

Fig. 4.16.1

Q **Describe the abnormality seen.**

A This man has bilateral ruptures of the proximal long-head of biceps, i.e. the bellies of the biceps muscles are lower and rounder.

Q   **What is the mechanism of injury?**

A   The tendon of the long-head of biceps, like that of the supraspinatus tendon usually ruptures near its scapular origin. The mechanism of injury is a gradual fraying and degeneration of the tendon on the underside of the acromion usually secondary to a repetitive movement.

Q   **How does the condition present clinically?**

A   The usual presentation is in a male aged over 50 years. While lifting, he feels a snap in a previously normal shoulder. The shoulder and arm aches for a while and is commonly bruised, due to subcutaneous bleeding. The pain resolves after a few days. On examination, the arm usually appears normal until the patient flexes his elbow to produce a prominent lump.

Q   **How is this condition treated?**

A   Rupture of the long-head of biceps proximally, results in near normal flexion and only 10–15% reduction in power as the short head of biceps continues to function and hypertrophies. Therefore, treatment is usually unnecessary, however, surgical repair may be offered to sportsmen, e.g. weightlifters.

Q   **What other injuries can occur to this structure?**

A   A rare injury is a tear to the distal biceps tendon. This results from a flexion injury in a previously healthy tendon. The patient reports pain in the lower forearm with local bruising and reduced flexion and supination of the elbow. The tendon is repaired surgically if the diagnosis is made early.

Case 4.17 Below-knee amputation

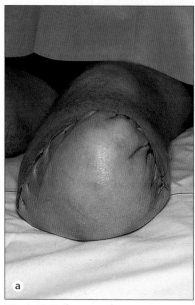

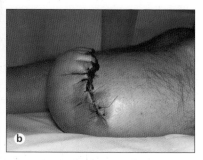

Fig. 4.17.1a,b

Q   **Describe what you see.**

A   This is a patient with a left below-knee amputation.

Q   **What are the indications for a below-knee amputation?**

A   Indications for a below-knee amputation include: ischaemia secondary to peripheral arterial disease, gangrene of the leg due to any cause, thrombo-angiitis obliterans (Buerger's disease), trauma causing severe multiple bony injuries, extensive full-thickness burns, untreated compartment syndrome, malignancies including connective tissue and bony tumours, severe spreading soft tissue infections refractory to conventional treatment, meningococcal septicaemia, chronic osteomyelitis, severe painful neuropathy as in diabetes mellitus, vasculitis secondary to connective tissue diseases, arteriovenous aneurysms, major ulceration in the limb and defective wound healing. In many instances, one or more of the above factors may be involved (neuropathy due to diabetes mellitus causing undetected trauma leading to ulceration; infection may supervene leading to non-healing and gangrene). However, the commonest causes are critical ischaemia from an acute arterial occlusion, acute-on-chronic ischaemia, and failed arterial reconstruction.

Q   **How would you perform a long posterior Burgess flap?**

A   The Burgess technique uses a long posterior flap which employs the posterior calf muscles to cover the transected bones. The incision extends from the medial border of the tibia horizontally across the front of the leg to the lateral border of the leg, approximately, 15 cm below the tibial tuberosity. Another method of arriving at the correct level of amputation is to measure 1 inch below the tibial tubercle for every foot of the patient's height. This leaves a reasonable stump to fit a prosthesis without leaving it too long, which can make subsequent limb fitting difficult. The incision then extends vertically down the leg on either side and joins across the calf just above the origin of the Achilles tendon. If the posterior flap is too long, this can be trimmed later when the muscles are thinned.

Q   **What are the complications of a below-knee amputation?**

A   The common complications could be divided into early, intermediate and late:

    Early complications include: Bleeding from the suture line, wound haematoma, wound infection (particularly in diabetics), flap breakdown and wound pain.

    Complications during the *intermediate period* include: Joint pain, joint contracture at the level of the knee, wound pain, phantom sensation and phantom pain.

    Late complications include: Knee joint pain, joint contracture, joint instability, pain due to pressure from ill-fitting prosthesis, phantom pain, stump neuroma, stump oedema due to proximal venous constriction, bulbous stump, unstable stump due to too much soft tissue left behind, stump fracture, skin maceration, blisters, abrasion, callosities, follicular hyperkeratosis, bone spur formation due to periosteal bone formation, osteoporosis, severe scarring in the stump or other cosmetic problems.

Case 4.18 Hallux valgus

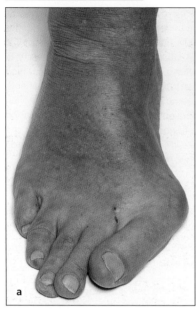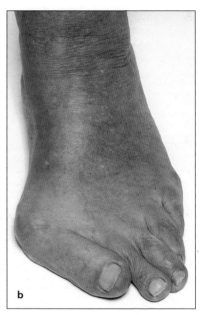

Fig. 4.18.1a,b

Q   **Describe what you see.**

A   There are bilateral hallux valgus deformities.

Q   **What is hallux valgus?**

A   Hallux valgus denotes the lateral deviation of the great toe. It is due to the prominence of the medial eminence of the first metatarsal head with or without an overlying bursa (the bunion); an osteophyte may also accompany this. Hallux valgus causes pain at the first metatarsophalangeal joint and the patient has difficulty in obtaining appropriate footwear; although inappropriate footwear may often lead to hallux valgus. This condition is more common in females with a 10:1 female to male ratio.

Q   **What is the aetiology of hallux valgus?**

A   The aetiology of hallux valgus is not clear. It may be hereditary since there is a strong familial predisposition. Systemic diseases such as rheumatoid arthritis, gouty arthritis and psoriatic arthritis may predispose to the formation of hallux valgus. However, the vast majority of cases are due to environmental factors, such as poorly fitting footwear (as in pointed shoes) and constant friction over the first medial metatarsal joint.

Q   **What changes do you expect to see radiologically?**

A   Radiological examination should be carried out in full weight bearing and in two planes. The first metatarsal head may be deviated medially and dorsally. As the first metatarsal splays dorsally, greater stress is placed on the central metatarsals, especially the second, leading to hyperostosis and occasionally stress fractures. The other main feature seen on a plain radiograph is medial exostosis (bunion).

Q   **How would you manage this condition?**

A   The factors to be considered while deciding the management options include the patient's level of activity, the state of their peripheral vasculature and their ability to cope with the treatment. The management is divided into conservative and surgical. Conservative management consists of: (1) adequate rest; (2) application of moist heat; (3) relieving pressure over painful bunion prominence; (4) correcting any functional factors such as excessive pronation and Achilles tendon tightness; (5) providing properly fitted, low-heeled stiff-soled shoes; (6) providing functional foot orthosis to be worn 5–6 hours a day and (7) splinting to separate first and second toe.

   Surgery includes: metatarsal osteotomy, exostectomy, excision arthro-plasty (Keller's operation) and arthrodesis (joint fusion). Metatarsal osteotomy corrects the deformity by moving the whole toe and metatarsal head laterally, and is the most common operation performed in young patients. Fusions are sound enough to allow free function after 6 or occa-sionally 8 weeks. About 5% of arthrodeses fail, but even then a painless, non-union is deemed to be successful. If the joint remains painful, the procedure may be repeated using an intramedullary bone graft across the joint, which should be kept protected for 6–8 weeks.

Case 4.19 Osteoarthritis of the hands

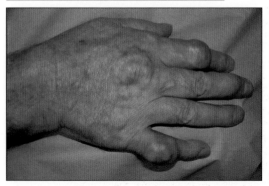

Fig. 4.19.1

Q   **Describe the changes you can see in this patient's hand.**

A   Bouchard's nodes are seen on the index and little finger. These are consistent with a diagnosis of hand osteoarthritis.

Q   **What is the origin of these changes?**

A   Heberden's nodes occur at the distal interphalangeal joints in familial generalised osteoarthritis. Bouchard's nodes occur at proximal interphalangeal joints. Both of these nodules result from osteophytes and synovial thickening at the margins of an osteoarthritic joint. The square thumb deformity is also seen in osteoarthritis of the hand and results from a deformity of the thumb carpometacarpal joint.

Q   **What is the usual clinical presentation?**

A   Osteoarthritis of the hands is a very common condition in post-menopausal women. The condition usually starts with pain and swelling in one or two fingers. Initially the distal joints are affected first with the proximal joints affected later. Eventually all the fingers on both hands are affected. On examination, there is reduced movement in the joints.

Q   **What changes would you expect to see on a plain radiograph?**

A   Narrowing of the joint spaces and osteophyte formation.

Q   **How is the condition managed?**

A   Patients are initially treated conservatively with analgesia, reduction of movements and thumb splints. If patients remain symptomatic, then surgical intervention may be undertaken. Surgery usually takes the form of joint arthrodesis.

Case 4.20 Rheumatoid hands

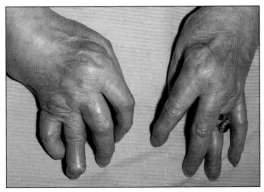

Fig. 4.20.1

Q   Describe the abnormalities in these hands.

A   There is bilateral ulnar deviation of all the fingers with synovial thickening around the metacarpophalangeal joints. There is also a boutonnière deformity of the left ring finger. These changes represent rheumatoid arthritis in the hands.

Q   Explain the underlying nature of these deformities.

A   Rheumatoid arthritis affects the synovium resulting in synovitis of the joints and is particularly common in the hands and wrists due to the numerous joints. The extensor tendon sheaths are affected producing the characteristic deformity of radial deviation at the wrist and ulnar deviation of the fingers. The tendons over the involved joints erode and may rupture producing a boutonnière (button hole) deformity (central slip of the extensor expansion detaches from its insertion at the base of the middle phalanx allowing the two slips to fall sideways and the proximal interphalangeal joint to protrude between them). A swan-neck deformity occurs by flexion at the metacarpophalangeal joint, proximal interphalangeal joint extension and flexion at the distal interphalangeal joint.

Q   What signs would you expect to see on a plain radiograph?

A   Early radiological signs are osteoporosis and soft tissue swelling. Later there is loss of joint space with small periarticular erosions. A late sign is joint deformity and dislocation.

Q   How is this condition managed?

A   Initial management is aimed at controlling the systemic disease and local synovitis by the use of oral anti-inflammatories and immunosuppressants and intra-articular injection of steroids. Pain is controlled with analgesia and splints. Disease progression may warrant surgical intervention. The choice of surgical intervention is based on a careful assessment of the patient's disability and likely benefit. Synovectomy is occasionally performed for uncontrolled synovitis. Isolated tendon ruptures are treated with primary repair or tendon transfer (extensor indicis proprius). Joint involvement is treated with arthrodesis or replacement arthroplasty.

Case 4.21 Fracture of the clavicle

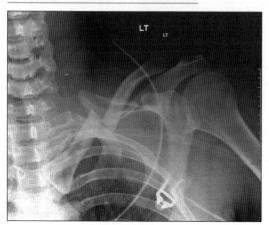

Fig. 4.21.1

Q **What is the diagnosis?**

A A displaced fracture of the mid-shaft of the left clavicle.

Q **What is the usual mechanism of injury?**

A A fracture of the clavicle is one of the most common fractures in all age groups. The usual mechanism of injury is a fall, landing on the tip of the shoulder causing a large upwards and backwards force causing the clavicle to fracture. This results in the outer fragment being pulled down by the weight of the arm, while the inner half is held up by the sternocleidomastoid muscle. Patients present clinically with swelling and tenderness at the fracture site, a bone spike may be palpable if it has not pierced the skin. Fractures which are displaced cause the shoulder to become displaced anteriorly and inferiorly.

Q **How is this injury classified?**

A Clavicular fractures are divided into:
- mid-shaft (80%)
- lateral to coracoclavicular ligament (15%) and further subdivided into:
- undisplaced, displaced and intra-articular extension
- medial (5%).

Q   **What is the treatment of this injury?**

A   Accurate reduction is not possible therefore the treatment consists of analgesia and a broad arm sling for support. The sling should be worn by children for 3–5 weeks and adults for 6 weeks. Displaced fractures lateral to the coracoclavicular ligament usually require surgical fixation with a tension band wire or plate and screws. Mid-shaft fractures may require open reduction and internal fixation if there is a neurovascular injury, open fracture or an associated scapular fracture.

Q   **What potential complications can occur?**

A   *Malunion:*   is inevitable because the fragments are displaced by the weight of the arm. In children, the bone soon remodels but in adults a slight angulation usually persists.

Non-union: occurs in 1–2% of clavicular fractures and is usually asymptomatic. Internal fixation with bone grafting is required if symptomatic.

Neurovascular injuries: Splinters of bone can penetrate the subclavian vessels or brachial plexus. Displaced fractures may also cause a direct lung injury or pneumothorax.

Callus formation: Prolific callus formation especially in children can cause a lump at the fracture site which can interfere with school bag straps. The lump reduces in size with bone remodelling over time.

Q   **What other injuries may occur by the same mechanism of injury?**

A   *Acromioclavicular dislocation:*   results from disruption of the fibrocarti-laginous disc. These injuries are usually treated with broad arm slings. Marked dislocation may require surgical fixation.

Sternoclavicular dislocation: These injuries are treated conservatively. The patient should be warned of the risk of subsequent subluxations.

Case 4.22 Supracondylar fracture

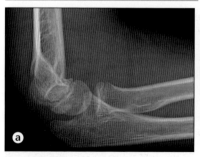 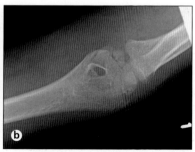

Fig. 4.22.1a,b

Q   **What is the diagnosis?**

A   A supracondylar fracture of a right humerus in a child.

Q   **What radiological signs corroborate this diagnosis?**

A   The distal fragment is tilted anteriorly, the anterior fat pad is elevated and a posterior fat pad is also present in addition to the fracture line. The radiographs in a child should be compared with those from the non-affected elbow.

Q   **Describe the usual mechanism of injury.**

A   Supracondylar fractures of the humerus are most frequently seen in children. The usual mechanism of injury is a fall on the out-stretched hand or from a direct blow to the elbow. A fall on the outstretched hand results in hyperextension of the elbow, with the olecranon impacting against the posterior aspect of the humerus to produce the fracture.

Q   **What complications may develop from this injury?**

A   Complications with this type of fracture are common and can be divided into vascular, nerve injury, compartment syndrome or malunion. Vascular injuries occur in 5% of fractures and result from the brachial artery becoming kinked over the anterior prominence of the proximal fragment, or from laceration. The distal circulation should be checked carefully and recorded in the patient's notes. Nerve injuries occur in 7% of fractures and can affect the radial, median or ulnar nerves. Muscle swelling in the anterior compartment can result in a compartment syndrome and is characterised by increasing excessive pain and finger paraesthesia. Missed compartment syndromes result in Volkmann's ischaemic contracture (necrotic muscle replaced with fibrous scar tissue). If the fracture is not reduced into a good anatomical position then malrotation or sideway angulation results in a permanent deformity.

Q   **What is the management?**

A   Displaced fractures require urgent reduction under general anaesthetic with traction and counter-traction, followed by correction of any side-ways, tilt, flexion of the elbow and correction of posterior tilt. It is important to check the distal pulses following reduction. Reduction is confirmed on radiograph and the arm held in a collar and cuff.

Case 4.23 Ankle fracture

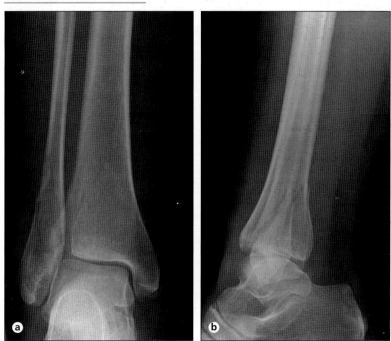

Fig. 4.23.1a,b

Q   **What is the diagnosis?**

A   There are undisplaced fractures of the right distal tibia and fibula.

Q   **What is the usual mechanism of injury?**

A   The usual mechanism of injury is a stumble over an obstacle or a fall from a height, twisting the ankle with respect to the leg. These mechanisms produce fractures at the medial malleolus of the tibia, distal fibula (lateral malleolus) or the posterior margin of the tibia (posterior malleolus). Bruising and swelling usually appear rapidly and there may be a marked deformity.

Q   **What other structures may be affected?**

A   The ligaments around the ankle joint may also be torn. The three ligaments at risk of injury are: the inferior tibiofibular ligament, the medial ligament and the lateral collateral ligament.

Q   **How is this injury classified?**

A   Ankle fractures are classified by the Danis–Weber classification. This classification is based on the level of the fibular fracture. Type A: the fracture is below the syndesmosis (tibiofibular ligament); Type B: the fracture is at the syndesmosis; Type C: the fracture is above the syndesmosis causing disruption of the syndesmosis resulting in an unstable fracture.

Q   **How is this injury managed?**

A   Swelling is rapid, if the fracture is not reduced within a few hours; definitive treatment is deferred while the swelling subsides with elevation. Most Type A and Type B fractures are treated with closed reduction and plaster casting. Large medial malleolar fragments require open reduction and placement of a screw. Type C fractures are unstable and require accurate replacement by open reduction and internal fixation with a long oblique screw.

Case 4.24 Head of humerus fracture

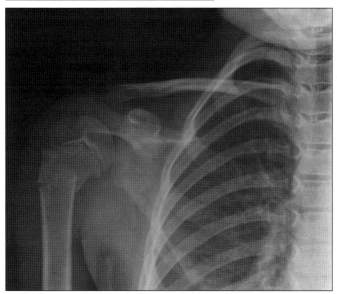

Fig. 4.24.1

Q   **What is the diagnosis in Figure 4.24.1?**

A   There is a minimally displaced fracture through the surgical neck of the right humerus in a child.

Q   **What is the mechanism of injury?**

A   Proximal humeral fractures are one of the most common fractures. They occur more commonly from middle age onwards in osteoporotic bones. They result from a fall on the outstretched hand or a fall onto the shoulder. Proximal humeral fractures in children result from similar mechanisms of injury in previously healthy bones.

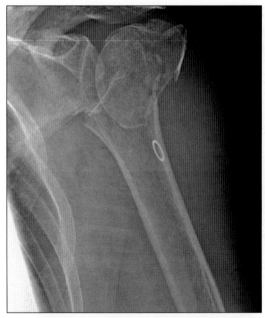

Fig. 4.24.2

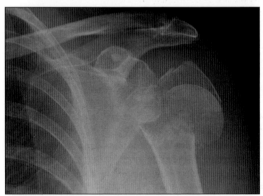

Fig. 4.24.3

Q   **How are these injuries classified?**

A   Neer's classification of proximal humeral fractures is used to provide a
guide for management and is as follows:

> ***One part fracture:***   undisplaced/impacted.
> ***Two part fracture:***   displaced >1 cm or angulated >45° (see Fig. 4.24.1).
> ***Three part fracture:***   displaced fracture plus one displaced tuberosity
> (see Fig. 4.24.2).
> ***Four part fracture:***   displaced fracture plus two displaced tuberosities
> (see Fig. 4.24.3).

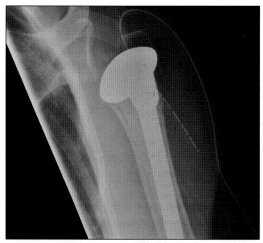

Fig. 4.24.4

Q **What complications may occur with this injury?**

A Neurovascular injuries from displaced bone fragments, i.e. axillary nerve, brachial plexus.

Rotator cuff injuries and shoulder dislocation.

Avascular necrosis in three and four part fractures.

Q **How is this injury managed?**

A Children are mostly treated conservatively even with marked angulation or displacement as they have a greater ability for remodelling. Support is provided with a collar and cuff sling for 4 weeks followed by mobilisation. With a collar and cuff sling the hand should be held as high as possible, this allows the elbow to hang, enabling the weight of the arm to produce traction on the fracture keeping it in alignment. Most fractures in adults are also treated conservatively with a collar and cuff. Surgical intervention is indicated in two part fractures if there is neurovascular injury or significant displacement. Most surgical interventions involve closed manipulation under anaesthetic. Occasionally open reduction and internal fixation is required. Three and four part fractures require fixation with K-wires or cannulated screws. Hemiarthroplasty is usually recommended in elderly patients (see Fig. 4.24.4).

Case 4.25 Forearm fracture

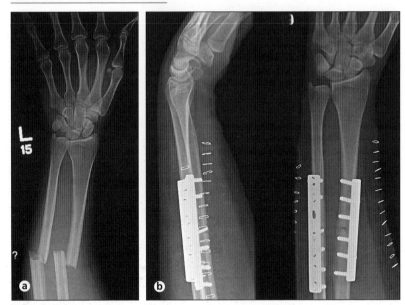

Fig. 4.25.1a,b

Q   **What is the diagnosis?**

A   There are displaced fractures of the mid-third of the left ulna and radius.

Q   **What is the usual mechanism of injury?**

A   Forearm fractures commonly involve both the radius and ulna, which fracture at different levels. Isolated fractures of the ulna or radius are unusual. They usually result from a twisting or fall on the outstretched hand, or from a direct blow. Single forearm bone fractures are commonly associated with a fracture dislocation as the force of the injury is usually transmitted to the proximal or distal radioulnar joints. These fracture dislocations are known as:

   Monteggia: ulnar fracture with proximal radioulnar (radial head) dislocation.
   Galeazzi: radial fracture with distal radioulnar dislocation.

   Forearm fractures usually present with an obvious deformity with pain and swelling over the fracture site.

Q   **What are the potential complications of this injury?**

A   **Compartment syndrome:** results from bleeding and oedema around the fracture resulting in an increase in pressure within the fascial compartment. Failure to recognise the condition results in a Volkmann's ischaemic contracture.

Malunion: Failure to reduce the fracture satisfactorily results in malunion and a loss of supination.

Cross union: Fracture of the ulna and radius may unite as healing progresses resulting in a loss of supination and pronation.

Non-union: results if rotation of the fracture is allowed to occur.

Persistent dislocation: usually results from a failure to recognise the dislocation at the time of injury.

Q How is this injury managed?

A Greenstick fractures with no obvious deformity are treated conservatively with a below elbow cast. Any deformity requires a closed manipulation under general anaesthetic and a full-length cast (axilla to hand). Adult fractures are inherently unstable and require open reduction and internal fixation with plates and screws (Fig. 4.25.1b). A full-length cast is usually also applied to abolish potential rotation. Fracture dislocations require open reduction, internal fixation and relocation of the joint.

Case 4.26 Osteoarthritis of the knee

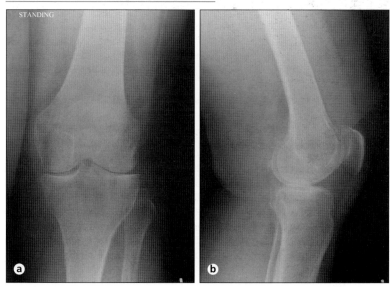

Fig. 4.26.1a,b

Q Describe the features on the radiographs in Fig. 4.26.1a and b.

A There is narrowing of the joint space with sclerosis of the weight-bearing surface. The lateral compartment is worst, although there is involvement of all three compartments of the knee. These changes are consistent with a diagnosis of osteoarthritis. Other radiological changes which can occur include: osteophyte formation around the joint margins and subchondral cyst formation.

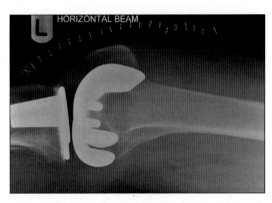

Fig. 4.26.2

Q   **What is the pathophysiology of this condition?**

A   Osteoarthritis is a degenerative joint disease resulting from a failure of the articular surface to regenerate. Direct or indirect trauma causes a breach in the articular cartilage resulting in a rough surface. Friction on the rough surfaces generates particles of cartilage, which act as foreign bodies when shed into the synovium. Clinically, the inflammatory response causes stiffness and aching of the joint after exercise. Eventually cartilage erosion exposes the subchondral bone. Bone moving on bone causes pain and micro-fractures (abnormal weight distribution within the joint) which heals by callus formation and gives the bone a sclerotic appearance on radiograph. Cysts are produced by synovial fluid being pushed into the exposed cancellous bone under pressure. Remodelling of the bone at the margin of the joints causes osteophyte formation.

Q   **How is this condition treated?**

A   Initial management of osteoarthritis is conservative by explanation and reassurance, analgesia (non-steroidal anti-inflammatory drugs), increased joint mobility (exercises and physiotherapy) and load reduction (walking stick). If symptoms worsen despite conservative measures then surgery is recommended. Younger patients may be offered realignment osteotomy to avoid joint replacement. The indications for joint replacement (hemi- or total) (Fig. 4.26.2) are unrelieved pain and progressive disability.

Q   **Describe the procedure of total knee replacement.**

A   The skin is incised in the midline from the quadriceps to the tibial tubercle. The incision is deepened through the medial side of the patella in the knee joint while rotating the patella to expose its articular surfaces. The infra-patella fat pad and meniscus are excised. The femoral and tibial surfaces are then cut to size using jigs supplied for the chosen prosthesis. The tibia is retracted, and the proximal and distal components are inserted into the femur and tibia respectively following the insertion of cement. The patella is trimmed and reduced to its anatomical position. The joint capsule and extensor apparatus are closed over two suction drains with interrupted absorbable sutures. Postoperative radiographs are taken to check the position and the patient is encouraged to mobilise following removal of the drains.

Vascular cases

Case 4.27 Varicose veins

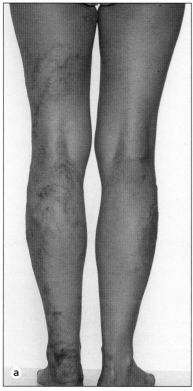

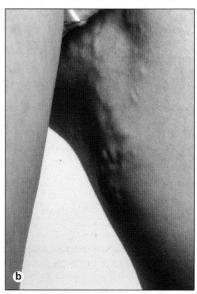

Fig. 4.27.1a,b

Q   **This 35-year-old woman has presented with prominent varicose veins of her left leg. Describe the clinical examination of varicose veins.**

A   The patient is examined standing in a warm room. The whole of the lower limb and abdominal wall are examined, to define the pattern of varices, skin changes and signs of chronic venous insufficiency. A tourniquet test (Brodie–Trendelenburg) or hand-held Doppler is used to define the source and level of the incompetence. Other useful clinical manoeuvres which are not commonly performed are: (1) the cough impulse test (Morrissey's test) – when a thrill is elicited on coughing with fingers placed over the region of an incompetent saphenofemoral junction; (2) the percussion or tap sign (Schwartz test) – tapping the varicosity in the lower leg causes the wave to be conducted uninterruptedly in the presence of valvular incompetence and be felt by the observing finger placed in the groin; (3) Perthes' test for deep vein patency – superficial veins are occluded by a tourniquet around the thigh and the patient asked to walk around for 5 minutes. If deep veins are not patent, the manoeuvre causes severe pain and prominence of the varicosities; (4) Fegans' method of location of perforators – the veins are decompressed with the patient supine and leg elevated. Palpation with a finger along the path of the varicosities reveals depressions with sharp margins corresponding to the site of perforators. Arterial pulses are palpated and if absent ankle-brachial pressure indices (ABPI) are performed.

Q   What is the most likely underlying disorder?

A   Varicose veins are due to valvular failure due to degeneration or developmental weakness. The most common type is incompetence of the saphenofemoral junction with or without perforator incompetence. The venous hypertension that ensues underlies the clinicopathological manifestations. Rarely an intra-abdominal mass compressing the major veins or an arteriovenous fistula may be contributing to the venous hypertension.

Q   What complications may occur if left untreated?

A   If varicose veins are left untreated, the patient may develop 'chronic venous insufficiency'. This condition is characterised by mild to moderate swelling, skin changes (varicose eczema, pigmentation due to haemosiderin deposits and fibrosis leading to lipodermatosclerosis) and ulceration.

Q   What are the indications for surgery?

A
- cosmetic appearance
- symptoms (swelling, aching, cramps, itching, tingling)
- recurrent superficial thrombophlebitis
- bleeding
- eczema
- ulceration.

Q   What are the contraindications for surgery?

A   Previous deep vein thrombosis (with demonstrable loss of patency of the deep venous system) is a contraindication as the patient maybe relying on the superficial venous system for venous return.

Q   Describe the surgical management.

A   The varicosities are marked preoperatively with the patient standing up. For isolated saphenofemoral incompetence the patient is positioned supine with 10° head down to partially decompress the varicose veins. A groin crease incision is made, centred over the saphenofemoral junction. The saphenofemoral junction is identified. Initially the venous tributaries (superficial circumflex iliac, superficial external pudendal, superficial epigastric and others) are ligated and divided. The long saphenous vein is ligated at the saphenofemoral junction ('flush ligation', 'high tie'). The long saphenous vein thus disconnected is stripped to the level of the knee or upper third of the leg. Multiple phlebectomies are then performed through stab incisions over the pre-marked varicosities ('stab avulsions').

Q   What is the recurrence rate?

A   The recurrence rate is quoted at 20%. However, the majority of these patients have persistent varicose veins, which were never adequately removed at the first operation. Recurrence rates are higher in short saphenous varicosities compared to long saphenous.

Case 4.28 Venous ulcer

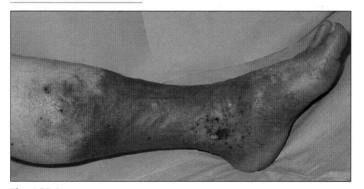

Fig. 4.28.1

Q   This 68-year-old man has presented with recurrent ulceration on the medial aspect of his left lower leg, what is the most likely aetiology?

A   There is a superficial ulcer with an irregular margin and sloping edges centred over the left medial malleolus. There is also surrounding lipo-dermatosclerosis. These findings would make a venous aetiology most likely.

Q   Describe the pathophysiology of this type of ulceration.

A   The underlying cause is impairment of venous return from the limb due to reflux, obstruction or calf pump failure. This leads to sustained venous hypertension and ultimately ulceration.

Q   **Describe the usual skin changes which the skin goes through prior to ulceration.**

A   Ulceration is usually preceded first by the formation of dry scaly skin (varicose eczema). This skin is friable and may become infected with scratching. Deposition of haemosiderin in the tissues produces the characteristic brown discoloration. The skin also becomes oedematous which with time becomes fibrotic and non-pitting. This fibrosis along with the haemosiderin deposition is known as lipodermatosclerosis. Ulceration usually results on the background of these skin changes from minor trauma. Ulceration predominately occurs on the medial aspects of the lower legs.

Q   **How should this ulceration be assessed?**

A   These patients need to be assessed to verify if the ulceration is of a purely venous origin (80%) or is due to a mixed arteriovenous origin. This is performed through clinical assessment and by assessing the ankle-brachial pressure index (suspect an arteriovenous origin if the ABPI <0.9). It is also important to exclude other possible aetiological causes, i.e. diabetes, rheumatoid arthritis. A venous Duplex is usually performed to exclude obstruction of the venous system if there has been a history of deep venous thrombosis, and to ascertain the presence of deep or superficial venous reflux.

Q   **How should this ulcer be treated?**

A   The ulcer is assessed clinically for evidence of infection and treated with topical antimicrobials or systematic antibiotics if present. A skin punch biopsy may be taken for microbiological assessment if there is any doubt. Eczema is treated with topical steroid ointments. The patient is advised on rest and elevation of the limb, to reduce oedema. Graduated elastic compression is applied to the affected limb by means of either bandages or stockings. These systems should apply pressure of 40 mmHg at the ankle graduated to 18 mmHg at the knee.

     NB Graduated compression should not be applied in the presence of arterial disease or obstruction of the venous system due to previous deep vein thrombosis.

Q   **What measures can be taken to lower the risk of recurrence?**

A   To lower the risk of recurrence (>70%) following healing, patients are advised to continue to wear graduated compression stockings. These patients should also be offered superficial venous surgery as this has also been shown to reduce the risk of recurrence.

Case 4.29 Thoracic outlet syndrome

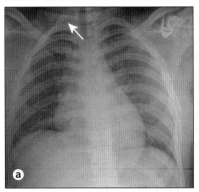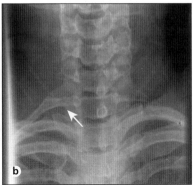

Fig. 4.29.1a,b

Q   **What do these radiographs show?**

A   A well-developed right cervical rib and a rudimentary left cervical rib.

Q   **What symptoms may be produced?**

A   The symptoms of thoracic outlet syndrome are due to compression of the vascular structures or nerves transversing the cervico-axillary canal. Arterial compression produces a spectrum of symptoms from mild aching through to painful ischaemia. Symptoms are precipitated by movement of the upper arms. Compression of the lower trunk of the brachial plexus produces ulnar nerve paraesthesia. Deep vein thrombosis may also result from compression.

Q   **What is the aetiology of the condition?**

A   The neurovascular structures become compressed between the clavicle and a rudimentary cervical rib, band or the scalenus anterior muscle.

Q   **How is the condition diagnosed?**

A   A full history is obtained including the impact on the patient's quality of life and trigger factors. The patient is examined in the sitting and standing positions. The supraclavicular fossa is palpated for a cervical rib, band or aneurysm. Tests performed at physical examination may be grouped into three categories: (1) shoulder girdle manipulation tests (Adson's test, hyperabduction test and military position or bracing manoeuvre); (2) exercise stress test (Roos' test); (3) brachial plexus palpation precipitating neurological symptoms (Spurling's sign). In the Roos' test, the fingers are opened and closed slowly with the arms held above the head. Roos' test is considered positive if the patient's symptoms are precipitated within 3 minutes. Duplex ultrasonography of the subclavian artery while performing Roos' test helps to confirm the diagnosis.

Q   Describe the treatment of this condition.

A   Patients with mild symptoms are given an explanation of the condition and advice on how to avoid provocative movements. Physiotherapy with exercises designed to lengthen the scalene muscles may also help. If symptoms are more severe then surgery is recommended. Surgery is aimed at decompressing the cervico-axillary canal. The thoracic outlet is approached through a supraclavicular incision. The clavicular fibres of sternocleidomastoid are divided. The phrenic nerve is retracted off scalenus anterior, prior to dividing this muscle. The subclavian artery sheath is divided and the artery retracted upwards to identify the cervical rib. The rib is then divided with bone-nibblers close to the vertebral articulation.

Case 4.30 Neuropathic ulcer

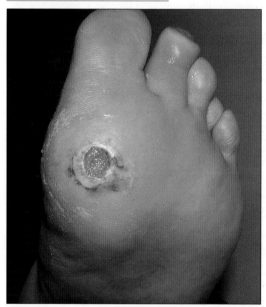

Fig. 4.30.1

Q   Figure 4.30.1 is a photograph of a 71-year-old male who has presented with a new ulcer on the plantar aspect of his left foot, what is the most likely aetiology?

A   This ulcer has most likely resulted from diabetic neuropathy.

Q   Describe the aetiology of this type of foot ulceration.

A   Diabetic foot ulceration is due to neuropathy in 45–60% of cases, 10% are due to arterial ischaemia and the rest are due to both neuropathy and ischaemia. The prevalence of neuropathy is approximately 20% in diabetic patients, with the majority of these being asymptomatic. Diabetic patients with neuropathy may also have autonomic neuropathy which results in a warm foot with bounding pulses and dry cracked skin. The majority of patients with diabetes develop arterial disease, with the distribution being more frequently below the knee. Neuropathy itself does not lead to spontaneous ulceration. Ulceration of the insensitive foot occurs when the ischaemic skin is subjected to trauma.

Q **What steps can be taken to prevent the 'at risk' foot proceeding to ulceration?**

A It is important to identify patients at risk of ulceration. Patients with diabetes should be screened annually by a nurse or doctor. This process requires an examination of the foot looking for: dry cracked skin (sign of autonomic neuropathy); ulceration; neuropathy (tuning fork, mono-filament); ischaemia (absent pulses, poor capillary refill, ABPI <0.9); and foot deformities. The management of diabetic foot problems requires a multidisciplinary team (diabetologist, diabetic nurse specialist, foot surgeon, vascular surgeon, chronic pain specialist, podiatrist, orthoptist and tissue viability nurse) approach. Patient education remains a central plank of treatment, as most risk factors are modifiable

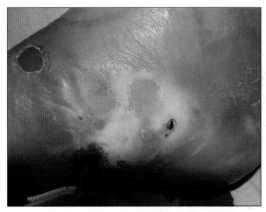

Fig. 4.30.2

Q **How should diabetic foot ulceration be managed?**

A When a diabetic patient presents with foot ulceration it is important to identify the aetiology, e.g. neuropathic, neuroischaemic etc. and whether infection is present. The patient should be assessed for ischaemia and neuropathy. A plain radiograph of the foot should also be performed if the ulcer is deep, to identify possible osteomyelitis. The size and shape of the ulcer should be recorded and any surrounding callus should be excised. Neuropathic ulcers require pressure relief by the use of appropriately prescribed footwear, worn in- and outdoors. More extensive neuropathic ulcers require bed rest or off-loading, e.g. total contact casting. Purely ischaemic or neuroischaemic ulcers require vascular intervention where appropriate. Ischaemia may result in necrosis and gangrene if the foot is not re-perfused. Local infections (red, swollen, malodorous) are treated with oral antibiotics and antiseptic dressings. More severe infections (Fig. 4.30.2) (abscess formation, crepitus, gangrene) require surgical de-bridement and a prolonged course of intravenous antibiotics. Osteomyelitis requires prompt diagnosis (isotope bone scan, MR scanning) and prolonged treatment with antibiotics with good bone penetration, e.g. Clindamycin, Ciprofloxacin. Unfortunately, even with aggressive treatments limb loss still occurs.

Q **What is Charcot neuroarthropathy?**

A This is a condition which affects up to 10% of diabetic patients with neuropathy and is characterised by bone and joint destruction, fragmentation and remodelling. The condition is thought to develop when an unnoticed trauma, followed by weight bearing results in a fracture and joint destruction. Typically, the patient presents with a relatively painless swollen foot. Treatment with a total contact cast is aimed at minimising bone and joint destruction. Corrective surgery may be attempted at a later stage.

Case 4.31 Raynaud's syndrome

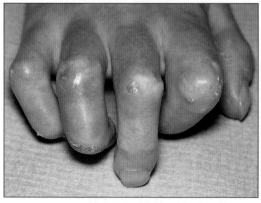

Fig. 4.31.1

Q **Describe the appearance of this patient's hand in picture Fig. 4.31.1.**

A There is tight, shiny, smooth skin on the hand. Telangiectasia can also be seen. These changes are seen in severe Raynaud's phenomenon.

Q **Describe the classification of Raynaud's phenomenon.**

A Raynaud's phenomenon describes the sequence of pallor, cyanosis and rubor in the extremities, triggered by cold or emotional stimuli. It is classified as primary or secondary Raynaud's phenomenon. Primary Raynaud's phenomenon is also known as Raynaud's disease or idiopathic Raynaud's phenomenon. A person diagnosed with Raynaud's disease has no identifiable underlying secondary disease or condition that may cause the vasospasm. Secondary Raynaud's phenomenon is more complex and is associated with other diseases such as connective tissue disorders and thoracic outlet syndrome. Secondary Raynaud's phenomenon is also known as Raynaud's syndrome.

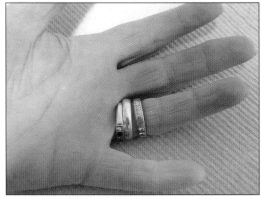

Fig. 4.31.2

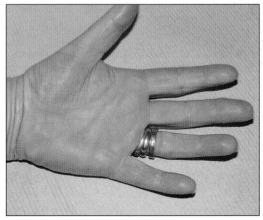

Fig. 4.31.3

Q   **Describe the classical presentation of Raynaud's phenomenon.**

A   The classical presentation of Raynaud's phenomenon in which digital ischaemia is produced by cold (Fig. 4.31.2) or emotion and is manifested by pallor (vasospasm) followed by cyanosis (deoxygenation of static venous blood) and finally rubor (reactive hyperaemia) (Fig. 4.31.3) due to the return of blood flow. However, a classical history is not essential to diagnose Raynaud's phenomenon. A history of cold-induced blanching with reactive hyperaemia may be sufficient to make the diagnosis.

Q   **What parts of the body may be affected by Raynaud's phenomenon?**

A   In addition to the digits, the vasospasm may also affect the nose tongue and ear lobes. Other organs may also be affected, e.g. brain, oesophagus and myocardium producing migraine and angina like symptoms when exposed to cold. The prevalence of Raynaud's phenomenon is 10%, with a male to female ratio of 1:9.

Q   **What is the pathophysiology of Raynaud's phenomenon?**

A   The precise pathophysiology of Raynaud's phenomenon is not completely understood, but is thought to be due to a combination of the peripheral nervous system abnormalities (α and β receptors in peripheral vessels are increased), abnormal blood cell–endothelium interactions and abnormal inflammatory and immunological responses.

Q   **How is the diagnosis made?**

A   Most cases of Raynaud's phenomenon are diagnosed on history and examination during an attack. It is important to differentiate primary and secondary Raynaud's phenomenon. The diagnosis may be confirmed by performing a baseline test using thermal imaging, or Doppler ultrasound and then exposing the patient's hands to a thermal challenge (placing the hands in luke-warm water) and then repeating the measurements.

Q   **How should the condition be managed?**

A   Patients with mild symptoms should be given an explanation of the condition and be reassured. The patients should also be advised to stop smoking and be given advice on cold avoidance. Medication, e.g. calcium channel blockers should be reserved for patients with more severe disease. In very severe cases in which the patient is at risk of losing a digit, intravenous prostaglandin therapy or chemical sympathectomy may be considered.

Case 4.32 Chronic limb ischaemia

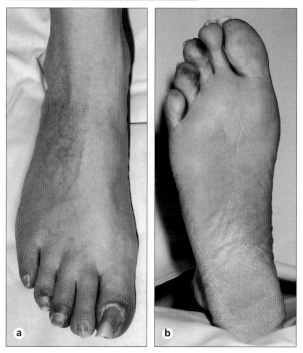

Fig. 4.32.1a,b

Q   Describe the appearance of this patient's foot and explain the significance of this investigation.

A   The right foot is pale and has trophic changes (shiny skin, hair loss and brittle nails). These changes occur in chronic lower limb ischaemia. The CT angiogram shows multiple stenoses of the right and left superficial femoral artery with occlusions of both origins. Bilaterally there is reconstitution distally and three vessel run-off. These clinical and radiological findings are likely to be the cause of symptoms of peripheral arterial disease, e.g. intermittent claudication or rest pain.

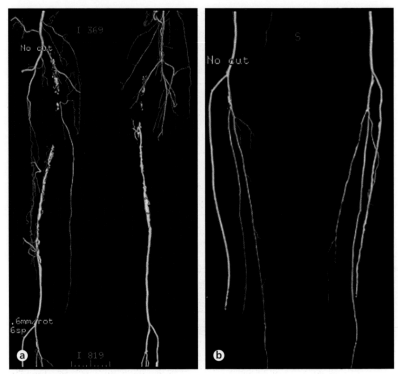

Fig. 4.32.2a,b

Q How should intermittent claudication be managed?

A Patients presenting with symptoms of peripheral arterial disease should be assessed by history, examination, ABPI, and arterial Duplex ultrasound as well as an assessment of the impact of these symptoms on the patient's quality of life. Initial management involves risk modification including smoking cessation; and optimal medical management of hypertension, hyperlipidaemia and diabetes. The patient should be prescribed an anti-platelet agent, e.g. aspirin. Patients who are not considered appropriate for surgery, should be reviewed by a vascular nurse specialist and given a structured exercise programme. These patients should be followed up by the nurse at regular intervals, to assess for concordance and improve-ments. When intermittent claudication has a major impact on quality of life, e.g. unable to carry on with employment, then medication (phosphodiesterase inhibitors), angioplasty or bypass surgery may be considered.

Q   **What are the potential complications of arterial angioplasty?**

A   Complications of angioplasty are divided into access site and distant complications. Access site complications include:

- bleeding from puncture site (ensure INR <1.5 prior to procedure, following removal of the sheath adequate pressure should be applied to the groin for at least 10 minutes)

- false aneurysm formation (small aneurysms usually resolve with compression with an ultrasound probe, while larger aneurysms require injection of fibrin or surgical closure).

Distant complications include:
- sub-intimal dissection (usually requires emergency bypass surgery)
- distal embolisation (usually requires emergency embolectomy).

Q   **What options are available for a patient presenting with critical ischaemia?**

A   Patients with critical ischaemia are at risk of limb loss in the short term. An assessment of the site of disease should be made with Duplex ultrasonography and/or intra-arterial/CT angiography. Short segment stenosis is best treated with balloon or sub-intimal angioplasty ± stent placement. Aorto-iliac segments have the best outcomes followed by femoro-popliteal interventions. For angioplasty to have a good outcome there must be a good inflow and run-off. If the pattern of disease is unsuitable for angioplasty then surgical intervention will be required. However, these patients also tend to have major co-morbidities and these should be optimised prior to surgical bypass. Patients with major co-morbidities may be best served with early amputation.

Q   **What procedure should be considered in critical ischaemia if there are no reconstructable options?**

A   As an alternative to amputation some patients may be treated with an intravenous infusion of prostacyclin (PGI_2), e.g. Iloprost. However, this tends to be poorly tolerated by some patients due to the vasodilation causing headaches and nausea. Lumbar sympathectomy (surgical or chemical) may also be attempted.

Case 4.33 Abdominal aortic aneurysm

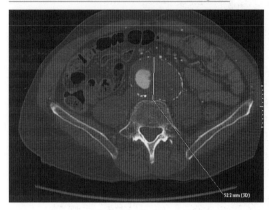

522 mm (3D)

Fig. 4.33.1

Q   **What abnormality can you see on this CT scan?**

A   There is an abdominal aortic aneurysm.

Q   **What are the risk factors for aortic aneurysm formation?**

A   The risk of developing an abdominal aortic aneurysm is greater in males (male to female ratio 4:1), advancing age, tobacco smoking, hypertension, chronic obstructive pulmonary disease; and in patients also affected by coronary, carotid or peripheral occlusive arterial disease.

The prevalence of abdominal aortic aneurysm in elderly males is 5% and has a mortality rate of 1.5% in all males over 55 years.

Q   **How should abdominal aortic aneurysm be detected and managed?**

A   Due to the high incidence of mortality for ruptured abdominal aortic aneurysm, there are moves to develop a national ultrasonographic screening programme to identify asymptomatic aneurysm in the high-risk groups. The decision to repair an abdominal aortic aneurysm should be made on an individual basis (risks of operation vs. risk of death from rupture). Most surgeons advise surgery to a patient with an aneurysm diameter >5.5 cm (if medically fit), as the risk of rupture is greater than the operative risks in aneurysms of this size.

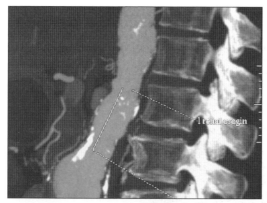

Fig. 4.33.2

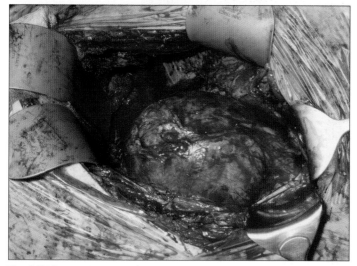

Fig. 4.33.3

Q   **Describe the operation of open abdominal aortic aneurysm repair.**

A   Preoperatively patients require optimisation of pre-existing co-morbidities (cardiac, respiratory). The morphology (i.e. neck of the aneurysm, iliac involvement) of the aneurysm is assessed by CT scanning (Fig. 4.33.2). An epidural is placed and at induction of general anaesthetic prophylactic antibiotics are administered. The patient is conventionally placed supine for a transperitoneal approach (or on the left side for a retroperitoneal approach, Fig. 4.33.3). A long midline incision is used for the transperitoneal approach. The small bowel is packed into the right upper quadrant with wet packs and the peritoneum over the aneurysm incised. The neck is dissected proximally and iliac vessels distally. The iliac vessels are clamped initially (to prevent embolisation), followed by the clamp to the aortic neck (below the left renal vein). The aneurysm sac is opened longitudinally and back bleeding controlled by over sewing the patent lumbar or inferior mesenteric arteries. A straight or bifurcated graft is anastomosed (inlayed in the aneurysm sac) with double-ended 2/0 or 3/0 Prolene sutures. The clamps are removed slowly (observing for hypotension and reapplied if there is a dramatic drop in blood pressure). The aneurysm sac is closed over the graft with 2/0 absorbable sutures.

Q **Briefly describe the technique of endovascular aneurysm repair.**

A Endovascular delivery of a vascular graft (affixed to a metallic stent) into an aneurysm, results in less trauma (no aortic cross clamping and reduced blood loss) and less pain (avoids long abdominal incision). The procedure is performed by passing the compressed graft through a small cut-down in the femoral artery and positioning it under radiological guidance in the aorta. The graft is then expanded to bridge the diseased segment. However, not all patients are suitable for endovascular repair due to the shape of the aorta (insufficient length of aorta proximally and distally to fix the graft). Complications include endoleaks (blood flow outside the graft in the aneurysm sac), graft migration and failure. Patients who have undergone an endovascular repair require annual CT scans as part of their follow-up.

Case 4.34 Popliteal aneurysm

Q **A 68-year-old male has presented with an ischaemic left foot. On examination, there is a pulsatile mass in the popliteal fossa. What is the diagnosis?**

A Popliteal aneurysm.

Q **What is the epidemiology of this condition?**

A Popliteal aneurysms are the most common peripheral aneurysm. One-third of patients with a popliteal aneurysm also have an abdominal aortic aneurysm. Half will have bilateral popliteal aneurysms. Some 95% occur in men over 65 years.

Q   **What is the clinical presentation of this condition?**

A   The normal diameter of the popliteal artery is 0.7 cm. The artery is considered to be aneurysmal if the diameter is >2 cm. Most popliteal aneurysms are asymptomatic until the patient presents with acute thrombosis, distal embolisation, rupture or local pressure effects. Acute thrombosis is the most common outcome with the patient presenting with a cold, painful leg in a previously asymptomatic limb. Outcome is variable with 20% of patients with thrombosis eventually requiring limb amputation. Distal embolisation is also a common presentation and may be acute or chronic. Rupture accounts for 4% of all presentation. It is rarely life threatening as the blood loss is tamponaded by the popliteal fossa but may cause a deep vein thrombosis due to pressure effects. Large popliteal aneurysms may impede knee flexion or press on the tibial nerve causing paraesthesia or foot drop.

Q   **Describe the treatment of this condition.**

A   All symptomatic popliteal aneurysms and asymptomatic aneurysms >2 cm should be treated surgically. Most surgeons advocate prophylactic treatment of asymptomatic popliteal aneurysms to prevent future complications. Asymptomatic aneurysms are treated with a femoro-popliteal bypass using a vein graft or prosthesis, combined with proximal and distal ligation of the aneurysm. Aneurysms causing compression are treated with resection of the aneurysm sac and anastomosis of a vein graft to the proximal and distal cut ends. Aneurysms presenting with embolisation require balloon embolectomy prior to repair. Thrombolysis performed the day prior to surgery improves the outcome for thrombosed aneurysms.

Case 4.35 Iliac occlusion

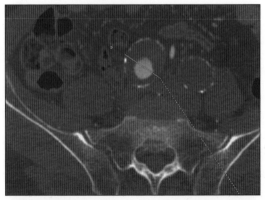

Fig. 4.35.1

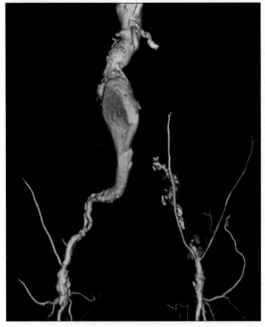

Fig. 4.35.2

Q   **What type of investigation is shown and where is the lesion?**

A   Figure 4.35.1 is a CT scan showing an aneurysm of the right common iliac artery and an occluded left common iliac artery. Fig. 4.35.2 is a reformatted CT angiogram showing an occlusion of the origin of the left common iliac artery.

Q   **Describe how this condition presents clinically.**

A   Most cases of aorto-iliac stenosis present with chronic symptoms, however a small proportion may present acutely. The typical presentation is with claudication of the lower limb (buttock, thigh or calf). Men may also present with Leriche's syndrome (diminished femoral pulses, claudication in the lower limbs and impotence). Patients may present acutely with thrombosis of the aorto-iliac segment or with distal embolisation.

Q   **How is the diagnosis made?**

A   A history and examination are taken to accurately assess the impact on the patient's quality of life and to differentiate the symptoms of aorto-iliac disease from those of femoro-popliteal disease. It is also important to exclude symptoms from a non-vascular cause, e.g. nerve root irritation. Duplex ultrasound is used to image the aorto-iliac segment, but may be obscured by bowel gas. Digital subtraction intra-arterial angiography remains the gold standard investigation, but due to the associated complications CT/MR angiography is increasingly used.

Q   **How is the condition treated?**

A   If symptoms impact on the patient's quality of life then intervention is recommended. Intervention is divided into endovascular techniques or surgery. Endovascular techniques usually involve balloon angioplasty introduced percutaneously on the contralateral side. In an attempt to prevent re-stenosis it is usual to place an endoluminal stent-graft at the same time. Surgery takes the form of aorto-iliac reconstruction, axillo-femoral or femoro-femoral bypass. Aorto-iliac reconstruction takes the form of aorto-bifemoral grafting or endarterectomy. Aorto-bifemoral bypass grafting has the best long-term patency rates but has a mortality rate of 5%. Axillo-bifemoral grafting is an extra-anatomic bypass and is indicated in patients who are unlikely to withstand aorto-bifemoral bypass grafting. Unilateral iliac disease is best treated with an extra-anatomic femoro-femoral cross-over graft.

Case 4.36 Thoracic aortic dissection

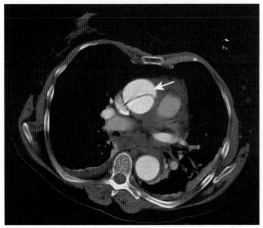

Fig. 4.36.1

Q   **What is the diagnosis?**

A   Thoracic aortic dissection.

Q   **How is this condition classified?**

A   Dissections are classified by distribution:

Type A: ascending aorta
Type B: aortic arch and distal aorta.

Q   **How does this condition usually present?**

A   Most patients with aortic dissection present with sudden, excruciating chest pain that radiates through to their back. One-quarter of patients have an audible murmur due to aortic regurgitation.

Q   **What is the pathophysiology of the condition?**

A   Acute aortic dissection results when blood enters the media through an intimal tear. As a result of hypertension and cystic medial degeneration, the tear propagates longitudinally through the aortic wall. Most intimal tears occur just above the aortic valve. Dissections are acute if they have occurred in the previous 14 days. Left untreated, 50% of patients will be dead at 48 hours. Death usually results from rupture into the mediastinum, pleura or abdomen. Other causes of death result from extension of the dissection into branch vessels producing myocardial infarction, stroke, limb ischaemia and renal ischaemia.

Q   **How is the condition managed?**

A   Emergency surgery is indicated for proximal dissections as these carry a worse prognosis. Uncomplicated distal dissections are treated medically with peripheral vasodilators. Initial management involves stabilisation of vital signs, and reduction of systolic blood pressure to approximately 120 mmHg using β-blockade. When the patient is stable they should be imaged with CT. Surgery is usually performed using cardiac bypass and circulatory arrest. Surgical repair usually necessitates the use of a tube graft to replace all of or part of the aortic arch.

Case 4.37 Symptomatic carotid artery disease

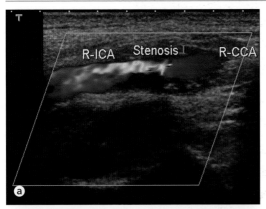

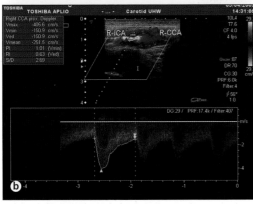

Fig. 4.37.1a,b

Q   **What do these images represent?**

A   This is a colour flow duplex and Doppler waveform of the right carotid bifurcation demonstrating a 90% stenosis of the right internal carotid artery. This is the modality of choice for assessing carotid artery stenosis, as it is accurate and non-invasive, but highly operator dependent.

Q **Which patients require investigation of suspected carotid artery stenosis?**

A The indications for investigation are transient ischaemic attacks (resolution within 24 hours of hemisensory or motor deficit affecting the face, arm and leg; homonymous hemianopia; and/or higher cortical dysfunction), amaurosis fugax (monocular visual loss) and patients with an evolving stroke. Both colour flow duplex of the carotid arteries and CT of the brain (to identify areas of infarction ± other cerebral pathologies) should be performed.

Q **Which patients should be offered carotid endarterectomy?**

A The risk of stroke increases with the severity of stenosis (the annual risk of stoke is 6% with a stenosis of 70–79%; 11% for 80–89%; and 18% for 90–99%). Large trials performed in Europe and the USA recommended that carotid endarterectomy should be performed in patients with symptomatic and asymptomatic stenosis of 70–99%. Carotid endarterectomy plus best medical treatment confers a six to ten-fold reduction in the long-term term risk of stroke in these patients. This must be compared with the perioperative risk of stoke of 4%. Recent trials have shown a benefit of carotid endarterectomy in asymptomatic stenosis of 70-99% in younger patients.

Q **Describe the operation of carotid endarterectomy.**

A The procedure is performed under local anaesthetic (cervical) block or general anaesthetic (with invasive monitoring of the internal carotid artery pressures). The carotid bifurcation is exposed through an oblique incision along the anterior border of sternocleidomastoid. The hypoglossal nerve is identified to avoid traction being applied with a retractor. Clamps are applied to the internal, common and external carotid arteries following a bolus infusion of heparin. A longitudinal arteriotomy is made across the stenosis and a shunt inserted if required. A plane is identified and developed between the plaque and the media. Once mobilised the plaque is divided proximally and distally with fine scissors. A distal intimal flap, if present, is tacked down with fine Prolene sutures. The arteriotomy is closed primarily with a running 6/0 Prolene suture or with a synthetic (Dacron) patch.

Postoperatively, the patient is assessed for neurological weakness or hypoglossal nerve injury (tongue deviates to the affected side).

Case 4.38 Deep vein thrombosis

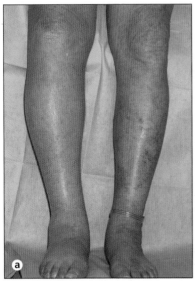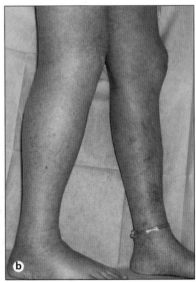

Fig. 4.38.1a,b

Q This 68-year-old man developed a low-grade pyrexia on the 5th postoperative day following repair of an abdominal aortic aneurysm. What is the diagnosis?

A Deep vein thrombosis.

Q How does this condition normally present?

A Deep vein thrombosis can present with a spectrum of symptoms ranging from being asymptomatic to causing limb threatening phlegmasia caerulea dolens. It most frequently occurs between the 5–10th postoperative days. Signs include swelling of the leg, dilatation of the superficial veins, warmth and tenderness. These signs are also often associated with a low-grade pyrexia.

Q What are the risk factors for this condition?

A Risk factors for deep vein thrombosis may be congenital (thrombophilia) or acquired. Hypercoagulability can result from thrombophilia, i.e. absence or reduction of natural anticoagulants which limit thrombosis. The naturally occurring factors include, antithrombin, protein C and protein S. Disorders of the fibrinolytic system and antiphospholipid syndrome also results in hypercoagulability.

Acquired causes include: operations causing immobility (e.g. pelvic and orthopaedic procedures), malignancy and the oral contraceptives/hormone replacement therapy.

Q   **What investigations should be performed?**

A   Clinical assessment of deep vein thrombosis is unreliable. A raised d-dimer on assay is non-specific but a useful test to exclude DVT when it is within normal limits (especially when there is a low clinical probability of DVT). Traditionally the diagnosis was confirmed with venography (injection of contrast into the distal superficial veins) but this has now been superseded by Duplex ultrasonography which is presently the definitive investigation of choice. However, false negatives are higher with Duplex, and the iliac veins are difficult to visualise due to overlying bowel gas. CT scanning with intravenous contrast is used to visualise the inferior and superior vena cava.

Q   **Describe the management of this condition.**

A   Initial management involves elevation of the limb and treatment with low molecular weight heparin (LMWH) or unfractionated heparin (UFH) to prevent thrombus propagation and pulmonary embolism. The dose of LMWH (given subcutaneously) is the equivalent that provides a total of 200 U/kg per day of anti-Xa activity. The dose in milligrams or millilitres will vary depending upon the type of LMWH chosen and the body weight of the patient. If unfractionated heparin is chosen, then a loading dose of 5000 units given intravenously is followed by an infusion of about 1000 units hourly with monitoring of APTT. Warfarin may be begun on the first day and heparin should be continued until INR is in the therapeutic range. Following initial management the patient will require 3 months of warfarin. Recurrent thrombosis will require life-long warfarin therapy.

Case 4.39 Haemodialysis access

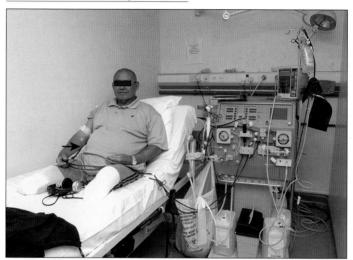

Fig. 4.39.1

Q   **What type of access is used for haemodialysis in this patient?**

A   Radio-cephalic arteriovenous fistula.

Q   **Why is it necessary to form this?**

A   Haemodialysis requires the insertion of two single bore catheters into the artery and the vein respectively, or the insertion of a double lumen catheter into a large vein. Blood is then transported from the patient to the haemodialysis membrane and then returned to the patient. Short-term haemodialysis can be provided with a double- lumen-catheter placed in a large vein, e.g. subclavian, jugular. However, due to the risk of line sepsis and thrombosis, long-term haemodialysis requires the formation of an arteriovenous fistula or the insertion of a long-term percutaneously tunnelled double-lumen central line. When an arteriovenous fistula is formed the increased pressure in the vein results in dilatation. Veins which were previously difficult to cannulate become enlarged and ideal for repeated cannulation. Once developed the fistula can remain patent indefinitely.

Q   **Describe the procedure for forming this type of access.**

A   Arteriovenous fistula can be performed between any vein and artery lying close to each other, which are of moderate size. Radio-cephalic fistulas are preferred. Prior to performing surgery the patency of both the ulnar and radial arteries are assessed by Allen's test or Duplex ultrasonography. The procedure is performed under local anaesthetic on the non-dominant arm. The patient is placed supine with the arm extended on an armrest. A single longitudinal incision is made between the two vessels at the wrist. The artery and vein are mobilised so that they will easily lie side-to-side without tension. Small bulldog clamps are placed proximally and distally on both vessels. Matching longitudinal incisions (7–10 mm) are made in the artery and vein. The vein is flushed with heparinised saline. The artery and vein are anastomosed with a 7/0 non-absorbable monofilament suture.

Q   **Following the procedure what steps can be taken to improve patency rates?**

A   Maintenance of adequate hydration and a warm limb are important for successful fistula formation. Glyceryl trinitrate patches may also be placed over the fistula to encourage vasodilatation of the venous limb.

Q   **What complications can occur?**

A
- thrombosis
- distal embolisation
- high output cardiac failure due to high flows
- infection at cannulation sites.

Abdominal and gastrointestinal

Case 4.40 Barrett's oesophagus

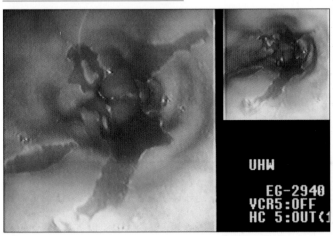

Fig. 4.40.1

Q   **Describe the lesion seen on this endoscopic picture of the lower oesophagus. What is the lesion pathologically?**

A   The endoscopic picture shows a tongue (or tongues) of smooth, velvety, orange-red mucosa above the gastro-oesophageal junction and extending proximally, consistent with Barrett's oesophagus.

Barrett's oesophagus is a premalignant complication of reflux disease and is a result of metaplastic change of the normal squamous epithelium of the lower oesophagus to a specialised intestinal type of columnar epithelium (incomplete type III intestinal metaplasia).

Q **What are the factors involved in the causation of Barrett's oesophagus?**

A Long standing gastro-oesophageal reflux is thought to result in the meta-plastic adaptation to a columnar epithelium which is more resistant to the effects of acid. However, only about 10% of patients with reflux disease ever develop Barrett's. Genetic factors are involved. Other risk factors include Caucasian origin, male gender, obesity, smoking, low dietary fruit and fibre and low dietary selenium.

Q **How would you diagnose Barrett's oesophagus?**

A Barrett's oesophagus does not have any characteristic clinical manifestation. It is diagnosed at endoscopy performed for a range of upper GI symptoms or as part of surveillance or screening in high-risk patients. The diagnosis is ultimately confirmed by histopathological analysis of appropriate biopsies. Three types are recognised: classic long segment (>3 cm), short segment (<3 cm), and ultra-short segment; (endoscopically and macroscopically normal gastro-oesophageal junction but histologically goblet cells are detectable).

Specialised techniques for diagnosis include chromoendoscopy and high-resolution magnification endoscopy. Chromoendoscopy uses dyes such as Lugol's iodine, methylene blue or indigo carmine to identify metaplasia, dysplasia and carcinoma. For example, Lugol's iodine sprayed into the oesophagus at endoscopy stains intracellular glycogen in the squamous epithelium, leaving the metaplastic, dysplastic and malignant cells unstained, aiding targeted biopsy. Magnification endoscopy allows enlargement of 35 times or more, enhancing epithelial visualisation and revealing subtle changes in the mucosa.

Q **Why and how should Barrett's oesophagus be monitored and treated?**

A Barrett's oesophagus progresses to dysplasia (low grade, high grade) which may undergo malignant transformation to adenocarcinoma. The risk of high-grade dysplasia and adenocarcinoma is 30–125 times as in general population with the annual incidence of adenocarcinoma in Barrett's being about 1% (0.4–2%). Hence, endoscopic surveillance with four quadrant biopsies of the lower oesophagus at 2 cm intervals, with 'jumbo forceps' to ensure adequate yield, is recommended to identify early, good prognostic and treatable lesions. For *non-dysplastic Barrett's* the first two endoscopies are done annually after which the interval is every 3 years provided there is no dysplasia. Pharmacological acid suppression or anti-reflux surgery should be offered to optimise symptom control as for reflux disease. There is no clear evidence that treatment of reflux in the presence of Barrett's disease prevents progression to dysplasia.

Patients with *low-grade dysplasia* should undergo endoscopic assessment on an annual basis until clear for 2 years. *High-grade dysplasia* should be confirmed by an expert pathologist to exclude malignancy. Options include endoscopic surveillance (3 monthly for 1 year and then 6 monthly), endoscopic ablation (mucosal resection, laser ablation, argon beam coagulation, electrocoagulation and thermoablation) or oesophagectomy in fit patients.

Case 4.41 Gastric outlet obstruction

Q   **What are the causes of gastric outlet obstruction?**

A   Gastric cancer and chronic peptic ulcer (gastric and duodenal) are the most common causes in adults, accounting for more than 90% of patients. Pancreatic pseudocyst, acute and chronic pancreatitis, pancreatic, peri-ampullary and duodenal tumours are other causes in the adult. Infantile hypertrophic pyloric stenosis is the commonest cause in children.

Rare causes include: antral mucosal diaphragm, duplication cyst of pylorus, gastric stromal tumour, large gastric polyps, ectopic pancreas, annular pancreas, duodenal impaction of gallstone (Bouveret's syndrome), impacted gastrostomy bulb and granulomatous diseases (Crohn's disease, sarcoidosis, tuberculosis).

Q   **What clinical findings might one expect to find in an adult patient with gastric outlet obstruction?**

A   Findings depend on the underlying cause.

> **General examination:** emaciation, dry skin (loss of turgor), pallor, pedal oedema (due to hypoalbuminaemia), icterus, supraclavicular lymphadenopathy (malignancy).

> **Abdominal examination:** visible gastric peristalsis, succussion splash (demonstrable even after 4 hours from last oral intake), epigastric mass, hepatomegaly and rarely an umbilical nodule (sister Joseph's nodule) or pelvic mass on rectal examination from metastasis (Blumer's shelf).

Q   **What metabolic abnormalities may occur in gastric outlet obstruction?**

A   Classically, a hyponatraemic, hypochloraemic, hypokalaemic metabolic alkalosis is seen. Vomiting of gastric secretions results in depletion of H^+ and Cl^- leading to a hypochloraemic metabolic alkalosis. Sodium and fluid loss leads to contraction of the extracellular fluid compartment and hyponatraemia. In an effort to retain sodium, renal mechanisms incur an obligatory loss of potassium and H⁺. This results in hypokalaemia and paradoxical aciduria in the face of alkalosis. Hypokalaemia is mainly due to urinary loss though, vomiting is contributory.

Q   **Describe the management of gastric outlet obstruction.**

A   Patients should be kept 'nil by mouth' with nasogastric aspiration (which helps to reduce bacterial colonisation, rehydrated with normal saline and have their hypokalaemia corrected.

Definitive treatment depends on the underlying cause which needs to be established by a combination of endoscopy (± biopsy), upper gastrointestinal contrast studies and CT scanning as appropriate. Benign obstruction caused by chronic peptic ulcer may be treated by endoscopic balloon dilatation. Surgical options (open or laparoscopic) include vagotomy and drainage (pyloroplasty or gastrojejunostomy); antrectomy; or distal gastrectomy.

Malignant obstructions, if operable and in fit patients, may need curative radical surgery (gastrectomy, pancreaticoduodenectomy as appropriate). Inoperable lesions may be palliated by endoscopic stenting or a gastrojejunostomy (open or laparoscopic).

Infantile hypertrophic pyloric stenosis is treated by Ramsted's pyloromyotomy.

Case 4.42 Pneumoperitoneum

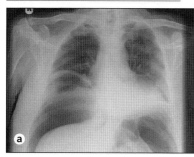

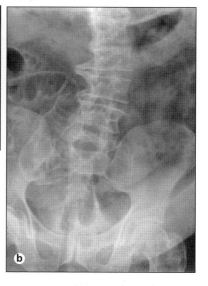

Fig. 4.42.1a,b

Q   **What is the abnormality demonstrated on these scans?**

A   The chest radiograph shows a large pneumoperitoneum below the diaphragm. On the abdominal radiograph, the bowel wall is outlined by air on both the inside and outside (Rigler's sign). In addition, air can be seen tracking along both medial umbilical folds and the falciform ligament.

Q **What are the causes of pneumoperitoneum seen on imaging?**

A The causes of pneumoperitoneum may be classified into three major groups, namely pathologic, iatrogenic and pseudopneumoperitoneum.

Pathologic causes:

1. Hollow viscus perforation is the most common cause. Examples are:

   Abdominal oesophagus: iatrogenic perforation at stricture dilatation

   Stomach: peptic ulcer, perforated tumour, endoscopic perforation

   Duodenum: peptic ulcer, post-ERCP perforation

   Small bowel: Crohn's disease, post-obstructive perforation, typhoid perforation, Meckel's diverticulum

   Large bowel: diverticular perforation, perforated tumour, ulcerative colitis.

2. Anastomotic leaks after surgery and penetrating trauma can cause perforation at all levels.

3. Other causes are pneumatosis cystoides intestinalis, jejunal diverticulosis (even without apparent perforation), tracking from a pneumothorax.

Iatrogenic pneumoperitoneum:

1. Open abdominal surgery (may persist for 1–24 days) or laparoscopic abdominal surgery.

2. Rarely, after gastric insufflation at endoscopy even without perforation.

3. Peritoneal dialysis.

4. Liver biopsy.

5. Uterine insufflation.

Pseudopneumoperitoneum:

1. Chilaiditi's syndrome: colonic interposition between the diaphragm and the liver.

2. Lipoperitoneum: fat under the diaphragm may cause a lucent shadow.

3. Subphrenic abscess: localised pocket of air in an abscess may mimic free peritoneal air.

4. Meteorism: in children excessive swallowed air may cause interposition of dilated, air-containing loops in close approximation to either diaphragm.

5. Artefacts: skin folds, rib margins overlapping diaphragm.

Q   **What are the ways of demonstrating pneumoperitoneum?**

A   An erect chest radiograph is the classical method of demonstrating pneumoperitoneum which may reveal as little as 1 ml of free air. Air under both diaphragms usually denotes a significant volume of free air and points to the stomach or large bowel as the source. Sitting the patient up for 10–20 minutes allows air to rise up and collect under the diaphragm increasing the chance of detection. However, this may be difficult in patients with poorly controlled pain.

In patients unable to sit up for an erect film, an abdominal left lateral decubitus film is useful. A supine abdominal film may reveal air, but is less sensitive.

Other potential methods include ultrasonography and CT. These imaging methods are rarely used to demonstrate pneumoperitoneum, but pneumoperitoneum is often an important additional finding when these are ordered to investigate other clinical conditions.

Q   **What are the signs of pneumoperitoneum on plain chest radiograph?**

A   A subphrenic crescent of air on an erect chest film is the classical sign found in up to 80% of patients with pneumoperitoneum. In addition, one or more of the following signs may be seen on a supine abdominal X-ray:

Subhepatic air

Rigler's sign (double wall sign):   both the inner and outer surfaces of the bowel wall are delineated clearly by air in contact with them.

Triangle sign: Air trapped between adjacent loops of bowel tends to form air triangles.

Silver's sign: Air demarcates the falciform ligament.

Football sign: In children in the presence of a large pneumoperitoneum the abdomen distends with air assuming a nearly spherical central lucency.

Dome sign: Large pneumoperitoneum raising both diaphragms like domes.

Cupola sign: Air in the median subphrenic space.

Inverted V sign: Delineation of the medial and lateral umbilical ligaments.

Urachal sign: Delineation of urachus in the midline by air.

Scrotal gas in children.

Case 4.43 Pseudocyst of pancreas

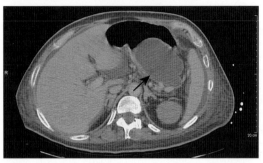

Fig. 4.43.1

Q   **What abnormality is seen on this CT scan?**

A   There is a pseudocyst of the pancreas protruding into the lumen of the stomach. The pancreas cannot be seen.

Q   **What are the complications of pseudocyst?**

A   ***Obstruction:***   Gastric outlet obstruction and duodenal obstruction are the usual forms of obstructive complications. However, on rare occasions pseudocysts can cause obstruction of the oesophagus, small and large bowel. Biliary obstruction is not uncommon with obstructive jaundice with a risk of cholangitis. Rarely, a pseudocyst may obstruct the vena cava, portal vein or the urinary tract.

Infection: Large cysts, prolonged observation and invasive intervention (such as ERCP in communicating cysts; needle aspiration) have an increased risk of infection.

Bleeding (5%):   Sudden and catastrophic haemorrhage may occur into the pseudocyst resulting in increasing pain and size of the cyst or from the gut wall due to erosion by the cyst. This may result in haemodynamic compromise and may need urgent intervention, either angiographic embolisation or open surgical haemostasis. The splenic artery, the gastroduodenal artery and the pancreaticoduodenal artery are the usual sources of bleeding.

Rupture (3%):   Cyst rupture may be acute or insidious. It may lead to pancreatic ascites or pleural effusion.

Malnutrition: Reduced oral intake due to anorexia, pain and or vomiting may lead to malnutrition over weeks.

Q What are the other cystic conditions of the pancreas that need to be differentiated from a pseudocyst?

A The most important condition to differentiate are the cystic neoplasms of the pancreas (serous and mucinous cystic neoplasms and teratomas). Rarer cystic pathologies are: congenital simple cysts (solitary or multiple), enterogenous cysts, dermoid cysts, lymphoepithelial cysts, fibrocystic disease (children) and echinococcal (hydatid) cysts.

Q What are the important considerations in planning the management strategy of pseudocysts?

A Presence of symptoms or complications warrants intervention, while asymptomatic cysts may be managed conservatively.

Type of cyst: Acute pseudocysts following acute pancreatitis often resolve, while chronic pseudocysts in the background of chronic parenchymal disease of the pancreas and ductal abnormalities rarely resolve.

Diagnostic uncertainty: Inability to rule out a neoplasm may warrant intervention.

Anatomical relation: Juxtaposition of luminal organs dictates the type of drainage chosen.

Ductal communication: External drainage of a communicating cyst can lead to a pancreatic fistula.

Maturity and wall thickness: Cysts with thin and friable walls are not amenable for internal drainage. Cysts take about 4–6 weeks to mature. Wall thickness of 0.5–1 cm or more is considered adequate.

The size of the cyst: Cysts more than 6 cm are less likely to resolve spontaneously. However, size alone does not dictate the need for intervention.

Q What are the management options for an acute pseudocyst?

A *Conservative management:* Uncomplicated, asymptomatic cysts may be managed with nutritional support and serial imaging. Octreotide may be of value in communicating cysts.

Percutaneous drainage: In patients unfit for surgery; as a temporising measure before more definitive surgery; cysts in an unusual location and not amenable for internal drainage.

Endoscopic drainage: Transpapillary or transmural drainage.

Laparoscopic drainage

Open surgical management: (a) internal drainage – cystogastrostomy, cystoduodenostomy or cystojejunostomy; (b) external drainage – for infected cysts; thin walled cysts; (c) resection – for cysts in the tail of pancreas.

Case 4.44 Incisional hernia

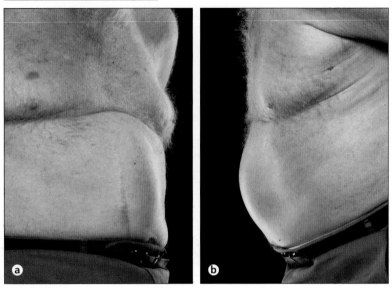

Fig. 4.44.1a,b

Q   **What are the factors that contribute to the formation of incisional hernia?**

A   Incisional hernias are multifactorial in origin. Patient-related factors, perioperative and wound-related factors, and technical factors are all contributory.

Patient related factors include: obesity, malnutrition, hypoproteinaemia and steroid therapy. Smoking (by influencing coughing) and the presence of significant co-morbidity (uraemia, uncontrolled diabetes, ascites, COPD) may also influence causation.

Perioperative and wound related factors are midline laparotomy, wound infection, anastomotic leak with fistula, ileus, postoperative chest infection, multiple re-laparotomies in the same admission and laparostomy.

Technical factors: surgeon's experience, closure under tension, inadequate tissue purchase due to poor bites of the tissue (ignoring Jenkins's rule of 4:1, suture length:wound length), poor choice of sutures, strangulation of tissue, poor haemostasis and breach of asepsis (deep surgical site infection).

Q   **What are the complications of incisional hernia?**

A   Irreducibility and pain, intestinal obstruction, strangulation, gangrene and perforation of intestine within the hernia are the more serious complications.

Other complications include development of adhesions between loops of bowel and the sac, and thinning and ulceration of overlying skin.

Q   **What are the risks that the patient should be informed about before surgery?**

A   *General risks:*
Chest infection, deep vein thrombosis

Specific risks:
Intraoperative: Inadvertent enterotomy, blood loss needing transfusion (in large hernias), need to remove umbilicus if necessary.
Short term: Wound infection, seroma, haematoma needing evacuation, skin necrosis, temporary or permanent sensory loss around the wound, excessive scarring and rarely synergistic gangrene and necrotising fasciitis. Need for postoperative ventilation in patients with large hernias.
Long term: Recurrence; late stitch sinus or abscess; prosthetic infection necessitating mesh removal; peritoneal adhesions with intestinal obstruction in transperitoneal repairs; rarely chronic neuropathic pain.

Q   **What should the patients be counselled to do in preparation for surgery?**

A   They should be advised to lose weight and stop smoking.

Q   **What are the options available for treating incisional hernias?**

A   Asymptomatic hernias which are wide-necked, especially in the elderly and poor surgical risk patients, may be observed.

Small hernias with a transverse diameter of <4 cm may be treated by simple closure using interrupted non-absorbable sutures, in a tension free manner, approximating healthy tissues. There are many variations in the techniques, such as layered closure (anatomical repair), overlapping Mayo repair (double breasting) and keel repair.

Hernias larger than 4 cm are best treated by a mesh placed pre-peritoneally (inlay) and overlapping the edges of the defect all around by 4 cm.

Hernias up to 10–15 cm in width may also be treated laparoscopically.

Very large hernias need specialised operations such as the Stoppa repair wherein a large piece of prosthetic mesh is placed in the pre-peritoneal space behind the defect, wrapping the viscera, or a procedure such as myofascial flap technique of separation of parts.

Case 4.45 Enteral nutrition

Q **How is this patient receiving nutrition?**

A This patient is being fed enterally by means of a jejunostomy.

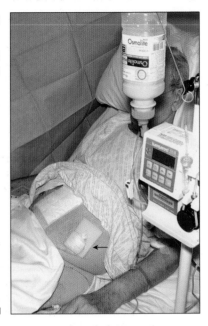

Fig. 4.45.1

Q **What are the indications for enteral feeding?**

A If it is anticipated that the patient cannot or will not eat enough, for a considerable period of time (usually 1 week), to meet their nutritional needs, but has a functioning gastrointestinal tract then enteral nutrition should always be considered first. Typical examples are patients with swallowing disorders, unconscious patients, complex gastro-oesophageal surgery, obstructing oesophageal lesions, patients with increased nutritional requirements (burns, trauma) and anorexic patients. The other important indication is in special situations when a specific type of enteral nutrition has a therapeutic value, such as the elemental diet in a relapse of Crohn's disease.

However, enteral feeding cannot be used in the presence of paralytic ileus, intestinal obstruction, perforation or high output intestinal fistula.

Q **What are the methods of enteral feeding?**

A Enteral feeding methods may be classified into nasoenteric and percutaneous methods. Nasoenteric methods use nasogastric feeding tubes (placed blindly) or nasojejunal feeding-tubes (placed endoscopically or radiologically). Percutaneous methods are percutaneous gastrostomy and percutaneous jejunostomy. The percutaneous tubes may be placed under endoscopic or fluoroscopic guidance or under direct vision at open surgery.

Q **What are the problems with nasoenteric methods?**

A They are uncomfortable (even if small bore) for the patient and may easily get displaced or pulled out. They should not be used for more than 4 weeks. The nasal route is contraindicated in patients who have a base of skull fracture. Pharyngeal, oesophageal and gastric obstructive lesions may preclude their use.

Q **What are the relative merits of gastrostomy and jejunostomy?**

A Gastrostomy is easier to establish than jejunostomy. However, gastrostomy is not appropriate if gastric emptying is delayed, if there is significant gastro-oesophageal reflux or abolition of gag reflex which leaves the airway unprotected. Jejunostomy is better tolerated and associated with a lower incidence of leak and pulmonary complications. The decrease in gastric and pancreatic secretions with jejunostomy is preferred particularly in conditions such as acute pancreatitis.

Q **What are the risks with enteral feeding?**

A Some of the risks lie with the access method chosen while others are due to the feeds themselves. Nasoenteric tubes may cause oesophageal ulceration, increase reflux and cause stricture. Percutaneous access-related complications or leaks, with peritonitis, or intra-abdominal abscess; exit site infection; bleeding and displacement resulting in intraperitoneal administration of feeds.

Feeding-related complications include reflux, aspiration, diarrhoea, constipation, fluid imbalance, hypo- or hyperglycaemia.

Case 4.46 Hydrocele

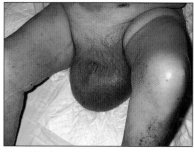 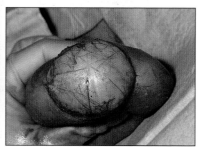

Fig. 4.46.1   **Fig. 4.46.2**

Q **What do these images of the scrotum show?**

A • There are bilateral scrotal swellings

• At operation, there are cystic swellings, with a thin translucent covering, arising from the scrotum anterior to the testis. The features represent hydroceles which are pathological collections of fluid in the tunica vaginalis.

Q　**What types of hydrocele are there?**

A　Hydrocele of the tunica vaginalis (vaginal hydrocele) may be classified into congenital and acquired types. Congenital hydroceles arise from non obliteration of the embryological connection between the greater peritoneal cavity and the tunica vaginalis, allowing fluid to accumulate. The acquired hydrocele may be of a primary (idiopathic) type or a secondary type which follows an identifiable locoregional pathological process such as chronic epididymo-orchitis or a testicular tumour. Classically, the acquired vaginal hydrocele collects between the testis and tunica vaginalis enveloping it from all sides especially anteriorly making the testis impalpable in most instances.

　Anatomical variants of hydrocele include funicular hydrocele, infantile hydrocele, encysted hydrocele of the cord, bilocular hydrocele and hydrocele of a hernial sac.

Q　**What are the salient clinical findings of a classical vaginal hydrocele?**

A　*Inspection:*　Swelling of the scrotum, loss of scrotal rugosity.
　Palpation:　Skin temperature not raised, the swelling is non-tender.
　Examination:　reveals a soft, smooth, fluctuant, transilluminant, irreducible, non-compressible, non-pulsatile, swelling whose upper limit can be reached. The testis is usually not palpable separately. There is no cough impulse.

　NB: Transillumination may be negative if the scrotum or sac is very thick or contents viscous (chylocele) such as in filariasis. Congenital and funicular hydroceles may be partly reducible as they communicate with the peritoneum. The testis may be palpable in small secondary hydroceles, funicular hydrocele, encysted hydrocele of the cord and hydrocele of the hernial sac. It may not be possible to get above the swelling in infantile hydrocele, congenital hydrocele, funicular hydrocele, bilocular hydrocele and hydrocele of the hernial sac which may either extend to or present entirely in the inguinal region.

Q　**What other conditions should a hydrocele be differentiated from?**

A　Inguinoscrotal hernia, testicular tumour, haematocele, large epididymal cyst(s), large spermatocele, large varicocele.

Q　**What clinical problems are posed by hydroceles?**

A　*To the patient:*　Heaviness, cosmetic disfigurement, infection (pyocele), bleeding (haematocele), pressure sores and maceration in bedridden patients with large hydroceles.

　To the surgeon:　Risk of missing an underlying testicular tumour; the loose tissue planes in the scrotum predispose to postoperative haematomas.

Q **How should hydroceles be treated?**

A Small vaginal hydroceles may be managed conservatively as long as an underlying testicular tumour can be ruled out. Large and symptomatic hydroceles need operative intervention. Options include drainage of fluid with eversion of sac (Jaboulay's procedure) or drainage and excision of sac with plication of redundant tunica (Lord's procedure).
Congenital hydrocele is treated by herniotomy.

Case 4.47 Inguinal hernia

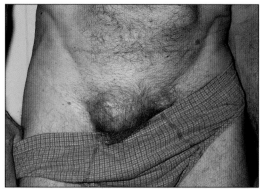

Fig. 4.47.1

Q **How would you go about examining this patient with a groin lump and what specific pieces of information would you expect to gather to help in your diagnosis?**

A The patient should be exposed from the upper abdomen to the knees and should be examined in the standing and supine positions by inspection, palpation, percussion and auscultation if necessary. Size, extent (scrotal or inguinoscrotal), position (in relation to the pubic tubercle, inguinal ligament, the surface marking of the deep ring, cord and testis), expansile cough impulse and reducibility (to confirm that it is a hernia), deep ring occlusion test; consistency, percussion and auscultation, if necessary, to assess the contents (bowel sounds may be heard).

Q **Does it matter if it is a direct or indirect inguinal hernia?**

A There are minor differences in the prognosis and operative steps between the two types of hernias. Direct inguinal hernias are usually diffuse and wide necked and are less likely to suffer obstructive complications when compared to indirect hernias. The sac in indirect hernias needs to be dissected from cord structures, transfixed and excised at the deep ring, whereas a direct hernial sac is simply reduced and held in position by plication of transversalis fascia if necessary. The deep ring in an indirect hernia may be stretched wide, needing a Lytle's repair, although this is not necessary in a direct hernia.

Q **What is the differential diagnosis?**

A Femoral hernia, enlarged inguinal or external iliac lymph node, lipoma of the cord, encysted hydrocele of the cord, varicocele, lymph varix, ectopic or undescended testis and an inguinal abscess.

Q **What are the treatment options?**

A The choice is usually between a herniotomy (excision of sac), herniorrhaphy (reinforcement by manipulating or suturing tissues) and hernioplasty (reinforcement using prosthetic material). Often, watchful observation is an option in the very elderly or unfit patients, with a wide mouthed reducible direct hernia. Surgery may be performed by a conventional open method (under local or general anaesthetic) or by minimal access techniques.

Herniotomy alone should suffice in children. There are many variations of herniorrhaphy for adults of which the Shouldice repair is the standard. Liechtenstein's tension free hernioplasty using a mesh (e.g. polypropylene) to reinforce the posterior wall is the standard hernioplasty procedure, with low recurrence rates and is the commonest technique used.

Minimal access procedures deploy a mesh from a posterior approach and are generally used for bilateral or recurrent hernias. There are three major variations in practice: (1) the transabdominal preperitoneal repair (TAPP); (2) the totally extraperitoneal repair (TEP) and (3) intraperitoneal on-lay mesh repair (IPOM).

Q **What risks would you counsel the patient of when consenting them for surgery?**

A In addition to the risks of anaesthesia and general complications such as chest infection and deep vein thrombosis, patients should be made aware of specific procedure related risks.

Intraoperative risks: Injury to the vas deferens, injury to testicular artery and veins; bleeding and nerve and bowel injury in laparoscopic repairs.

Short-term risks: Reactionary haemorrhage, haematoma (scrotal, inguinal) which may need surgical evacuation; seroma; wound infection (2–5%); skin necrosis; synergistic gangrene, necrotising fasciitis (rare); infected collection in the scrotum; infection of prosthesis; stitch sinus; inguinal and genital paraesthesia or loss of sensation.

Long-term risks: Recurrence (<1%), testicular atrophy and chronic neuropathic pain, which may be difficult to treat. The patient should be warned of adhesions and port site hernias in laparoscopic repairs.

Case 4.48 Obstructing rectal lesion

Q   What investigation is shown in Fig. 4.48.1? What does it show?

A   This is a double contrast enema examination. It shows a stricture in the upper rectum ('apple-core' lesion) with shouldering suggestive of a malignant obstructing lesion.

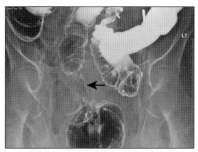

Fig. 4.48.1

Q   What investigation is shown in Fig. 4.48.2? What does it show?

A   This is a MR scan of the rectum and shows a locally invasive rectal tumour.

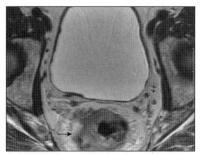

Fig. 4.48.2

Q   What investigation is shown in Fig. 4.48.3? What does it show?

A   This is a CT scan of the abdomen showing metastases within the liver. A histological diagnosis is required to confirm the diagnosis of liver metastases.

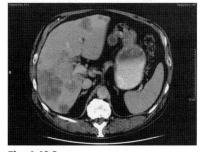

Fig. 4.48.3

Q ·   Is this a common presentation?

A   No. Obstructing cancers occur more frequently in the left colon than the right colon, obstructing rectal cancers are uncommon. This is because of the capacious nature of the rectum. However, annular cancers can occur in the recto-sigmoid junction and are more likely to present with obstruction because there is less accommodation. Rectal cancers more commonly present with rectal bleeding, tenesmus or altered bowel habit (particularly early morning bloody diarrhoea).

Q **What are the treatment options at emergency laparotomy for an obstructing rectosigmoid cancer?**

A The type of operation performed depends on the site of tumour, extent of disease, presence of perforation, fitness of the patient and experience of the surgeon. The following are the options available:

Resection with primary anastomosis with or without a proximal covering stoma: In a fit patient, with a localised resectable lesion in the upper rectum, without perforation, on-table lavage is performed to clean the proximal bowel with:

- anterior resection with colorectal anastomosis or
- subtotal colectomy with ileorectal anastomosis, if the viability of the proximal bowel (usually the caecum) is in question or when there are synchronous tumours making this the ideal option.

Resection without anastomosis:

- Hartmann's procedure: the proximal bowel is brought out as an end colostomy and the residual rectal stump closed
- subtotal colectomy with end ileostomy.

Proximal diversion alone, without resection:

- loop colostomy (are difficult to manage because of the size and complications, e.g. prolapse)
- end colostomy and mucous fistula.

This may be a definitive procedure in advanced unresectable disease or an initial temporising measure in a staged operation, with elective resection carried out later, it is not an acceptable alternative otherwise.

Q **If the patient has significant co-morbidity with a prohibitive risk for anaesthesia and surgery, are there any other options?**

A Self-expanding stents which can be deployed endoscopically offer good palliation. Endorectal laser canalisation or diathermy canalisation may help in the short term. Palliative or potentially curative radiotherapy may be considered in the medium term once the crisis of obstruction has passed and the patient is deemed fit.

Case 4.49 Crohn's disease

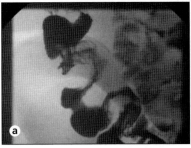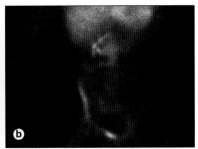

Fig. 4.49.1a,b

Q **What investigation is shown in Figs 4.49.1a and b? What do they show?**

A (a) is a small bowel enema showing the characteristic signs of ileal Crohn's disease, i.e. asymmetry, oedema, narrowing and ulceration; (b) is a radioisotope labelled white cell scanning showing accumulation of white cells in the region of the terminal ileum indicating active disease.

Q **When do patients with Crohn's disease need surgery?**

A Failed medical treatment and development of surgically treatable complications which threaten life are the two broad groups of indications for surgical intervention.

Intestinal obstruction, symptomatic fistulas not treatable by conservative management, perforation with intra-abdominal abscess or peritonitis, bleeding, fulminant colitis, intractable perianal sepsis and development of malignancy are the complications needing surgery. In children, failure to thrive may need resection of diseased bowel.

Q **What are the surgical options in Crohn's disease and general principles in applying them?**

A Surgery should be aimed to remove only the minimum segment of bowel as is absolutely necessary to treat the complication. This reduces the risk of developing short gut syndrome in the long term. A limited or segmental resection (such as an ileo-caecal resection for terminal ileal disease) is the usual procedure performed if the area causing obstruction is actively inflamed or incorporates a fistula with sepsis. It is not necessary to remove all macroscopically abnormal areas of Crohn's, nor is it necessary to aim for macroscopically disease free margins. In non-phlegmonous, fibrotic strictures, a bowel sparing option of stricturoplasty should always be considered.

In patients with pancolitis needing surgery, a proctocolectomy with permanent end ileostomy may be necessary. In intractable perianal Crohn's disease with sepsis, a proximal diverting stoma may be needed.

Q **What preventive measures may reduce the incidence of relapse after resectional surgery for Crohn's with no apparent residual disease?**

A Stopping smoking is probably the most important measure currently available. It halves the symptomatic recurrence at 10 years postoperatively. Among the medications, immunosuppressive agents (azathioprine, 6-mercaptopurine) and metronidazole hold some promise. Immunosuppressives should be considered in the high-risk group (ileocolic anastomosis, smoking females, perforating disease and repeated surgery). Oral metronidazole therapy loses its protective effect after 1 year postoperatively. Long-term aminosalicylates are not very effective with about 12 patients needing to be treated to prevent recurrence in one patient. Steroids are not recommended for preventing relapse.

Q **Crohn's disease is a remitting-relapsing condition with a wide range of clinical manifestations needing frequent tailoring of treatment. Are you aware of any scoring indices that will be useful in serial monitoring of patients with some objectivity?**

A The Crohn's disease activity index (CDAI) is a commonly used, composite scoring system which assesses patient-reported, general well-being, abdominal pain, number of liquid stools, need for opiates to control diarrhoea and the presence of fistula, arthritis, skin and eye manifestations. It also factors in the patient's body weight and haematocrit. A score of <150 indicates remission.

Other clinical scoring systems that have been developed include the Harvey–Bradshaw index and the Van Hees index (Dutch index). Endoscopic scoring systems include the Crohn's disease endoscopic index of severity (CDEIS) and the Rutgeert's ileitis score.

Q **Crohn's disease has many extraintestinal manifestations and complications. Would you be surprised if this patient has gallstones or renal stones?**

A No. Patients with Crohn's disease have a higher incidence of both gallstones and renal stones. Terminal ileal disease or loss of ileal length due to previous resections results in a reduced bile salt pool due to interference with the enterohepatic circulation. Reduced bile acids in bile decreases cholesterol solubility which results in stone formation (lithogenic bile).

Oxalate and uric acid stones in the urinary tract occur with a higher frequency in patients with Crohn's. Oxalate is poorly absorbed in Crohn's disease resulting in a high colonic load, from where it is reabsorbed, resulting in hyperoxaluria and stone formation. Patients who have had a colectomy are protected from oxalate stones. Uric acid stones occur with increased frequency in patients with an ileostomy. Low urine volumes, acidic urine, low urinary sodium and magnesium are thought to contribute.

Case 4.50 Change in bowel habit

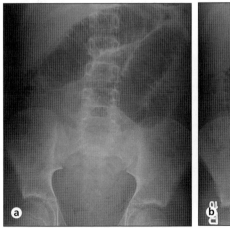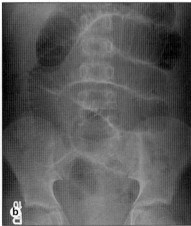

Fig. 4.50.1a,b

Q This patient presented with abdominal pain, vomiting and absolute constipation. What do these radiographs show?

A An evolving small bowel obstruction.

Q What different groups of conditions causing altered bowel habit would you keep in mind as you proceed through history taking and examination?

A *Conditions presenting with chronic diarrhoea (>4 weeks duration):*
Inflammatory diarrhoea: ulcerative colitis, Crohn's disease, infective colitis
Neoplastic causes: colonic polyps (villous adenoma), colorectal cancer
Osmotic diarrhoea: malabsorption syndromes (intestinal, pancreatic)
Secretory diarrhoea: neuroendocrine tumours, collagen vascular disease
Dysmotility: irritable bowel syndrome, autonomic neuropathy, hyperthyroidism
Drug induced: laxatives.

Conditions presenting with constipation:
Malignancy
Diverticular disease
Other causes of strictures: post-radiation, post ischaemic
Pelvic and anal conditions: prolapse, pelvic floor dysfunction
Metabolic: hypothyroidism, hypercalcaemia
Drugs: opiates, anticholinergics
Precipitated by lifestyle: poor diet, reduced water intake, immobility.

Conditions having a variable presentation of alternating diarrhoea and constipation:

Malignancies
Diverticular disease
Irritable bowel syndrome
Drugs: opiates (spurious diarrhoea).

Q **What are the important factors and clues in history that you would seek to explore to narrow down the differential diagnosis?**

A Details of the bowel habits of the patient prior to the onset of change, any pre-existing conditions such as haemorrhoids or fissure and the duration of alteration in bowel habit are important baseline characteristics which should be established initially. Other diagnostically helpful associations are:

Age: Malignancy is uncommon under the age of 40.

History: Travel and diet, medications and recent lifestyle changes.

Weight loss: Significant weight loss suggests malignancy, inflammatory disease or malabsorption.

Volume and frequency of stool: Large volume diarrhoea suggests small bowel or a right colonic cause, while small volume diarrhoea suggests a colonic cause. Frequent passage of small volume stool may be due to incontinence or, when associated with tenesmus, may be due to proctitis.

Timing of stool: Early morning diarrhoea may occur with rectal neoplasms; more frequent diarrhoea in the initial part of the day tending to taper off towards the evening suggests a functional cause (irritable bowel syndrome); diarrhoea only at night is common in autonomic neuropathy; diarrhoea which wakes up a patient from sleep more often than not has an organic cause.

Bleeding: While the characteristics of bleeding do not categorically differentiate the different causes, they may provide some useful clues. Blood in stools makes a functional cause less likely as opposed to neoplastic, infectious or inflammatory cause. Bright red blood points to a distal cause while altered or maroon coloured blood suggests a proximal cause. Blood only on toilet tissues suggests a local cause. Blood mixed with stools suggests inflammation or neoplasm. Painless bleeding is common in neoplasia (unless advanced) and haemorrhoids ('flash in the pan'). Severe sharp perianal pain with blood coating stool or dripping is typical of a fissure, which may be contributing to, or the result of constipation. Lower abdominal pain with bleeding occurs with infectious or inflammatory colitis.

Mucus: Large amounts of mucus in stools may occur with inflammation, neoplasm or rapid transit.

Q What are the principles and merits of the alternative ways of investigating a patient presenting with a few months' history of altered bowel habit, who you suspect, may have a large bowel cause?

A Probability of a serious or potentially treatable cause (such as carcinoma, polyps, inflammatory bowel disease); need for histopathological proof; availability of resources (technology, personnel and time); age, general fitness and wishes of the patient, influence the pathways that a particular patient might follow. However, the general principles are that the entire colon should be evaluated and that the risks, delays and need for repetition should be kept to the minimum.

Colonoscopy is ideal as it can visualise the entire colon and terminal ileum, offers the benefit of tissue sampling and therapy (e.g. polypectomy). However, it needs bowel preparation and sedation and carries a small but definite risk of morbidity. Simple change in bowel habit alone is a low yield indication, while age >50, associated iron deficiency anaemia, bleeding or positive faecal occult blood have a relatively high yield and are justifiable.

The alternative is to perform a rigid or flexible sigmoidoscopy and a double contrast barium enema. The sigmoidoscopy can be performed rapidly in un-sedated patients with minimal preparation. It complements barium enema which may miss small rectosigmoid lesions. Barium enema needs bowel preparation, exposes the patient to radiation, tends to over diagnose caecal abnormalities, does not provide tissue samples and may give an inconclusive verdict necessitating colonoscopy.

Case 4.51 Stoma complications

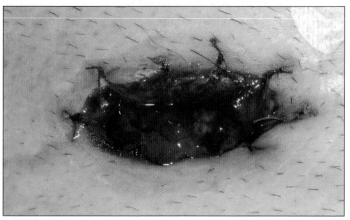

Fig. 4.51.1

Q **What type of stoma does this patient have? What is the complication?**

A The stoma is in the left iliac fossa and seems to have only one lumen. So it is likely to be an end colostomy (sigmoid or descending colon) after a Hartmann's procedure or an abdominoperineal excision of rectum. The edge of the stoma has retracted into the wound.

Q **What are the considerations in siting a stoma?**

A A stoma should be away from any bony prominences, scars and wounds. It should not lie on a skin fold. It should be in a position where the patient can see or care for it comfortably. It should ideally be brought out through the rectus muscle.

Q **What complications may occur with stomas?**

A ***Stomal and peristomal complications:***
Oedema and congestion in the immediate postoperative period are common and usually self- limiting, resolving in 48–72 hours. Ischaemia progressing to gangrene is rare.

Bleeding in the immediate postoperative period may result in a haematoma or bruising at the stomal site. Later, bleeding may occur due to trauma, ulceration, recurrent Crohn's, polyps or peristomal varices.

Infection: Cellulitis, wound infection and parietal abscesses may occur. Synergistic gangrene is rare.

Fistulas may occur between the emerging loop and the surrounding soft tissues. This may or may not be due to recurrent Crohn's disease.

Sinuses may be related to deep lying sutures or a mesh.

Skin problems include erythema, maceration, furrowing, ulceration, progressing to florid effluent (faecal) dermatitis.

Functional and obstructive complications:
Prolonged ileus may lead to delayed postoperative functioning of the stoma.

Obstruction due to too tight a parietal window or due to a volvulus may occur.

Ileostomy dysfunction syndrome describes a functional obstruction at the spout, which presents about 1 week postoperatively with abdominal pain, vomiting and irregular ileostomy action. It occurs almost exclusively in non-everted ileostomies.

Stomal stenosis is a late sequel.

Fluid/electrolyte imbalance: High ileostomy output (ileostomy flux) may lead to rapid dehydration, shock and renal failure. The imbalance may develop insidiously with chronic dehydration, hyponatraemia and hypokalaemia.

Problems with integrity:
Stomal gangrene
Stomal retraction: intraperitoneal leak, peritonitis
Parastomal hernia
Stomal prolapse.

Metabolic complications:
Higher incidence of gallstones and renal stones
Short gut syndrome: though not directly related to the stoma, an ileostomy may exacerbate or unmask a short bowel syndrome.

Q   **What are the types of hernia that can complicate a stoma?**

A   Anatomically, there are four types of hernias that can occur with stomas which may be grouped into two broad types: the parastomal hernias (interstitial, subcutaneous, intrastomal) and prolapse.

Interstitial hernia: the hernial sac lies within the layers of the parietes.
Subcutaneous hernia: the hernia lies in a superficial plane under the skin.
Intrastomal hernia: occurs with end ileostomies. The hernial sac dissects a plane alongside the stoma and lies under a dome between the everted layer of the stoma and the emergent bowel.
Peristomal hernia or prolapse: the prolapsing stoma is a type of herniation with the sac and contents propelling itself through the stoma or the stomal loop intussuscepting externally. There are two types of prolapse: fixed and sliding. Among all stomas, transverse loop colostomies have the highest rate of prolapse.

Q   **What are the ways of managing parastomal hernias?**

A   If the stomal hernia is small, asymptomatic and does not interfere with stoma care then it may be left alone. Symptomatic and complicated hernias may be managed in one of three ways. Simple repair involves reducing the hernia and strengthening the local musculo-aponeurotic components around the aperture, through which the stoma emerges, with non-absorbable sutures. However, this carries a high risk of recurrence. Mesh repair is more effective. The mesh may be incorporated in the preperitoneal or extraparietal plane. Re-siting the stoma in a healthier site is also a good option.

Case 4.52 Prostate cancer

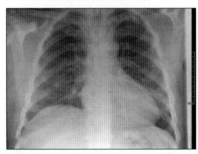

Fig. 4.52.1

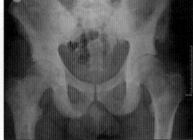

Fig. 4.52.2

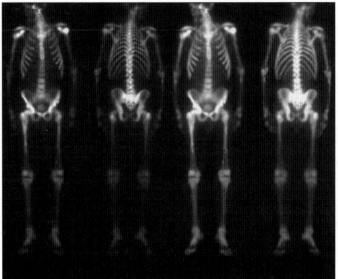

Fig. 4.52.3

Q   A 70-year-old man presented with a few weeks history of poor stream of urine, hesitancy and one episode of haematuria was found to have an enlarged nodular prostate. He underwent the above investigations during the course of his further evaluation. What do you infer from the tests and would you be able to justify requesting these tests?

A The chest and pelvic radiograph shows generalised bone sclerosis with lytic lesions in the clavicles, humeri and right femur. The isotope bone scan shows hot spots in the pelvis, sternum and long bones. The patient is most likely to have a prostatic cancer for which the chest radiograph and bone scan have been requested to stage the disease.

Bone metastases are present in up to 20% of patients at presentation and are typically sclerotic. They are commonly seen in the pelvis, spine and ribs. Lymphangitis carcinomatosa and pleural effusions may be seen on a chest radiograph in advanced disease. A bone scan using technetium phosphate isotope reveals metastases as hot spots. Unless there is bone pain or radical local treatment for the primary is being considered, a bone scan is not justified if the prostate specific antigen (PSA) is <10 ng/ml and Gleason score is <8.

Q **What are the various ways that prostatic cancer comes to light?**

A Prostatic cancer usually produces symptoms only when it is locally advanced or metastatic.

It may present in the following ways:

Asymptomatic/incidental: elevated PSA on screening, enlarged nodular prostate on digital rectal examination, metastatic nodule on physical examination or chest radiograph, unexplained deranged liver function tests, hypercalcaemia, unexpected malignant histology in prostatic specimens from surgery for benign hypertrophy and lastly, being discovered at autopsy.

Urological presentation:

- lower urinary tract symptoms (LUTS) which may be 'irritative' or 'obstructive' symptoms

- acute retention of urine

- chronic retention of urine

- haematuria

- renal impairment due to chronic retention or ureteric obstruction.

Symptomatic loco-regional or distant spread: Bone pain, pathological fracture, paraplegia, pedal oedema from pressure effects on veins/lymphatics, anaemia.

Q   **How is bladder outlet obstruction defined in simple terms? What are the other causes of bladder outflow obstruction apart from prostatic cancer?**

A   Objectively, a peak flow rate of <15 ml/second and a residual volume of >100 ml is indicative of bladder outflow obstruction.

Benign prostatic hyperplasia, bladder neck stenosis, bladder neck hypertrophy, functional obstruction due to neuropathy and urethral stricture are some of the causes of bladder outflow obstruction that may mimic the symptoms of prostate cancer.

Q   **How would you investigate a patient with an enlarged prostate on rectal examination who is otherwise asymptomatic?**

A   A PSA level should be requested. Normal levels depend on the age of the patient. In general, the upper limit of normal is 4 ng/ml in young and middle-aged adults and 6.5 ng/ml for men in their 70s. PSA levels over 10 ng/ml significantly increase the probability of cancer.

The prostate should be evaluated by transrectal ultrasound (TRUS). Suspicious areas should be biopsied under guidance. Ultrasound is also useful in quantifying prostatic volume, which is important in a clinically useful interpretation of PSA levels called PSA density. PSA density is the ratio of serum PSA in ng/ml to the weight of prostate in grams and should normally be <0.15.

Q   **In brief, what are the types of treatment that are on offer for prostatic cancer?**

A   The choice of treatment depends on the stage of the disease and the patient profile (fitness, symptoms, life expectancy and wishes).

For early potentially curable cancer in fit patients, radical retropubic prostatectomy or radiotherapy are equally viable options. Radiotherapy may be external beam radiotherapy or brachytherapy (the insertion of multiple radioactive (Iridium-125) seeds through the perineum into the prostate in carefully selected patients, i.e. those with minimal lower urinary tract symptoms).

For advanced local or metastatic disease, hormonal therapy is the choice. This takes one of three forms: (1) androgen deprivation (orchidectomy or chemical castration with luteinising hormone agonists); (2) anti-androgens: cyproterone, bicalutamide, flutamide, nilutamide; (3) combined androgen blockade using both the above options.

Palliative treatments include chemotherapy, e.g. docetaxel; radiotherapy (for bleeding, to control locally advanced disease; and for bony metastasis – external radiotherapy or strontium radionuclide); bisphosphonates for bone pain and to reduce skeletal related events, i.e. fractures, spinal cord compression; transurethral resection to relieve obstruction; ureteric stenting and hormonal treatment.

Case 4.53 Renal tract calculi

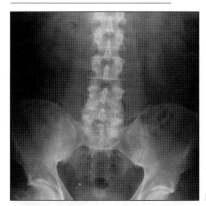

Fig. 4.53.1

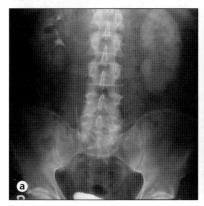
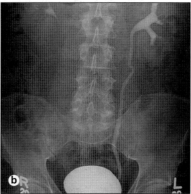

Fig. 4.53.2a,b

Q How would you interpret these radiographs which were performed on a 43-year-old man with a 4-hour duration of pain which was sudden in onset, severe and colicky, radiating from the left loin to the groin and tip of the penis. Urine dipstick showed haematuria.

A Figure 4.53.1 is a KUB (kidneys, ureters and bladder) radiograph. Figures 4.53.2a and b are intravenous urograms, radiographs taken in the early phase (15 minutes following the injection of intravenous contrast) and in the late phase (3.5 hours following injection of contrast). The KUB shows no obvious calculi in the ureters. The early phase film shows normal excretion from the right kidney with delayed excretion on the left. On the late phase radiograph, the left pelvicaliceal system and the left ureter are dilated up to the vesico-ureteric junction. A small amount of contrast is in the right renal pelvis. The picture is consistent with a left ureteric calculus causing obstruction at or near the vesico-ureteric junction.

Q   **What are the relative merits of the different diagnostic modalities used in a patient with ureteric colic?**

A   The investigation of choice to confirm the diagnosis of a calculus is an unenhanced helical CT of the abdomen and pelvis which has a sensitivity of 96% and a specificity of nearly 100%. The other advantage of CT in this situation is the ability of CT to reveal co-existing or alternative pathology in the abdomen.

An intravenous urogram (IVU) is a useful test in the absence of CT, but has a lower efficacy (sensitivity 87%; specificity 94%) and carries the risk of contrast anaphylaxis and nephrotoxicity. Ultrasonography has a high specificity (90%) but unacceptably low sensitivity (25%) for routine use. However, it is a valuable tool in evaluating pregnant patients. A plain radiograph (kidneys, ureters and bladder, KUB) is not routinely recommended. Although 75–90% of stones are radiopaque, overlapping bony and bowel shadows, similarity in appearances with phleboliths and calcified lymph nodes limits its clinical utility. It is useful to assess the radio-opacity of the stone before planning lithotripsy.

Q   **What analgesia would you prescribe for a patient with ureteric colic?**

A   Intravenous opiate analgesia (morphine, pethidine) has been the conventional method used for pain control. Provided renal function is not compromised, non-steroidal inflammatory agents (diclofenac 50 mg orally three times a day, or 100 mg rectally once a day; or ketorolac 30–60 mg loading dose parenterally, followed by 15 mg 6-hourly) are equally effective and better tolerated than opiates.

Desmopressin nasal spray has been used with some success as an adjunct in analgesia.

Avoiding overhydration also helps with pain control.

Q   **What would be your definitive management strategy for confirmed ureteric stones?**

A   The important issue is to identify patients who need urgent intervention. These are patients with an obstructed infected upper urinary tract, compromised renal function, anuria, obstruction of a solitary or transplanted kidney and patients with intractable pain or vomiting. These patients should undergo emergency decompression by either percutaneous nephrostomy or ureteric stenting. Patients with suspected infection should have parenteral antibiotics.

For patients not needing urgent intervention there are two courses of action available.

Observation: Small stones (5 mm or less) most often pass spontaneously and therefore may be observed for 1 month with follow-up imaging. Uric acid stones may be dissolved by alkalinising the urine (pH >6.5) with potassium citrate.

Intervention: Stones larger than 5 mm need intervention, the choice of which depends on availability and expertise. For proximal ureteric calculi (proximal to iliac vessels) which are less than 1 cm, extracorporeal shock wave lithotripsy (ESWL) is preferred. For larger stones, ureteroscopy or percutaneous nephrolithotomy (PCNL) are options. For distal ureteric calculi, ESWL or ureteroscopy are the choices. If none of the above facilities are available or if the stone is impacted, then open surgical removal (open ureterolithotomy) may be undertaken for stone at any level. Laparoscopy may also be used in selected instances.

In addition, patients should be encouraged to drink enough fluids to produce a urine output of 2 litres/day to reduce the chance of recurrence. Stone biochemistry should be performed whenever possible. Patients with recurrent stones should undergo metabolic evaluation.

INDEX